ANALYSIS MANUAL
FOR
HOSPITAL INFORMATION
SYSTEMS

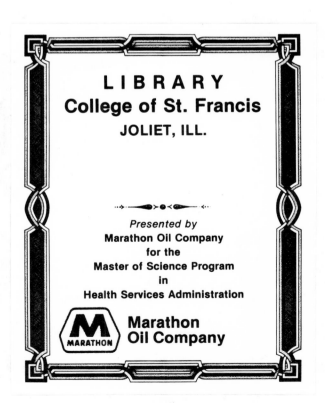

LIBRARY
College of St. Francis
JOLIET, ILL.

Presented by
Marathon Oil Company
for the
Master of Science Program
in
Health Services Administration

Marathon
Oil Company

AUPHA Press is an impriant of Health Administration Press.

Health Administration Press
M 2240 School of Public Health
The University of Michigan
Ann Arbor, Michigan 48109

313-764-1380

Association of University Programs
  in Health Administration
One DuPont Circle
Washington, D.C. 20036

202-659-4354

ANALYSIS MANUAL FOR HOSPITAL INFORMATION SYSTEMS

Owen Doyle
Charles J. Austin
and
Stephen L. Tucker

AUPHA PRESS
Washington, D.C. • Ann Arbor, Michigan

Library of Congress Cataloging in Publication Data

Doyle, Owen
  Analysis manual for hospital information systems.

  1. Hospitals – Administration – Data processing – Evaluation. 2. Hospital records – Evaluation. 3. Information storage and retrieval systems – Hospitals – Evaluation. I. Austin, Charles J., joint author. II. Tucker, Stephen L., joint author. III. Title. [DNLM: 1. Hospital administration. 2. Information retrieval systems. WX26.5 A935a]
RA971.6.A92   362.1′1′068   80-13875
ISBN 0-914904-41-8 (pbk.)

AUPHA PRESS
One DuPont Circle
Washington, D.C.
and
The School of Public Health
The University of Michigan
Ann Arbor, Michigan
1980

Table of Contents

Foreword

The three authors of the Analysis Manual have enjoyed the assistance of a number of talented and willing contributors in the Manual's development.

Thomas W. Butler, Chairman of the Board and Chief Executive Officer of NADACOM, Dallas, Texas, recognized the need for such a Manual, and provided the support for its development. Mr. Butler urged us to seek publication of the manual in the belief that its general availability would benefit hospital managers and students investigating the information and communication processes within hospitals.

Several sections of the Manual were drafted by persons with deep professional understanding of the elements of the organization which they addressed. Sections were developed by Robert T. Moore (cost considerations, general financial system), Nan Chandler (food service), Rita McIntyre (EKG/EEG services, surgical services), Robert Van Syke (medication distribution) and Greg Zobell (laboratory service).

Writing the Manual was greatly expedited by the editing of Marian F. Pfrommer and Rosario Padilla's patient and accurate typing.

We would like to dedicate the work in the Manual to our wives, Suzanne Doyle, Carroll Austin, and Lucy Tucker.

Owen Doyle
   Miami Valley Hospital
   Dayton, Ohio
   Administrative Health Management, Inc.
   Dayton, Ohio

Charles J. Austin
   Georgia Southern College
   Statesboro, Georgia

Stephen L. Tucker
   Trinity University
   San Antonio, Texas

1980

Introduction

Purposes of the Book

This book is designed to help hospitals conduct a comprehensive analysis of current information processing practices. It is based on the premise that major decisions related to developing automated information systems and/or acquiring computers and other data processing equipment should be preceded by a complete study of existing information-handling practices. The results of such a study will (1) document the existing information flows (2) determine current information-processing costs, and (3) determine problems, inefficiencies, gaps, and duplications in the existing procedures for processing information.

This information, gained with the aid of this Manual, should enable hospital management to set priorities for developing information systems and procuring computer hardware and software. It will also help to identify functional areas where improved communications are needed. The study results should prove beneficial regardless of whether or not any automated systems are implemented as a consequence of the analysis. A completed analysis, guided by this Manual, also can provide baseline information about the current state of information processes to be used in evaluating the need for proposed new information systems within the hospital.

Using the Manual

The Analysis Manual provides hospital management with a mechanism for accomplishing the following:

1. Assessing the effectiveness of current communications processes which occur among the functional elements of the organization.

2. Providing a model of the current communications processes to provide a basis for comparison with information systems which the hospital might consider for implementation.

3. Providing, especially through the use of the "standards" sections, models against which performance objectives can be established for use in managerial planning and control techniques such as management-by-objectives programs.

4. Establishing documentation of the operating and capital costs of communication systems in the organization. Through the use of similar methods of documentation throughout the organization, these cost determinants will have particular validity in comparing costs among the elements of the hospital.

5. Furnishing the hospital with a device for the orientation and education about the institution's communication processes for personnel new to the organization or new to the hospital setting.

Hospital administrators, institutional planners, management engineers, data processors, and department heads can choose the portions of the Manual appropriate to any of those listed above for their particular needs.

External to the hospital, the Analysis Manual provides a model and approach to the analysis of communications processes within hospitals for students in educational programs dealing with the services provided within the hospital, and in programs dealing with the management of these services.

Overall Structure of the Manual

The Manual provides a standard, guided approach to be followed in an information systems analysis of the major functions carried out in a typical acute care hospital. It is recommended that the study be conducted by a hospital systems analyst, industrial engineer, or administrator with some knowledge of system techniques. The person conducting the study should gather the information called for in the Manual by working with hospital management personnel, department heads, and other key departmental personnel.

The Manual is necessarily generalized, and some adaptations will be required to use it in any particular hospital. However, a basic premise is that acute, general hospitals are more alike than they are different and that a generalized format, such as the one presented in this Manual, can save the hospital much time and effort in conducting a comprehensive information systems analysis.

The book divides the hospital's information flow into 41 functional areas referred to as systems. A complete list of these systems is included as Figure 1. Note that the systems do not necessarily coincide with organizational lines in the hospital. Some systems may involve only one hospital department; others may include several departments. Also, many hospital departments appear in more than one system. Certain functions, which either are not directly related to patient care or generate a minimum amount of informational activity, have been excluded from this Manual. Examples of these functions are listed as Figure 2.

For each system included in the Manual, the following seven aids for analysis are included:

1. A narrative system description
2. An information flow chart
3. A list of typical input documents associated with the system
4. A list of master files typically utilized for storing information
5. A list of typical output reports produced in this system
6. A set of management standards for evaluating hospital performance in this functional area
7. A set of cost factors to aid in analyzing information costs associated with this system

How to Use the Manual

The Manual should be used on an *exception reporting basis.* System descriptions, flow charts, lists of input documents, master files, output reports, performance standards, and cost factors are presented for a *typical* hospital. These are on the left side of the page, with blank space on the right side for noting differences found at the hospital being studied (space for flow charts may be on the reverse).

For each system, the analyst using the book should follow these steps:

Step One: Read the description for the system being considered. This will give you an idea of how the system operates in a typical hospital.

Step Two: Determine which people you must interview in order to ascertain how this system operates in your hospital. Refer to the people listed in the Input, Master File, and Report inventories. For most systems, these individuals will be able to provide all needed information.

Step Three: As you gather information, identify the one key management person responsible for the overall operation of the system. Ask that person to describe the system and how it operates. When the hospital's approach differs from the approach presented in the system description, note the differences in the right-hand column of the system description pages. If the features described are essentially similar to what happens in your hospital, check block A. If there are minor variations, check B. If there are significant differences, check C.

Step Four: In the blank pages opposite the flow charts for the typical hospital, note your hospital's individual differences and construct new flow charts for your hospital. See Figure 3 for a glossary of flow-chart symbols used.

Step Five: The Input Inventory should include all forms that are originated as part of the system. Match the Input Inventory against forms actually used in your hospital and note differences and additions in the right column. Obtain copies of each form listed, and, working with the person who gave you the sample, complete an "Input Document Analysis Form" for each form you received. Attach the sample document to the Analysis Form. See Figure 4 for a sample Analysis Form.

Step Six: The Master File Inventory is a listing of all places where information is stored for this system. Match the Master File Inventory against files actually used in your hospital and note differences and additions in the right-hand column. Complete a "Master File Analysis Form" for each file so noted. See Figure 5 for a sample Analysis Form.

Step Seven: Match the Output Report Inventory against reports actually produced in your hospital; note differences and additions in the right-hand column. Obtain copies of each report listed in the revised Report Inventory. Working with the person who supplied you with each report, complete a "Report Analysis Form" for each report. See Figure 6 for a sample Analysis Form.

Step Eight: Working with the key management person identified in Step Three, complete a "Standards Analysis Form" for each listed standard.

If the answer to question one for any standard is "No," ask only questions three and six on the

Standards Analysis Form. See Figure 7 for a sample Analysis Form.

Step Nine: Complete the Cost Analysis Form for this system as shown in Figure 8. Because of the complex nature of cost analysis, a detailed set of instructions for completing this form has been included. It may be necessary to develop estimates of some of these costs if detailed, historical cost data is not available.

Figure 1
List of Systems for Analysis

Patient Services

1.0 Inpatient Services Systems
    1.1 Admissions, Discharge, Transfer/Census Control
    1.2 Medication Distribution
    1.3 Nursing Services
    1.4 Support Services Systems
        1.4.1 Patient Food Services
        1.4.2 Linen/Laundry
        1.4.3 Patient Transportation
        1.4.4 Housekeeping
        1.4.5 Social Services
        1.4.6 Patient Information Services

2.0 Ambulatory Care Services Systems
    2.1 Emergency Services
    2.2 Referred Outpatient Services
    2.3 Clinics

3.0 General Patient Services Systems
    3.1 Diagnostic Services Systems
        3.1.1 Laboratory
        3.1.2 Diagnostic Radiology
        3.1.3 Therapeutic Radiology
        3.1.4 Nuclear Medicine
        3.1.5 Respiratory Services
        3.1.6 EKG/EEG Services
    3.2 Rehabilitation Services
    3.3 Surgical Services

4.0 Patient Records Management Systems
    4.1 Transcription
    4.2 Indexing, Storage, and Retrieval
    4.3 Quality Assurance

Management Services

5.0 Financial Management Systems
    5.1 Patient Charging, Billing, and Accounts Receivable Systems
        5.1.1 Charging
        5.1.2 Credits
        5.1.3 Billing
        5.1.4 Accounts Receivable
    5.2 Budgeting
    5.3 Accounts Payable
    5.4 General Accounting
    5.5 Cash Management

6.0 Personnel Management Systems
    6.1 Timekeeping/Payroll
    6.2 Position Control
    6.3 Evaluation and Training

7.0 Materials Management Systems
    7.1 Capital Equipment
    7.2 Purchasing and General Stores
    7.3 Central Supply

8.0 Facilities and Equipment Management Systems
    8.1 Work Orders
    8.2 Scheduled Maintenance

9.0 Management Planning and Control Systems
    9.1 Internal Management Reporting
    9.2 External Reporting

Figure 2

The functions listed below which often constitute usual activity in hospitals are not included in this Manual.

Audio/Visual
Cafeteria
Chaplain
Coffee Shop
Disposal of Capital Equipment
Education and Research
Energy Management
Gift Shop

Investment Management
Library
Parking
Print Shop
Real Estate
Security
Vending
Volunteers

Figure 3
Glossary of Flow Chart Symbols

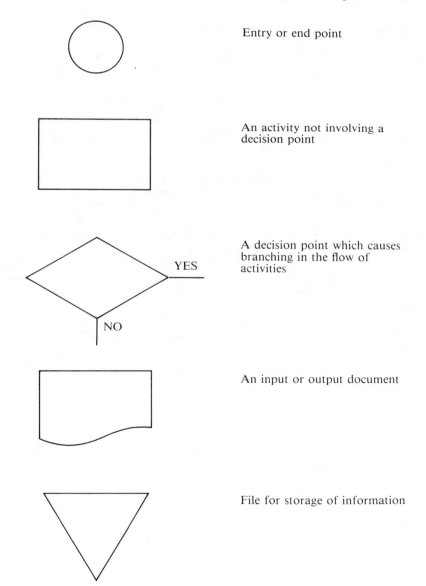

Entry or end point

An activity not involving a decision point

A decision point which causes branching in the flow of activities

YES

NO

An input or output document

File for storage of information

Instructions for Completing the
Input Document Analysis Form,
Master File Analysis Form, and
Report Analysis Form
(Figures 4, 5, and 6)

1. Fill in all blanks; right-hand justify and fill in leading zeros where necessary for numeric fields.

2. Fill in the System Number in Columns 1–4 using the codes shown in Figure 1.

3. Assign your own five-digit form/file number for columns 6–10.

4. Assign your own two-digit code for hospital departments in columns 12–13. A list of typical hospital departments is included in Figure 9.

5. Write the form/file name in columns 14–30 and provide an *abbreviated* description and purpose in columns 31–75.

6. Enter form usage information into columns 14–19, 20, and 21–23 of Card 2.

7. In columns 24–27 of Card 2, indicate the average hourly clerical salary cost in the department *or* as an alternative, use the salary cost for the person(s) most likely to be completing the form.

8. If possible, fill out the remaining columns of cards 2 and 3 with the detailed information requested. Some hospital departments may not be able to break down their activities into the nine categories shown. In this case, enter in columns 32–40 of card 31, the total time spent for this form, master file, or report.

9. Use the second page to record additional information in narrative form about the Input Form, Master File, or Report under consideration.

Figure 4
Input Document Analysis Form

SYSTEM: ☐☐☐☐ 1- -4

ID [1] 5

FORM NO: ☐☐☐☐☐ 6- -10

CARD [1] 11

DEPT NO: ☐☐ 12- -13

FORM NAME: ☐☐☐☐☐☐☐☐☐☐☐☐☐☐☐☐☐ 14- -30

DESCRIPTION AND PURPOSE:
31- ☐☐☐☐☐☐☐☐☐☐☐☐☐☐
☐☐☐☐☐☐☐☐☐☐☐☐☐☐
☐☐☐☐☐☐☐☐☐☐☐☐☐☐ -75

CARD [2] 11

VOLUME: ☐☐☐☐☐ 14- -19

FORMS PER: (CHECK ONE)
☐ 1-DAY
☐ 2-WEEK
☐ 3-MONTH
☐ 4-YEAR
20

NUMBER OF COPIES ☐☐☐ 21- -23

AVERAGE HOURLY SALARY IN DEPARTMENT: $☐☐.☐☐ 24- -27

SUPPLY COSTS: $☐☐☐ 28- -30

		HOURS SPENT	ANNUAL FREQUENCY
[1] 31	HOURS, DATA ACQUISITION	☐☐☐.☐ 32- -35	☐☐☐☐☐ 36- -40
[2] 41	HOURS, DATA TRANSCRIPTION	☐☐☐.☐ 42- -45	☐☐☐☐☐ 46- -50
[3] 51	HOURS, STORING DATA	☐☐☐.☐ 52- -55	☐☐☐☐☐ 56- -60
[4] 61	HOURS, RETRIEVING DATA	☐☐☐.☐ 62- -65	☐☐☐☐☐ 66- -70
[5] 71	HOURS, INFOR. DEVELOPMENT	☐☐☐.☐ 72- -75	☐☐☐☐☐ 76- -80

CARD [3] 11

		HOURS SPENT	ANNUAL FREQUENCY
[6] 31	HOURS, DISSEMINATING INFOR.	☐☐☐.☐ 32- -35	☐☐☐☐☐ 36- -40
[7] 41	HOURS, INFOR. ANALYSIS	☐☐☐.☐ 42- -45	☐☐☐☐☐ 46- -50
[8] 51	HOURS, INFOR. EVALUATION	☐☐☐.☐ 52- -55	☐☐☐☐☐ 56- -60
[9] 61	HOURS, CHECKING DECISION/RESP.	☐☐☐.☐ 62- -65	☐☐☐☐☐ 66- -70

Figure 4, continued
Input Document Analysis Form (Page 2)

ROUTING OF FORM:

COST FACTORS:

PROBLEMS:

COMMENTS:

Figure 5
Master File Analysis Form

SYSTEM: ☐☐☐☐ | ID ☐2 ☐ 5 | FILE NO: ☐☐☐☐☐ 6- -10 | CARD ☐1 11 | DEPT NO: ☐☐ 12- -13

SYSTEM: 1- -4

FILE NAME: ☐☐☐☐☐☐☐☐☐☐☐☐☐☐☐☐☐ 14- -30

DESCRIPTION AND PURPOSE:
31-
☐☐☐☐☐☐☐☐☐☐☐☐☐☐☐☐☐
☐☐☐☐☐☐☐☐☐☐☐☐☐☐☐☐☐
☐☐☐☐☐☐☐☐☐☐☐☐☐☐☐☐☐
-75

CARD ☐2 11 | FILE SIZE: (NO. OF RECORDS) ☐☐☐☐☐☐ 14- -19 | FREQUENCY OF UPDATING ☐☐☐ 20- -22 | TRANS. PER: ☐ 1-DAY ☐ 2-WEEK ☐ 3-MONTH ☐ 4-YEAR 23

AVERAGE HOURLY SALARY IN DEPARTMENT: $☐☐.☐☐ 24- -27 | SUPPLY COSTS: $☐☐☐ 28- -30

		HOURS SPENT	ANNUAL FREQUENCY
☐1 31	HOURS, DATA ACQUISITION	☐☐☐.☐ 32- -35	☐☐☐☐☐ 36- -40
☐2 41	HOURS, DATA TRANSCRIPTION	☐☐☐.☐ 42- -45	☐☐☐☐☐ 46- -50
☐3 51	HOURS, STORING DATA	☐☐☐.☐ 52- -55	☐☐☐☐☐ 56- -60
☐4 61	HOURS, RETRIEVING DATA	☐☐☐.☐ 62- -65	☐☐☐☐☐ 66- -70
☐5 71	HOURS, INFOR. DEVELOPMENT	☐☐☐.☐ 72- -75	☐☐☐☐☐ 76- -80

CARD ☐3 11

☐6 31	HOURS, DISSEMINATING INFOR.	☐☐☐.☐ 32- -35	☐☐☐☐☐ 36- -40
☐7 41	HOURS, INFOR. ANALYSIS	☐☐☐.☐ 42- -45	☐☐☐☐☐ 46- -50
☐8 51	HOURS, INFOR. EVALUATION	☐☐☐.☐ 52- -55	☐☐☐☐☐ 56- -60
☐9 61	HOURS, CHECKING DECISION/RESP.	☐☐☐.☐ 62- -65	☐☐☐☐☐ 66- -70

Figure 5, continued
Master File Analysis Form (Page 2)

PURGE CRITERIA:

COST FACTORS:

PROBLEMS:

COMMENTS:

Figure 6
Report Analysis Form

SYSTEM: ☐☐☐☐ 1- ☐ -4 ID 3 5 REPORT NO: ☐☐☐☐☐ 6- -10 CARD 1 11 DEPT NO: ☐☐ 12- -13

REPORT NAME: ☐☐☐☐☐☐☐☐☐☐☐☐☐☐☐☐☐ 14- -30

DESCRIPTION AND PURPOSE:
31- ☐☐☐☐☐☐☐☐☐☐☐☐☐☐☐
☐☐☐☐☐☐☐☐☐☐☐☐☐☐☐
☐☐☐☐☐☐☐☐☐☐☐☐☐☐☐ -75

CARD 2 11 VOLUME: (NO. OF PAGES) ☐☐☐☐☐☐ 14- -19 NUMBER OF COPIES ☐☐☐ 20- -22 FREQUENCY OF REPORTING
☐ 1-DAILY
☐ 2-WEEKLY
☐ 3-MONTHLY
☐ 4-QTRLY
☐ 5-ANNUAL 23

AVERAGE HOURLY SALARY IN DEPARTMENT: $☐☐.☐☐ 24- -27 SUPPLY COSTS: $☐☐☐ 28- -30

			HOURS SPENT	ANNUAL FREQUENCY
1 31	HOURS, DATA ACQUISITION		☐☐☐.☐ 32- -35	☐☐☐☐☐ 36- -40
2 41	HOURS, DATA TRANSCRIPTION		☐☐☐.☐ 42- -45	☐☐☐☐☐ 46- -50
3 51	HOURS, STORING DATA		☐☐☐.☐ 52- -55	☐☐☐☐☐ 56- -60
4 61	HOURS, RETRIEVING DATA		☐☐☐.☐ 62- -65	☐☐☐☐☐ 66- -70
5 71	HOURS, INFOR. DEVELOPMENT		☐☐☐.☐ 72- -75	☐☐☐☐☐ 76- -80

CARD 3 11

		HOURS SPENT	ANNUAL FREQUENCY
6 31	HOURS, DISSEMINATING INFOR.	☐☐☐.☐ 32- -35	☐☐☐☐☐ 36- -40
7 41	HOURS, INFOR. ANALYSIS	☐☐☐.☐ 42- -45	☐☐☐☐☐ 46- -50
8 51	HOURS, INFOR. EVALUATION	☐☐☐.☐ 52- -55	☐☐☐☐☐ 56- -60
9 61	HOURS, CHECKING DECISION/RESP.	☐☐☐.☐ 62- -65	☐☐☐☐☐ 66- -70

Figure 6, continued
Report Analysis Form (Page 2)

DISTRIBUTION OF REPORT:

COST FACTORS:

PROBLEMS:

COMMENTS:

Instructions for Completing the
Performance Standards Analysis Form
(Figure 7)

1. Code Columns 1–4, 6–10, and 12–13 as specified in the instructions for completing the Input Document Analysis, Master File, and Report Analysis forms.

2. Enter the appropriate numerical value of your standard in columns 15–18.

3. Use the list of suggested standards shown in the description of each hospital system in the Manual. Some hospitals may not have information system standards. The lists provided may serve as a starting point in developing these standards. The lists of standards included in this Manual were developed from the informed judgment and experience of the three authors assisted by various functional specialists in selected areas.

Figure 7
Performance Standards Analysis Form

| SYSTEM: ☐☐☐☐
1-　　-4 | ID
4
5 | STD. NO: ☐☐☐☐☐
6-　　　-10 | DEPT.
NO. ☐☐
12--13 |

| DOES YOUR HOSPITAL
HAVE A STANDARD? | ☐ 1-YES
☐ 2-NO
14 | WHAT IS YOUR
STANDARD? | ☐☐☐☐
15-　　-18 |

TO WHAT DEGREE IS THIS STANDARD
IMPORTANT IN MEETING OVERALL
HOSPITAL OBJECTIVES?
☐ 1-CRITICAL
☐ 2-VERY IMPORTANT
☐ 3-IMPORTANT
☐ 4-OF MINOR IMPORTANCE
19

HOW OFTEN IS THE
STANDARD MET?
☐ 1-ALWAYS
☐ 2-MOST OF THE TIME
☐ 3-OCCASIONALLY
☐ 4-NEVER
20

IF STD. IS MET ONLY OCCASIONALLY
OR NEVER MET, IS IT POSSIBLE
TO MEET THE STD.?
☐ 1-YES
☐ 2-NO
21

IF THERE ARE PROBLEMS IN
THIS AREA, DO THEY RELATE
TO (CHECK AS MANY AS
APPLICABLE):

☐ LACK OF TIMELINESS OF INFORMATION
22

☐ INACCURATE INFORMATION
23

☐ IRRELEVANT INFORMATION
24

☐ INEFFICIENCIES IN THE PROCESSING
25　OF INFORMATION

DESCRIPTION
OF
STANDARD:

31-
☐☐☐☐☐☐☐☐☐☐☐☐☐☐☐
☐☐☐☐☐☐☐☐☐☐☐☐☐☐☐
☐☐☐☐☐☐☐☐☐☐☐☐☐☐☐
　　　　　　　　　　　　　　　-75

COMMENTS:

Instructions for Completing
the Cost Analysis Form
(Figure 8)

In completing the Cost Analysis Form, each department head who is involved with the issuance or receipt of the forms and/or reports used in this sub-system should consider the following questions in addition to the previous responses in relation to standards of Hospital Systems Performance:

1. How much equipment is used primarily to facilitate communication systems, e.g., embossographs, flexowriters, terminal cathode ray tubes, dry copy reproducers, typewriters, filing cabinets, etc.?
2. What is the property book value of this equipment?
3. What data processing services are used in conjunction with this subsystem?
4. What are the costs of these services (either from in-house data processing department or external source)? Use an appropriate cost allocation formula for assigning data processing costs to this particular system.
5. How much of the equipment and furnished information services are dedicated to each of the information systems that impact on this department? How much to each subsystem of each system? What basis of allocation should be used to apportion these costs to each system and subsystem?
   a. Percent of departmental effort (estimated percent of time spent)?
   b. Workunits affected by each subsystem?
   c. Other?
6. How many times is it necessary to have some completed report, form, or file duplicated because another department or individual needs the information and did not get it, did not keep it, or lost it? How many pages of material is this in an average month? How much does it cost to duplicate one page?
7. How many times are incorrect decisions made because of incorrect, incomplete, or insufficient data available from the existing system? What are the types of incorrect decisions that are made?

Examples:
   a. Department not notified of an admission or transfer?
   b. Insurance company erroneously billed?
   c. Patient had to be placed in a bed other than the one specified on the admitting form?
   d. Patient told bed was not available that day?
   e. Insufficient consent forms secured from patient?
8. What does it cost to correct such erroneous decisions in terms of:
   a. Labor costs for the erroneous decision plus the time to make the correction?
   b. Supply costs?
   c. Lost revenue?
   d. Direct overhead costs?
9. How many times must an action already taken be duplicated because of an inadequate information system? What types of actions have to be repeated?
   Examples:
   a. Lab test, radiographic report, EKG, physical examination, etc., due to lost reports?
   b. Second meal sent to a different ward because department was not notified of the transfer?
   c. Midnight Census report must be revised?
10. What does it cost to duplicate these actions in terms of:
   a. Labor costs?
   b. Supply costs?
   c. Lost revenue?
   d. Direct overhead costs?
11. What opportunity costs are involved in the incorrect decisions or the duplicated actions, i.e., what was not done with the resources that were used in order to correct a decision or duplicate an action?

Figure 8
Cost Analysis Form

SYSTEM				

SYSTEM NO: ☐☐☐☐   ID ⑤   DEPARTMENT NO: ☐☐
1-   -4   5   12 - 13

EQUIPMENT COSTS: Enter the annual costs associated with the information and communications equipment used for this system (if equipment is used for more than one system, pro-rate annual cost to each system based upon percent of effort each system consumes).

EQUIPMENT LEASING CONTRACT CHARGES (NET)   _____
EQUIPMENT SERVICE AND MAINTENANCE COSTS   _____
DEPRECIATION EXPENSE ON OWNED EQUIPMENT   _____
TOTAL EQUIPMENT COSTS FOR YEAR $ ☐☐☐☐☐☐
25-   -30

DATA PROCESSING SERVICES: Enter the annual costs associated with either purchasing information services from another firm or the share of in-house information services furnished from this system. (Allocations of data processing services based upon the amount of data processing time experienced by the providing element).

PURCHASED DATA PROCESSING SERVICE $ ☐☐☐☐☐☐
35-   -40

DUPLICATING COSTS: Enter the annual costs associated with printing of forms and reproducing copies of completed forms and reports due to insufficient distribution.

PRINTING OF FORMS   _____
REPRODUCING COMPLETED FORMS, REPORTS   _____
TOTAL DUPLICATING COSTS PER YEAR $ ☐☐☐☐☐☐
45-   -50

DECISION CORRECTION COSTS: Enter the number of incorrect decisions which arise from incorrect, incomplete, or insufficient information available from the existing system at the time the decision must be made and the costs of correcting each decision. (Correction costs include labor cost of department staff, other direct costs and lost revenue). See Cost Consideration section for this system.

NO. INCORRECT DECISIONS/YEAR: ☐☐☐☐   COST TO CORRECT EACH DECISION: $ ☐☐☐☐☐☐
51-   -54   55-   -60

DUPLICATE RESPONSE COSTS: Enter the number of times an action, already accomplished, must be duplicated due to the failure of the existing system to provide timely information, and the costs associated with duplicating that action. See Cost Considerations section for this system.

NO. DUPLICATE RESPONSES/YEAR: ☐☐☐☐   COST TO DUPLICATE EACH ACTION $ ☐☐☐☐☐☐
61-   -64   65-   -70

Figure 9
Typical Hospital Departments

Departmental Identification

Administration and Staff
Administrative Offices
Planning
Management Engineering
Legal Affairs
Public Relations
Development
Personnel/Industrial Relations
Education and Training

Fiscal Affairs
General Accounting
Budgeting
Credit and Collections
Payroll
Internal Audit
Property Book
Cashier

Medical Staff Affairs
Medical Staff Office
Medical Education
Utilization Review
Medical Audit
Infection Control

Nursing and Patient Care Units
Nursing Units—Inpatient
Emergency Department
Clinics
Nursing Administration
Nursing, Professional Education
Nursing, Inservice Education
Anesthesia
Surgery (All sites)
Recovery Room
Labor and Delivery
Referred Outpatient

Diagnostic and Treatment Services
Laboratory—Clinical
Laboratory—Anatomical
Radiology—Diagnostic
Radiology—Therapeutic
Nuclear Medicine
Respiratory Therapy
EKG
EEG
Rehabilitation Medicine
Blood Bank

Service Departments—General
Admission
Telephone/Information
Patient Transportation
Mail Room
Dietary (Patient)
Data Processing
Maintenance
Security
Housekeeping
Laundry
Linen Service

Service Departments—Materials Management and Patient Support
Purchasing
Stores
Pharmacy
Central Supply Room
Social Service
Medical Records
Photography; Medical

Inpatient Services Systems

System 1.1: Admission/Discharge/Transfer and Census Control

Description 1.1

	A B C	Notes ↓
The flow of a patient through the hospital begins when the admission is scheduled.	☐ ☐ ☐	
The most common type of scheduling occurs when a physician's office contacts Admitting to schedule, or book, an admission. If the patient is to have surgery, Admitting schedules the admission for the first day when both a bed and surgical facilities will be available.	☐ ☐ ☐	
In judging when a bed will be available, Admitting, based on experience, estimates how many beds will be free on each particular day of the week. As each admission is scheduled, one bed is subtracted from the estimated number available on that day.	☐ ☐ ☐	
Once the admission date is selected, Admitting enters information about the patient on a Booking Sheet. This information includes expected date of admission, patient name and telephone number, admitting physician, and admitting diagnosis.	☐ ☐ ☐	
Another type of scheduling is the emergency admission. In life-or-death situations, patients are admitted right away. If a bed is not immediately available, the patient is held in the Emergency Department (ED) Room until one is found.	☐ ☐ ☐	
In the event a bed is not available for a scheduled admission, Admitting will call the patient and cancel the admission. Such a cancellation is usually caused by one of two factors – fewer beds are available than Admitting had estimated, or an expected patient discharge does not materialize, meaning a bed will be occupied for another day.	☐ ☐ ☐	

Preadmission

After a patient has been scheduled for admission, preadmission can begin. This involves contacting the patient to gather as much admitting information as possible before the patient

---

actually arrives at the hospital. Contact can be by a mailed questionnaire or a telephone call.

A B C
☐ ☐ ☐ _____

Admission

When the patient arrives to be admitted, an Admitting Form is completed. In addition to stating the reason (i.e., admitting diagnosis) for the admission, this form also contains two other types of information: demographic (name, age, sex, date of birth, etc.) and payment related (information on the person who is financially responsible for the bill, names of insurance companies involved, credit information, etc.).

☐ ☐ ☐ _____

The Admitting Form has eight or more copies. It is the prime document used to notify all affected departments that this particular patient has arrived and will be in a certain bed.

☐ ☐ ☐ _____

One copy of the form goes to the Nursing Station for insertion in the patient's chart. This copy becomes a permanent part of the patient's medical record.

☐ ☐ ☐ _____

Another copy goes to the Business Office, which then establishes an account for the patient.

☐ ☐ ☐ _____

Other personnel who may receive copies are Dietary, Information Desk, Surgery (to give surgeons and anesthesiologists information), and the hospital's Utilization Review Committee.

☐ ☐ ☐ _____

In addition, other notifications, such as index cards with selected information about the patient, are prepared and sent to such departments as Social Service, Medical Records (to allow the Department to enter the patient into the locator file), and Housekeeping.

☐ ☐ ☐ _____

Reports

Once the patient is admitted, he or she will appear on the Midnight Census, a daily listing of patients sorted by Nursing Station. This is accurate as of midnight, and is distributed before 7 A.M. to a large number of hospital departments. The Midnight Census shows, among other things, room and bed number, patient number, and date of admission.

☐ ☐ ☐ _____

Another common census report is the A/D/T list, which shows in alphabetical order all patients admitted, discharged, and transferred on the previous day.

☐ ☐ ☐ _____

A = essentially similar   B = minor variations   C = significant differences

Census information is compiled by Medical Records for the purpose of generating statistical reports. The most common is the Nursing Section's daily report on hospital occupancy.

A B C
☐ ☐ ☐

Tests

The final part of the admission process is rendering admission tests. For most admissions, this involves collecting samples for lab work and taking x-rays. For some surgical admissions, an EKG is often part of the normal workup. Other admitting tests may also be part of the admissions process.

☐ ☐ ☐

These procedures are conducted in one of two ways – either the patient is sent to the appropriate departments before being sent to his or her room or the patient is taken to his or her room and then transported to the appropriate departments.

☐ ☐ ☐

Transfer

When a patient is transferred from one bed to another, the Nursing Station is responsible for notifying all departments that need to know the patient's location. To do this, the Nursing Station completes a transfer notification which goes to such departments as:

☐ ☐ ☐

1. Admitting – to list the vacated bed as available and assure that the transfer will be noted on the next Midnight Census and A/D/T Report.

☐ ☐ ☐

2. Business Office – to update the account in cases where the patient is being transferred between rooms with differing daily charges.

☐ ☐ ☐

3. Housekeeping – to alert the staff to prepare the vacated room for the next patient.

☐ ☐ ☐

In addition, many other departments need to know about the transfer. Some get copies of the transfer notice; others must wait until the next Midnight Census is available.

☐ ☐ ☐

Other departments which may need to know about a transfer include:

1. Dietary – to make sure meals are sent to the correct room.

☐ ☐ ☐

2. Information Desk.

☐ ☐ ☐

A = essentially similar   B = minor variations   C = significant differences

3. Laboratory, Radiology, and other clinical departments – to assure that phlebotomists and transporters are sent to the right room.

A B C
☐ ☐ ☐ _____

Discharge

When the patient is discharged, the Nursing Station advises the same departments that are notified in room transfer situations.

☐ ☐ ☐ _____

The discharge notice signals the Business Office to begin preparing the patient's bill.

☐ ☐ ☐ _____

It also notifies Admitting that a particular bed can be put back into use and signals Admitting to remove the patient from the Midnight Census.

☐ ☐ ☐ _____

Preparing the Census

Admitting prepares the Midnight Census. The previous day's census is used as a master sheet. As patients are admitted, and as transfer and discharge notices are received, the master is marked up to reflect the hospital's current occupancy pattern. In addition, the Nursing Stations telephone in corrections after reviewing the last day's census.

☐ ☐ ☐ _____

At midnight, the new census is printed.

☐ ☐ ☐ _____

With a computerized census – batch or online – an alphabetic census can be generated. This report contains the patient's bill to date. The Business Office uses this report to monitor patient balances, particularly when the patient has little or no insurance coverage.

☐ ☐ ☐ _____

A = essentially similar   B = minor variations   C = significant differences

Flow Chart 1.1a

Inpatient Admissions – Booking

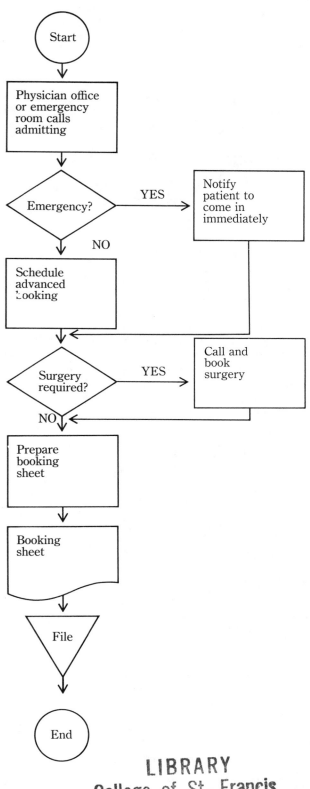

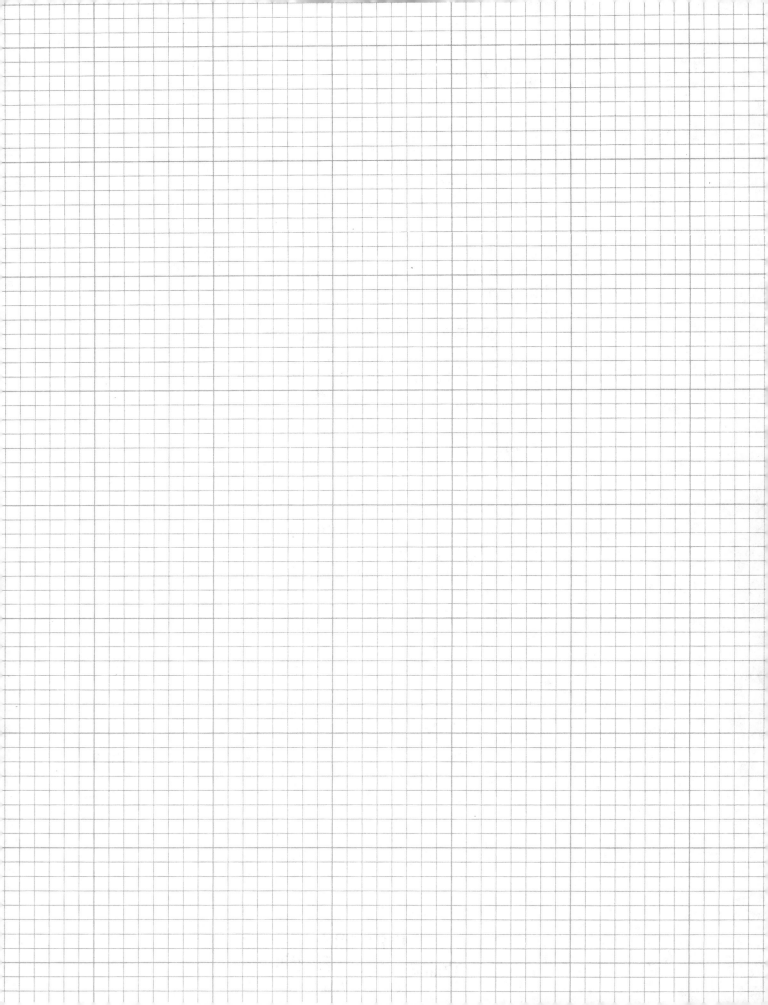

Flow Chart 1.1b

Inpatient Admissions Process

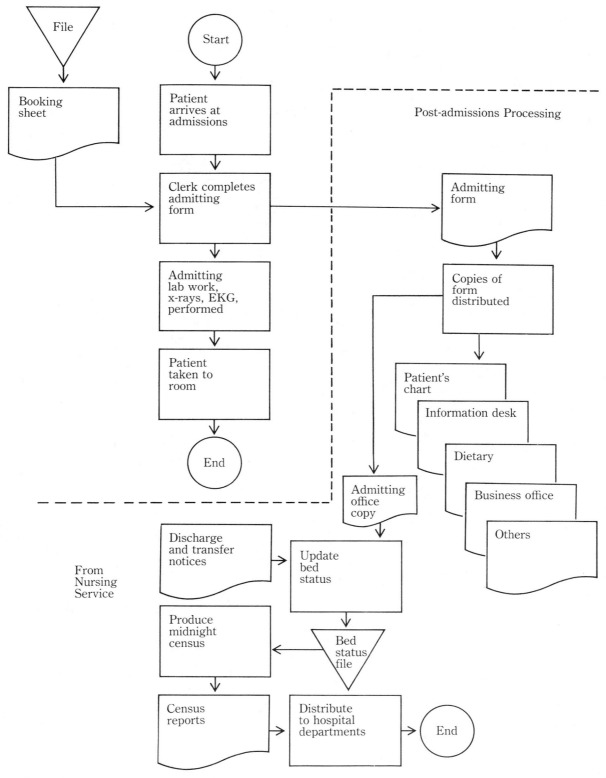

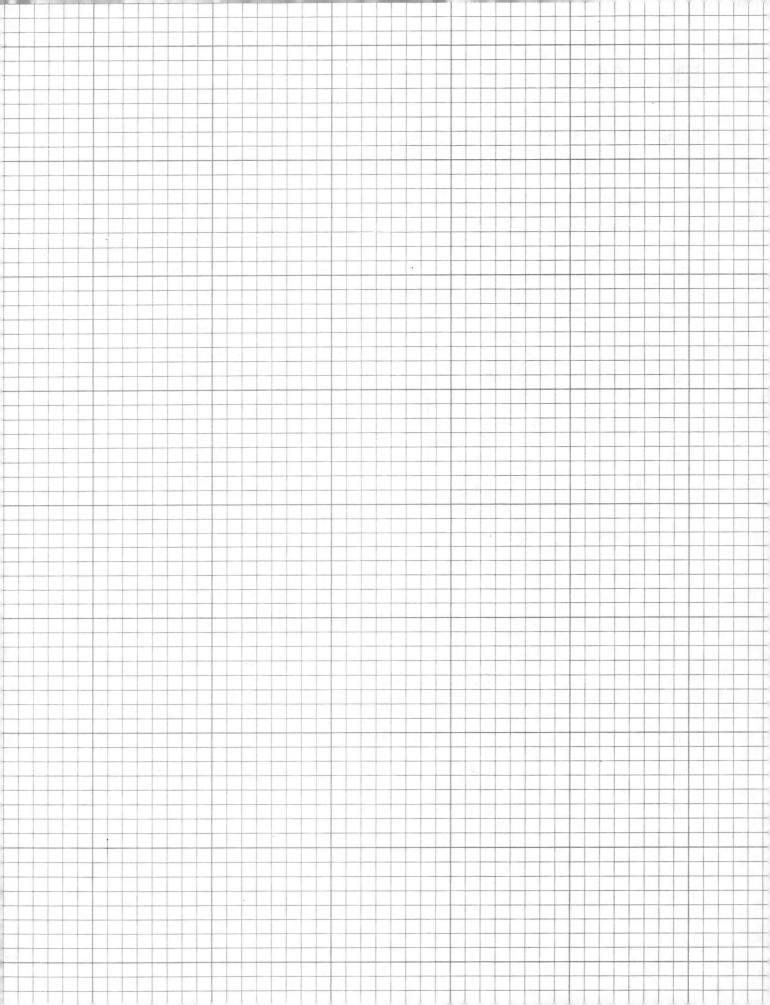

Input Inventory 1.1

A. Admitting Department Head

your document title
↓

	A	B	C	
1. Booking Sheet.	☐	☐	☐	_____
2. Preadmission questionnaire.	☐	☐	☐	_____
3. Admitting Form.	☐	☐	☐	_____
4. Form or forms used to notify departments of a patient's admission.	☐	☐	☐	_____
5. Special requisition used for ordering x-rays, lab work, and/or an EKG at the time of admission.	☐	☐	☐	_____
6. Insurance forms that accompany a copy of the admitting form to the Business Office. Determine which of these forms the patient is required to sign.	☐	☐	☐	_____
7. Consent forms.	☐	☐	☐	_____
8. Any other form the patient is required to sign at the time of admission.	☐	☐	☐	_____

B. Head Nurse

	A	B	C	
1. Transfer notification form.	☐	☐	☐	_____
2. Discharge notification form.	☐	☐	☐	_____

USE INPUT DOCUMENT ANALYSIS FORM

A = same document title	B = minor variations	C = significant differences

Master File Inventory 1.1

A. Admitting Department Head

Notes
↓

	A	B	C	
1. Booking sheet file.	☐	☐	☐	_____
2. Midnight Census file.	☐	☐	☐	_____
3. Log of admission.	☐	☐	☐	_____

4. Bedboard. This usually is a marked-up copy of the current Midnight Census, or a cardex arrangement.

A B C
☐ ☐ ☐ _____

5. Physician roster.

☐ ☐ ☐ _____

USE MASTER FILE ANALYSIS FORM

A = essentially similar   B = minor variations   C = significant differences

Report Inventory 1.1

your document title
↓

A. Admitting Department Head

A B C
1. Midnight Census.

☐ ☐ ☐ _____

2. Other types of census reports, including alphabetical census.

☐ ☐ ☐ _____

3. Admission/Discharge/Transfer report.

☐ ☐ ☐ _____

B. Medical Records Department Head

Statistical census reports such as occupancy compiled by nursing unit.

☐ ☐ ☐ _____

USE REPORT ANALYSIS FORM

A = essentially similar   B = minor variations   C = significant differences

System Performance Standards 1.1

	Units	A	B
1. What proportion of hospital inpatients are preadmitted?	percent _____	☐	☐
2. How long does it take to admit a patient?	minutes_____	☐	☐
3. How many transfers occur?	daily average _____	☐	☐
4. How long does it take to effect a transfer?	minutes_____	☐	☐
5. How many admissions does the hospital have to cancel?	daily average _____	☐	☐
6. What is the accuracy of the Midnight Census?	percentage of total beds inaccurately reported as to name and number of occupant _____	☐	☐

7. How long does it take to deliver the Midnight Census   A   B
   to all people on the distribution list?   minutes_____   ☐   ☐

USE PERFORMANCE STANDARDS ANALYSIS FORM

A = we have a standard   B = we do not have a standard

System Cost Factors 1.1

1. If Nursing is late in notifying Admitting of discharges, Admitting may cancel
   admissions because it erroneously believes that beds are not available.

   What is the monthly loss in revenue due to late notifications? $ _____

2. What percentage of the hospital's bad-debt write-offs could be prevented by a
   preadmission/financial screening program? $ _____

3. How much surgical suite time is wasted because of cancelled admissions? $ _____

4. When a patient is admitted through the Emergency Room, the admission time
   should be the time that patient arrives for service. However, the Admitting
   Clerk may record the admission at the time the form is completed. If the patient
   arrives before midnight, but the admission time is recorded as being after
   midnight, the hospital loses one day's worth of room-rate revenue.

   How often does this error occur? $ _____

5. How many surgeries must be cancelled or delayed because admission workup
   results are late? $ _____

6. How much time is spent and how many people are involved in distributing
   census reports? $ _____

7. What is the dollar value of meals prepared for patients who have already been
   discharged or transferred? $ _____

8. How much nursing time is spent preparing discharge and transfer forms? $ _____

USE SYSTEM COST ANALYSIS FORM *(also see Instructions, p. 15)*

System 1.2: Medication Distribution

Description 1.2

Notes
↓

Inventory

Pharmacy has direct control over the medication inventory. Levels are inspected daily, weekly, or monthly by either the pharmacy staff or drug manufacturer representatives, depending on the type and usage of the drug in question. It is from this inspection process that periodic purchase orders are generated to replenish depleted stock levels.

A B C
□ □ □ _____

Medications are purchased via a variety of sources – local wholesalers, drug manufacturers, and specific contractual arrangements. The process begins when a purchase order (PO) is initiated. One copy is forwarded to the vendor, and two copies are held in an on-order file in Pharmacy. When the ordered medications are delivered, a copy of the purchase order, the packing slip, and the items themselves are inspected to insure accuracy. Once the invoice has been received and scrutinized, it is forwarded to Accounts Payable, together with one copy of the purchase order and any notations. The remaining copy of the purchase order is filed in Pharmacy for reference.

□ □ □ _____

In some hospitals, Purchasing plays a role in medication purchases. However, the Pharmacy almost always has primary control over the drug-purchasing mechanism.

□ □ □ _____

Most hospitals have a formulary list of the drugs available for use in the hospital. This hospital formulary serves both as a descriptive and restrictive tool for medication utilization. The Pharmacy and the Therapeutics Committee of the medical staff generally define the criteria for admission to the formulary and act on specific written requests.

□ □ □ _____

Medication Order Transmittal

Medication distribution begins when the physician enters the medication order on the patient's chart. This medication order infor-

_____

A = essentially similar   B = minor variations   C = significant differences

32

mation is then transmitted to Pharmacy by one of two means. In some hospitals, a requisition is prepared by Nursing and sent to Pharmacy. Another approach involves transmitting a copy of the physician's order. In some states, this second method is mandated.

STAT (immediate) orders are usually transmitted to Pharmacy via telephone, with follow-up documentation required.

Dispensing and Distributing

Two general systems exist for dispensing and distributing medications – the traditional system and the unit-dose system.

Traditional System

The order is visually screened by the pharmacist for any inconsistencies, incompatibilities, or inadequacies. In some hospitals, a patient-specific profile may be utilized at this stage. This profile is a card that lists all medications ordered for a specific patient, along with pertinent drug-related information including patient-related drug sensitivities, current status of the medication orders, and drug administration information. If a profile is used, the dispensing process is carried out using the profile as the reference document. Without a profile system, the reference document is the physician order copy or nursing requisition.

Once the order screening and transcription procedures are completed, the actual dispensing process begins. A label showing the patient's name, room and bed number, and identifying medication information is prepared. The medication itself is retrieved and/or prepared, and the label is attached to the appropriate container. Then a final inspection is made. With this traditional system, a three-to-ten day supply of medication is dispensed. The exact amount depends on a number of factors, such as the dosage form of the medications, the therapeutic categorization of the drug, and the average length of stay for patients.

The packaged medication is then delivered to the Nursing Station.

The refilling process requires the nursing unit to either return the empty container to Pharmacy or specifically reorder the medication.

Notes
↓

A B C
□ □ □

A = essentially similar   B = minor variations   C = significant differences

33

Unit-dose System

The concept of unit dose implies both a packaging system and a distribution process. Unit-dose packaging means that a single dose of medication is completely labeled and ready to be administered to the patient.

A B C
☐ ☐ ☐

The requisition screening is no different than in the traditional system; however, a profile is necessary for the unit-dose system.

☐ ☐ ☐

Once the order is transcribed to the profile, the dispensing of initial doses takes place in a manner similar to that described for the traditional system. The only exceptions are that ready-to-administer unit doses are used, and labeling requirements are unique. The physical distribution of these initial doses also is accomplished in the same manner as described before.

☐ ☐ ☐

The primary difference between the unit-dose concept and the traditional system is in the dispensing and distribution of subsequent or refill doses. This system involves a cart exchange process. Two sets of carts containing patients' medication containers or cassettes are in use at all times – one in the patient care unit and one in Pharmacy. These carts are exchanged at least once every 24 hours. The cart in Pharmacy is refilled, using the patient profile as a reference document. The carts are generally exchanged by pharmacy personnel, and a reconciliation process sometimes is instituted in the nursing unit by comparing the nursing medication record with the pharmacy cart inventory record.

☐ ☐ ☐

Medication Administration

As part of each chart, the Nursing Station keeps a patient-medication profile which lists all ordered drugs and verifies actual administration. Each time the physician writes an order, the nurse enters this order on the profile. These profiles are then used to prepare medication-administration schedules. In a traditional system, the medications are placed in a patient tray, which may be part of a cart. With the unit-dose system, the initial doses are placed in a patient-specific cassette on a movable cart.

☐ ☐ ☐

The nurse administers the medication according to the medication-administration schedule and then documents the administration on the patient medication profile.

☐ ☐ ☐

A = essentially similar   B = minor variations   C = significant differences

Charging

There are many ways for Pharmacy to charge patients for medications. The most common approach involves either using a copy of the requisition as a charge document or initiating a charge document in Pharmacy. The proper charge is entered by Pharmacy, and the charge form is then sent to the Business Office.

A B C
☐ ☐ ☐ _____

System Variations

The basic traditional and unit-dose systems described accommodate the vast majority of medications dispensed in the typical hospital pharmacy inpatient setting. However, certain specific categories of drugs are distributed through specialized mechanisms. These will be identified and described here.

☐ ☐ ☐ _____

Floor Stock

Medication items that are both nonprescription and frequently used by a given nursing unit are often designated as floor stock. Such items are requisitioned from Pharmacy in accordance with predetermined inventory levels for the nursing unit. Floor stock often presents billing problems, since nurse-initiated charge documents are required in a charging system otherwise controlled by Pharmacy.

☐ ☐ ☐ _____

Controlled Substances

The federal and state governments have strict requirements for the control and distribution of certain medications. These regulations usually result in a system of locked floor-stock, with rigid requisition, inventory, and administration procedures.

☐ ☐ ☐ _____

Intravenous Admixtures

Many pharmacies have instituted intravenous (IV) admixture services designed to provide the proper environment and control for such critical care preparations. This service requires somewhat elaborate scheduling, preparation, and distribution mechanisms and usually necessitates the use of separate patient IV profiles and direct medication order copies.

☐ ☐ ☐ _____

A = essentially similar   B = minor variations   C = significant differences

Flow Chart 1.2

Traditional or Unit-Dose Medication System with Profile

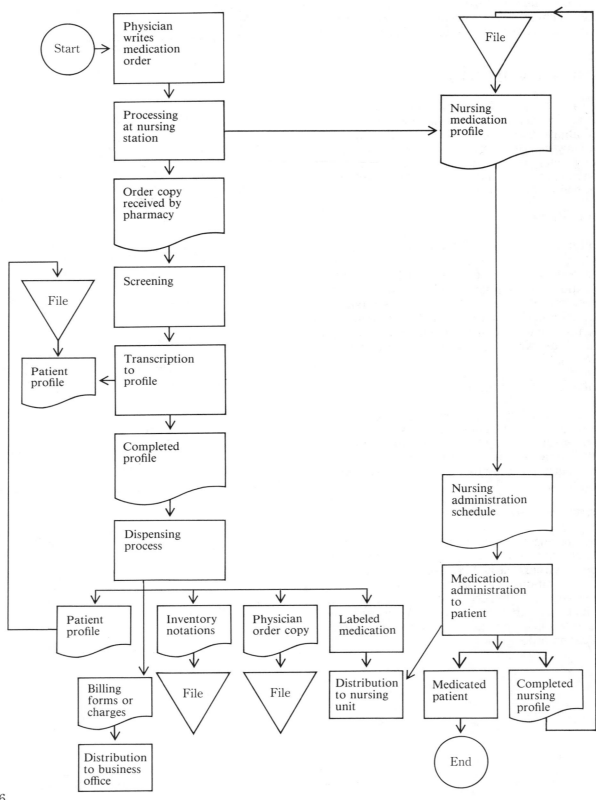

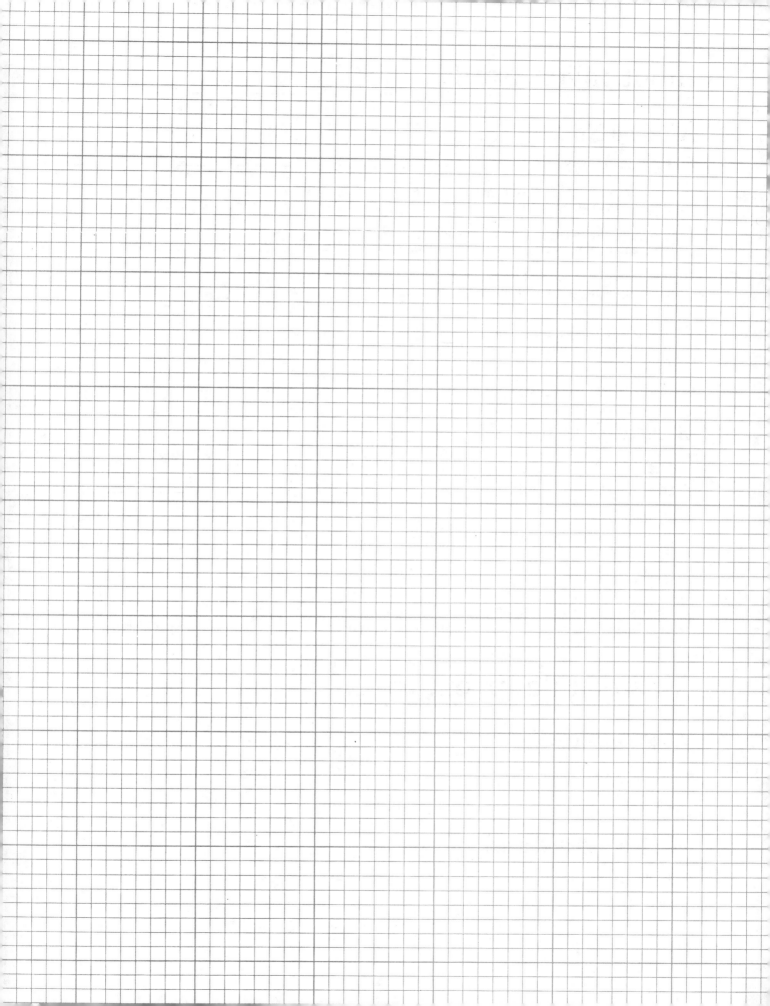

Input Inventory 1.2

A. Head Nurse

A B C

1. Medication order form. ☐ ☐ ☐ _____

2. Medication-order copies – only when original order system is in use. ☐ ☐ ☐ _____

3. Nursing patient medication profiles – for documentation of medication administration. ☐ ☐ ☐ _____

4. Administration schedule forms – for coordination of medication administration in a nursing unit. ☐ ☐ ☐ _____

5. Specialty requisition forms – including floor stock, controlled substances, and IV admixtures. ☐ ☐ ☐ _____

6. Controlled-substance log. ☐ ☐ ☐ _____

B. Head Pharmacist

1. Patient profile. ☐ ☐ ☐ _____

2. Medication label. ☐ ☐ ☐ _____

3. Charge form. ☐ ☐ ☐ _____

4. Inventory control sheet. ☐ ☐ ☐ _____

5. Purchase order. ☐ ☐ ☐ _____

USE INPUT DOCUMENT ANALYSIS FORM

A = same document title   B = minor variations   C = significant differences

Master File Inventory 1.2

A. Head Nurse

A B C

1. Nursing medication profile files. ☐ ☐ ☐ _____

2. Formulary. ☐ ☐ ☐ _____

B. Head Pharmacist

1. Patient profile file. ☐ ☐ ☐ _____

2. Physician-order copy files. ☐ ☐ ☐ _____

		A	B	C	Notes
3.	Formulary.	☐	☐	☐	_____
4.	Physician roster.	☐	☐	☐	_____
5.	Inventory status file.	☐	☐	☐	_____
6.	Price book.	☐	☐	☐	_____
7.	Purchase order file.	☐	☐	☐	_____

USE MASTER FILE ANALYSIS FORM

A = essentially similar   B = minor variations   C = significant differences

Report Inventory 1.2

A. Head Nurse

your document title ↓

		A	B	C	
1.	Current medication administration schedules.	☐	☐	☐	_____
2.	Medication error reports.	☐	☐	☐	_____

Head Pharmacist

		A	B	C	
1.	Inventory status report.	☐	☐	☐	_____
2.	Periodic purchasing reports – by dollars, by vendor, by drug category.	☐	☐	☐	_____

USE REPORT ANALYSIS FORM

A = essentially similar   B = minor variations   C = significant differences

System Performance Standards 1.2

		Units	A	B
1.	How much time elapses between the time a physician writes an order and the delivery of the order to Pharmacy?	minutes_____	☐	☐
2.	How much time elapses between the receipt of an order by Pharmacy and the delivery of the medication?	minutes_____	☐	☐
3.	How many STAT orders are received?	number of STAT orders weekly divided by total number of medication orders weekly _____	☐	☐

4. How many prescriptions are filled per patient day?

number of prescriptions filled
monthly divided by patient
days per month _____ A B □ □

number of prescriptions filled
monthly divided by patient
days per month _____ A B □ □

5. How many prescriptions are filled per pharmacy employee?

prescriptions filled yearly
divided by Pharmacy full-
time equivalents (FTEs) ____ □ □

6. Does Pharmacy have a formulary?

yes or no _____ □ □

7. How many medication errors are reported monthly?

number per month _____ □ □

8. What is the value of Pharmacy's inventory?

dollars _____ □ □

9. What is the value of all floor stock inventory?

dollars _____ □ □

USE PERFORMANCE STANDARDS ANALYSIS FORM

A = we have a standard   B = we do not have a standard

System Cost Factors 1.2

1. How much time is spent by Pharmacy discussing orders with physicians and nurses? $ _____

2. How many people are employed to deliver medications to Nursing Stations? $ _____

3. How much medication is stolen yearly? $ _____

4. How much nursing time is spent preparing medication for distribution? $ _____

USE SYSTEM COST ANALYSIS FORM *(also see Instructions, p. 15)*

System 1.3: Nursing Services

Description 1.3

Nursing is the hub of all hospital activity. It is the major contact point with patients; coordinates and carries out physician-originated treatment plans; interfaces between the physician and the patient; and, to an increasing degree, is involved in teaching the patient self-care.

Nursing's impact on the rest of the hospital is also significant. In one way or another, the department interacts with every other part of the institution. The flow charts below show the major areas of information flow into and out of Nursing.

Each hospital is divided into Nursing Stations. Each Nursing Station is classified according to the type of patient it handles. Medical and General Surgical are the two most common categories, usually accounting for up to 80 percent of the hospital's total bed complement.

Other types of Stations commonly encountered are:

A. Intensive Care.

B. Cardiac Intensive Care.

C. Surgical Intensive Care.

D. Labor and Delivery.

E. Maternity.

F. Pediatrics.

G. Nursery.

H. Gynecology.

I. Mental Health.

J. Stepdown.

K. Disease-Specific Stations, such as Oncology Stations.

L. Specialist-Specific Stations, such as Orthopedic Stations.

Notes

A B C

A = essentially similar   B = minor variations   C = significant differences

41

Each type of Station differs in terms of the number of people assigned, the skills required of Nursing personnel, and the mix of job titles needed for the Station. In addition, some types may require special forms. But the basic flow of information and responsibility is about the same for all types of Stations.

A B C

☐ ☐ ☐ _____

The figure which follows shows the typical organization of a Nursing Department. The number of levels of management may vary, depending on the size of the hospital, but the basic structure remains the same. Flow charts 1.3a, 1.3b, 1.3c, and 1.3d present a view of how nursing interacts with various departments.

☐ ☐ ☐ _____

A = essentially similar   B = minor variations   C = significant differences

Figure 10
Organization of a Typical Nursing Department

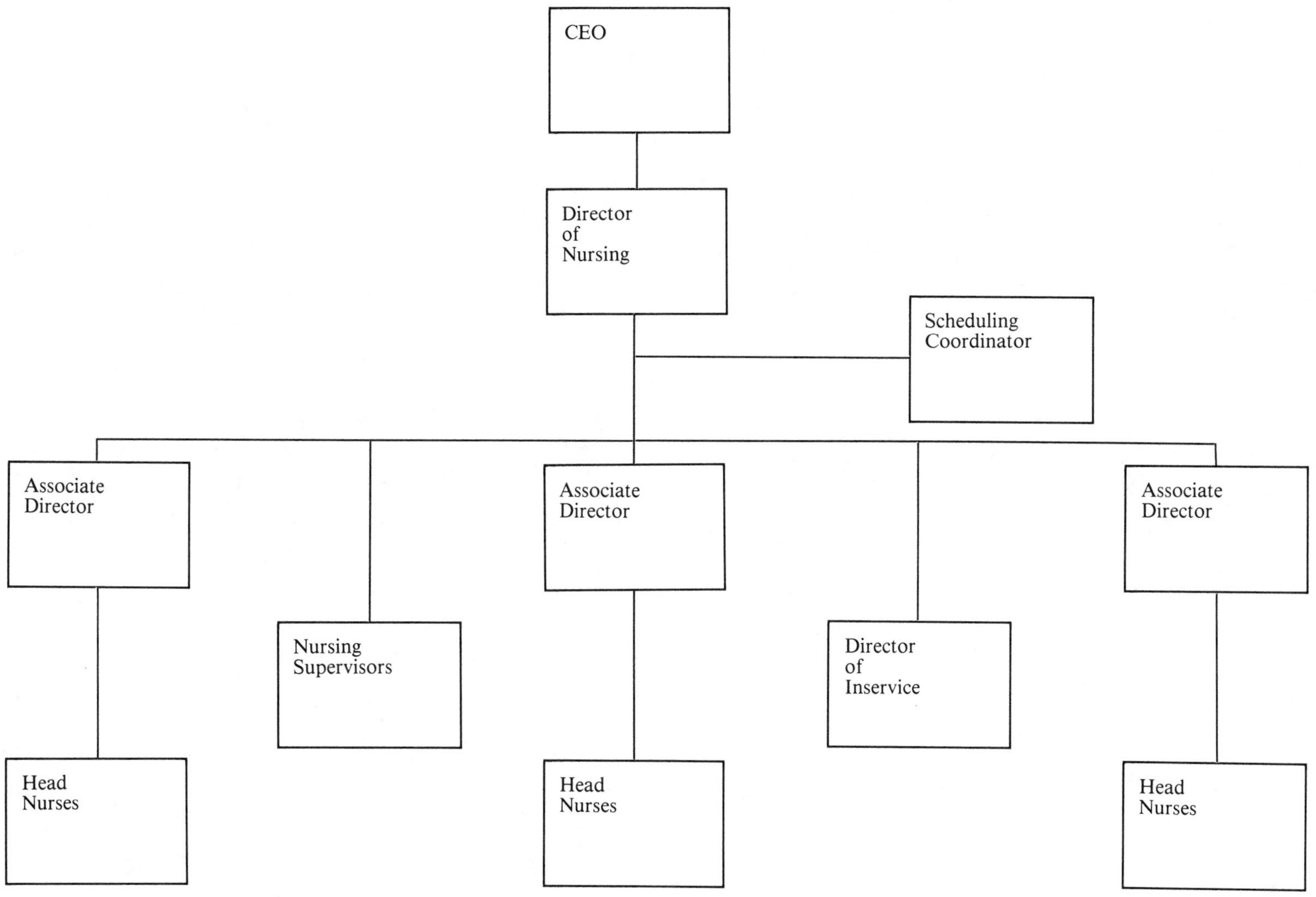

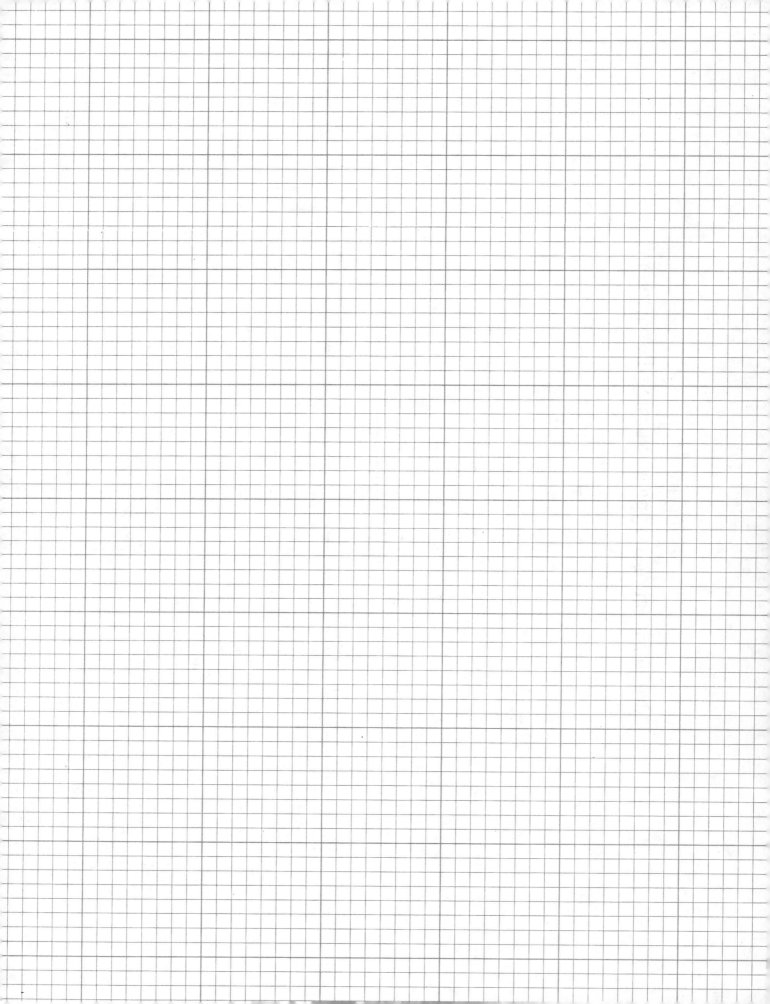

The Flow

The movement of a patient through a Nursing Station is described below. It should be kept in mind that Nursing interacts in some way with practically all other systems and subsystems in the institution. The flow charts following the description broadly indicate how these relationships work. For more detail, consult the sections dealing with the individual non-Nursing departments.

A B C
☐ ☐ ☐ _____

A patient comes to the Nursing Station from Admitting, the Emergency Department, or another Nursing Station.

☐ ☐ ☐ _____

When the patient arrives a nurse performs an initial evaluation of the patient's condition, makes sure that the patient has been placed in the right bed and room, and obtains orders from the patient's physician. The orders, which the physician writes in the patient's chart, are transcribed – converted into requisitions for services and treatments.

☐ ☐ ☐ _____

After this initial activity is completed, the Nursing Staff prepares a treatment plan. In some institutions, this becomes part of the Medical Record; in others, it is filed alphabetically by Nursing. In conjunction with the physician's orders, the plan establishes the treatment regimen for the patient.

☐ ☐ ☐ _____

The Nursing Station is responsible for a large number of ongoing activities.

☐ ☐ ☐ _____

The patient's condition is continually evaluated, with modifications being made to the treatment plan as required.

☐ ☐ ☐ _____

Physician orders are carried out promptly and accurately.

☐ ☐ ☐ _____

Nurses record information about the patient's condition and about related items in the Nursing Notes portion of the patient's chart.

☐ ☐ ☐ _____

Vital signs (i.e., temperature, blood pressure, and pulse) are recorded periodically.

☐ ☐ ☐ _____

Medications are administered and custodial care is rendered.

☐ ☐ ☐ _____

When the physician writes a discharge order, the Nursing Station is responsible for preparing the patient for discharge. This responsibility may include patient training.

☐ ☐ ☐ _____

A = essentially similar   B = minor variations   C = significant differences

Scheduling

Traditionally hospitals may take either of two approaches to scheduling Nursing Personnel. One method is to assign a relatively large number of people to each Station. Then, as patient load and employee attendance dictate, Nursing administration reassigns (i.e. pulls) these people on a temporary basis to the Stations that need the most help.

A B C
□ □ □ _____

The second approach is to establish a float pool, made up of Nursing personnel who are not permanently assigned to a particular Station. Instead, they are moved about by the Staffing Coordinator on a day-by-day basis.

□ □ □ _____

Some hospitals are now trying to staff on the basis of how much care patients at each Nursing Station need. In one variation the total number of care units (or level of patient acuity) is computed on the basis of the patient's diagnosis, length of stay to date, and age. Another approach is to compute care units needed by having the Nursing Stations complete question-naires about each patient each day.

□ □ □ ____ _____

The staffing-by-need approach has two theoretical advantages. First, more precise staffing, in terms of the number of Nursing personnel assigned, results. Second, better staffing, in terms of skill levels, results.

□ □ □ _____

Nurse Audit

Many hospitals have a committee of nurses with the responsibility of monitoring the quality of the nursing care rendered in the institution.

□ □ □ _____

It is usually called the Nurse Audit Committee. It reviews the charts of patients with specific diagnoses and compares the treatment rendered with the treatment called for by contemporary nursing standards.

□ □ □ _____

A = essentially similar   B = minor variations   C = significant differences

Flow Chart 1.3a

Nursing Interactions/Patient

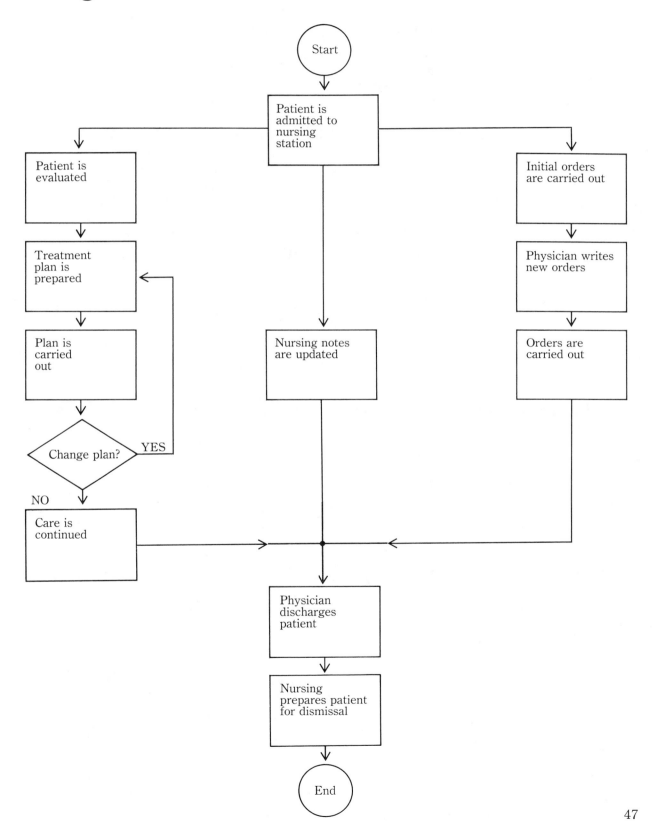

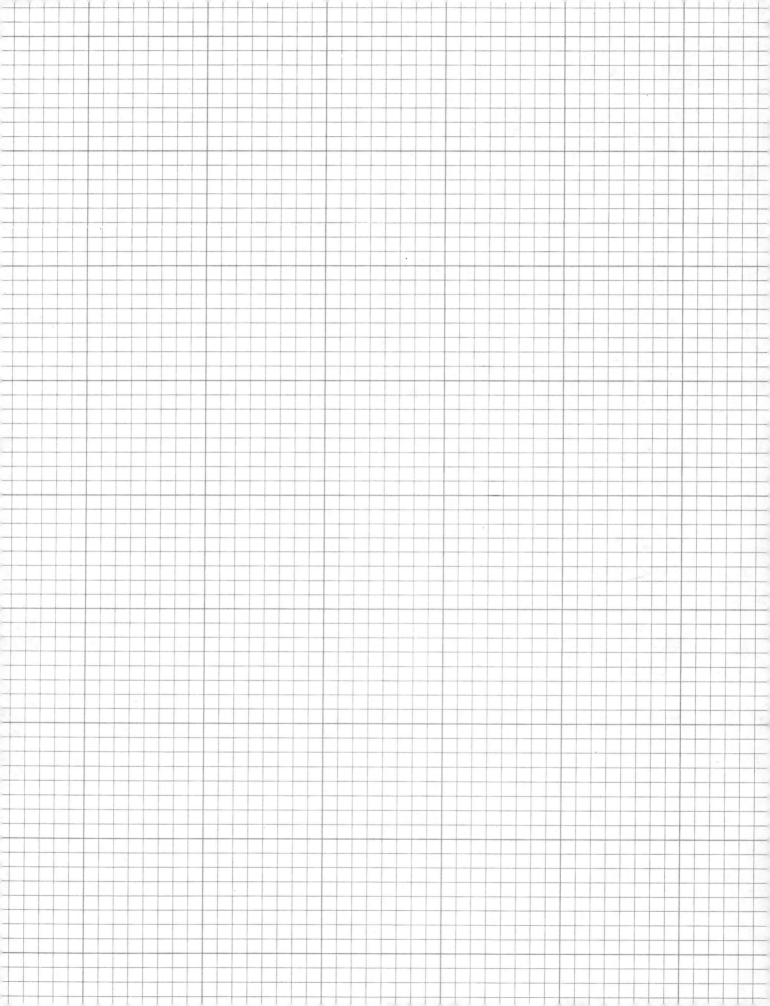

Flow Chart 1.3b

Nursing Interactions/Support Departments

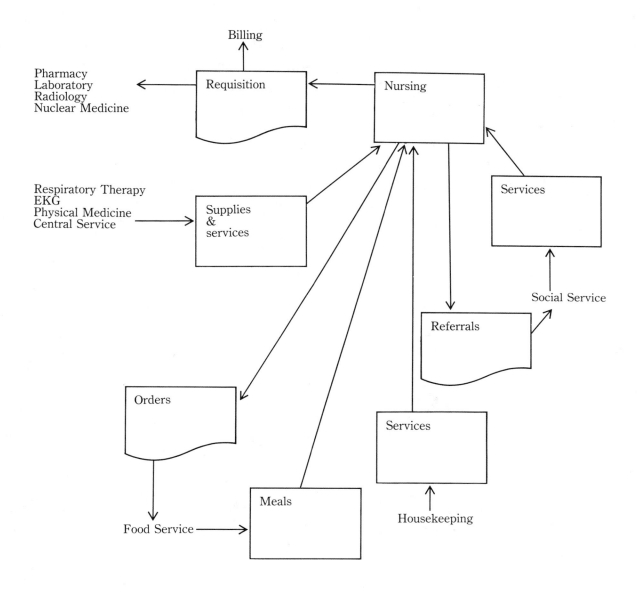

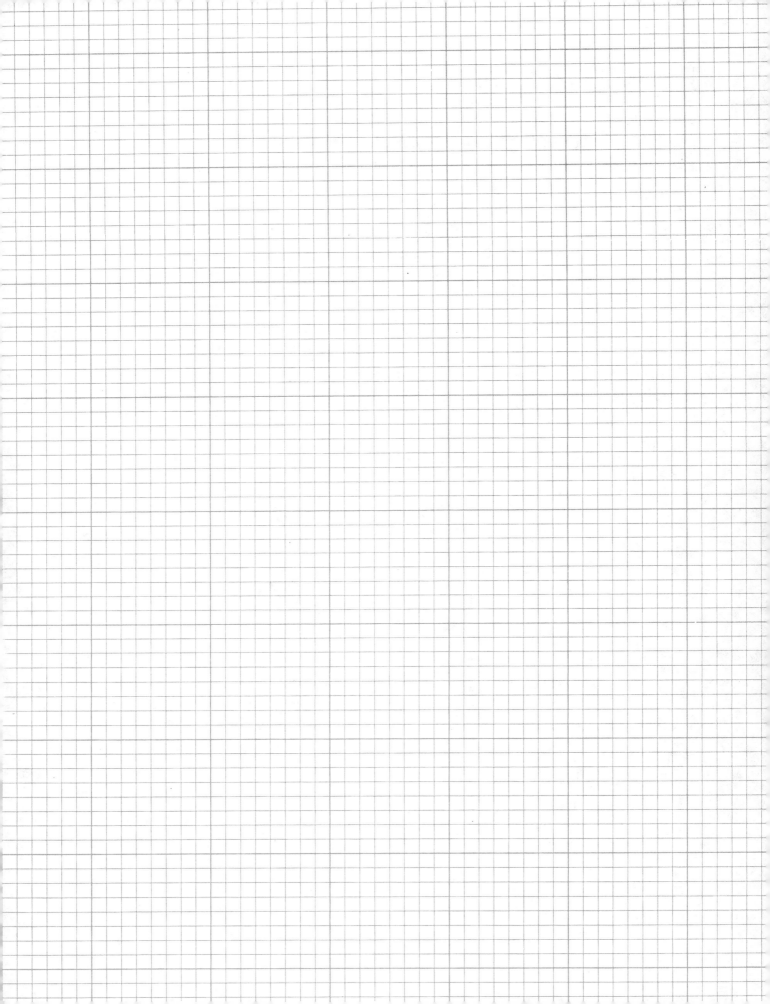

Flow Chart 1.3c

Nursing Interactions/Patient Movement

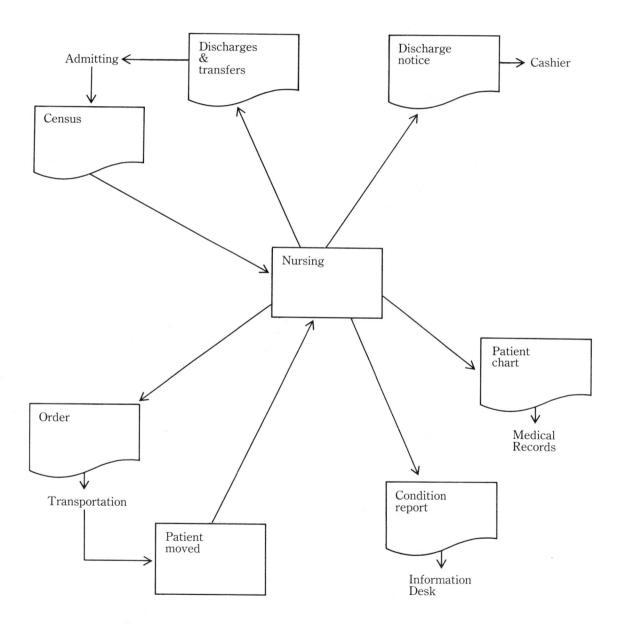

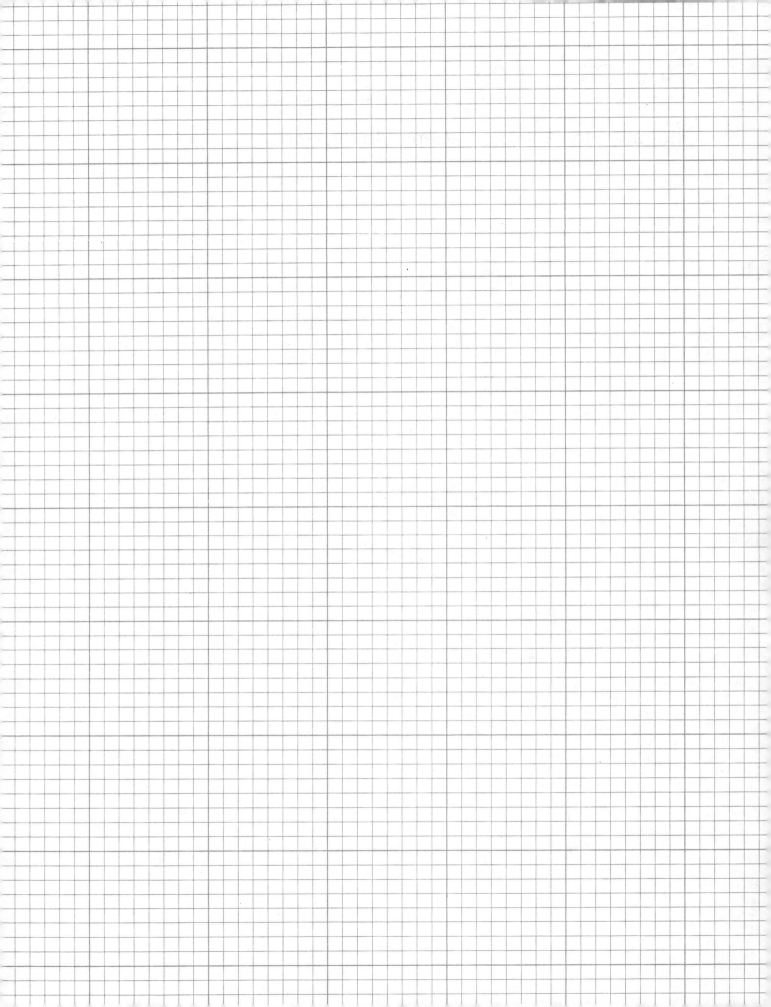

Flow Chart 1.3d

Nursing Interactions/Nonpatient Services

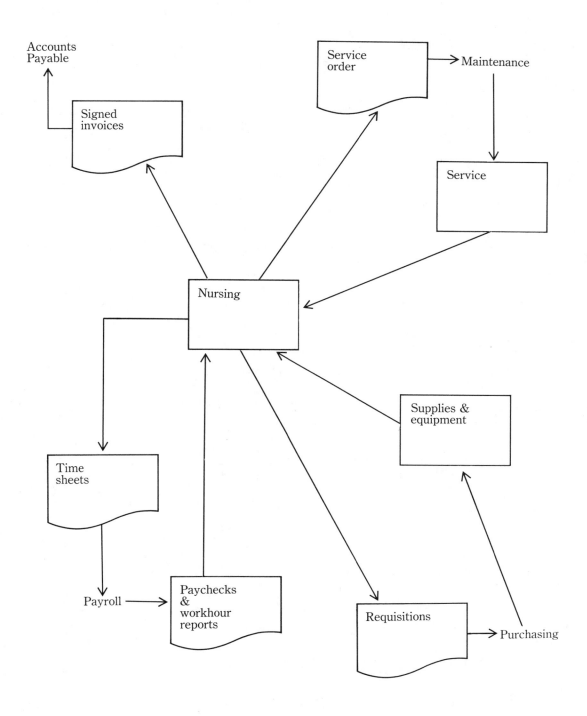

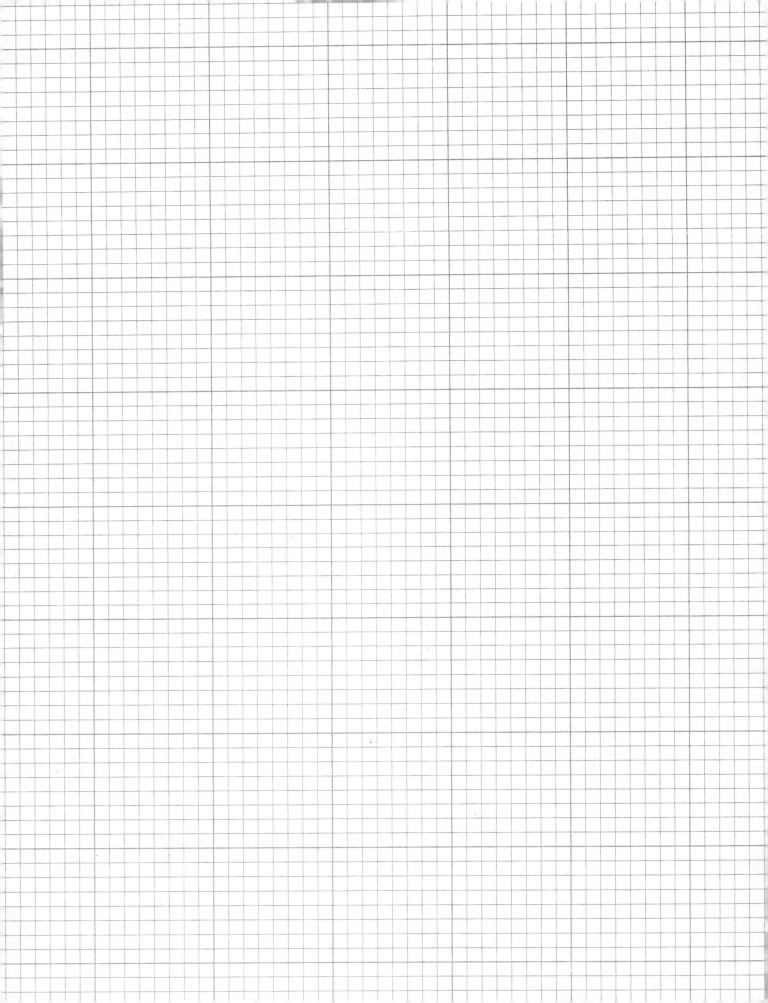

Input Inventory 1.3

A. Director of Nursing

your document title
↓

      A B C

1. Treatment Plan.   □ □ □ _____

2. Scheduling Worksheet.   □ □ □ _____

B. Head Nurse/Specialty Units

(Obtain copies of all special forms.)   □ □ □ _____

USE INPUT DOCUMENT ANALYSIS FORM

A = same document title	B = minor variations	C = significant differences

Master File Inventory 1.3

A. Director of Nursing

Notes
↓

      A B C

Treatment plans.   □ □ □ _____

USE MASTER FILE ANALYSIS FORM

A = essentially similar	B = minor variations	C = significant differences

Report Inventory 1.3

(none)

System Performance Standards 1.3

	Units	A	B
1. What percentage of physician orders are transcribed within 30 minutes?	percent _____	□	□
2. Are Nursing Notes up-to-date (i.e., the last entry was made less than eight hours ago)?	yes or no _____	□	□
3. Is there a treatment plan for each patient?	yes or no _____	□	□
4. Is there a Nurse Audit Committee?	yes or no _____	□	□
5. Are test results arranged in the chart in a way that allows the physician and the nurse to easily spot trends?	yes or no _____	□	□

6. What is the ratio of nursing hours to patient days?

nursing workhours for a two-week period divided by the product of 14 and the average census for those two weeks _____

A B
□ □

7. How much overtime does nursing work?

nursing overtime hours divided by total hours worked _____

□ □

8. Are Nursing Notes timed, dated, and signed?

yes or no _____

□ □

9. How much time does each Nurse spend in continuing education (i.e. inservice) conducted in the hospital?

hours per year per nurse ____

□ □

10. How much time to RNs spend in "charting" activities?

hours per shift _____

□ □

11. How many medication errors are made?

ratio of medication errors yearly to annual patient days _____

□ □

USE PERFORMANCE STANDARDS ANALYSIS FORM

A = we have a standard

B = we do not have a standard

System Cost Factors 1.3

1. How much Nursing time is spent preparing requisitions? $ _____

2. How much Nursing time is spent performing all clerical functions? $ _____

3. What is the dollar value of all forms stored at a typical Nursing Station? $ _____

4. What is the dollar value of all floor stock stored at a typical Nursing Station? $ _____

5. What is the turnover rate for Nursing? $ _____

6. How many medical records do Nursing Stations send to Medical Records without the records having all test results posted? $ _____

7. Does the amount of non-floor-stock medication stored at Nursing Stations correspond to that shown on patient medical records and Pharmacy records of medications issued? $ _____

USE SYSTEM COST ANALYSIS FORM *(also see Instructions, p. 15)*

System 1.4.1:
Patient Food Services
Description 1.4.1

The Food Service Department has four main roles – to provide meals to patients, carry out dietary orders from physicians, provide patients with nutrition and diet education, and consult with physicians on nutritional problems.

A B C
□ □ □ _____

Meal Service

The flow begins when the head of the Food Service Department develops a Master Menu. This document lays out the items that will be served each day for a fixed period of time (normally two weeks). When that period is over, the department recycles the Master Menu. The Master Menu approach provides predictability to the department and variety to the patient.

□ □ □ _____

Working from the Master Menu, the Food Preparation Supervisor requisitions needed food items from the department's inventory area. In addition, each day the supervisor prepares a production schedule for the next day. This schedule shows how much of each item (e.g., how many tossed salads, how many slices of bacon) should be prepared and who is responsible for which item. The Master Menu determines what is to be made, and the hospital census determines the quantity. Admissions routinely routes this census to the Food Preparation Department.

□ □ □ _____

Once all needed items have been readied, tray preparation begins. The exact composition of each tray depends on two factors – the menu dictated by the Master Menu and the dietary restrictions invoked by the patient's physician.

□ □ □ _____

The Tray Preparation Supervisor is responsible for preparing a specific layout for each tray. Information on dietary restrictions comes from the Clinical Nutritionist.

□ □ □ _____

Some hospitals allow patients to select their meals from a menu that offers two or three choices. Most hospitals prepare selective menus for each major dietary regimen. Under this system, menus are passed out to patients, who then mark their selections. These menus are

---

A=essentially similar   B=minor variations   C=significant differences

delivered to the Tray Preparation Supervisor, who incorporates the patient selections into his or her tray-layout instructions.

The patient-selection system is compatible with the Master-Menu approach. It just results in a more complicated Master Menu.

☐ ☐ ☐

Once trays are prepared, Food Service technicians deliver them to the Nursing Stations. In some hospitals, the technicians also serve the meals. In others, Nursing is responsible for this task.

☐ ☐ ☐

At a fixed time after the meal hour, the Food Service technicians return to the Nursing Stations to retrieve the trays. The trays are returned to the department, where the garbage is disposed of, and the trays, flatware, and utensils are cleaned.

☐ ☐ ☐

Clinical Activities

The physician personally writes the dietary order. Nursing Stations are then responsible for providing the order for special therapeutic diets. In some cases, the dietary order is part of a standing order relating to a patient who is going to surgery or being scheduled for a specific diagnostic procedure.

☐ ☐ ☐

The Unit Secretary transcribes the order onto a Diet-Change form. In some institutions, codes have been developed for the most common orders (low sodium, liquid, etc.)

☐ ☐ ☐

The Diet-Change form is sent to the Nutritionist, who puts the information on an index card, which is kept in an alphabetical file. If a patient has been under prior dietary orders, a card for the patient will be in a file. In this case, the Nutritionist reviews the patient's dietary history and adds the new information to the card.

☐ ☐ ☐

Once the Nutritionist examines the Diet-Change Form, he or she notifies the Tray Preparation Supervisor of the type of diet the patient is to receive. This information is used to establish a tray-preparation worksheet for that patient.

☐ ☐ ☐

The Nutritionist may also meet with the patient to discuss the physician's dietary prescription.

☐ ☐ ☐

A = essentially similar   B = minor variations   C = significant differences

Census Information

The Food Service Department should receive copies of discharge and transfer notices as well as notification of admissions.

A B C
□ □ □ _____

When the department is told of an admission, it adds the patient's name to the list of those who will receive a tray at the next meal hour.

□ □ □ _____

Transfer notices allow the department to bring the proper meal to the proper room.

□ □ □ _____

Discharge information allows the department to discontinue service. In addition, it alerts the Nutritionist to remove the cards of certain discharged patients from the special-diet file.

□ □ □ _____

Other Services

The Food Service Department also provides meals on a nonscheduled basis in circumstances such as late admissions.

□ □ □ _____

In most hospitals, the department also has responsibility for operating the hospital's cafeteria.

□ □ □ _____

Inventory

The Food Service Department is one of the few departments handling its own purchasing. (Pharmacy is usually the only other.)

□ □ □ _____

Purchasing procedures are similar to those followed by the hospital's Purchasing Department. In some hospitals, Purchasing assigns a block of PO numbers to Food Service, and then monitors the flow of purchase orders. In other institutions, Food Service operates entirely independent of Purchasing.

□ □ □ _____

The department's own Inventory Supervisor places orders based on the Master Menu. The items are stocked in a central area and distributed to the Food Preparation Area on the basis of requisitions submitted by the Food Preparation Supervisor.

□ □ □ _____

A = essentially similar   B = minor variations   C = significant differences

Flow Chart 1.4.1

Meal Preparation

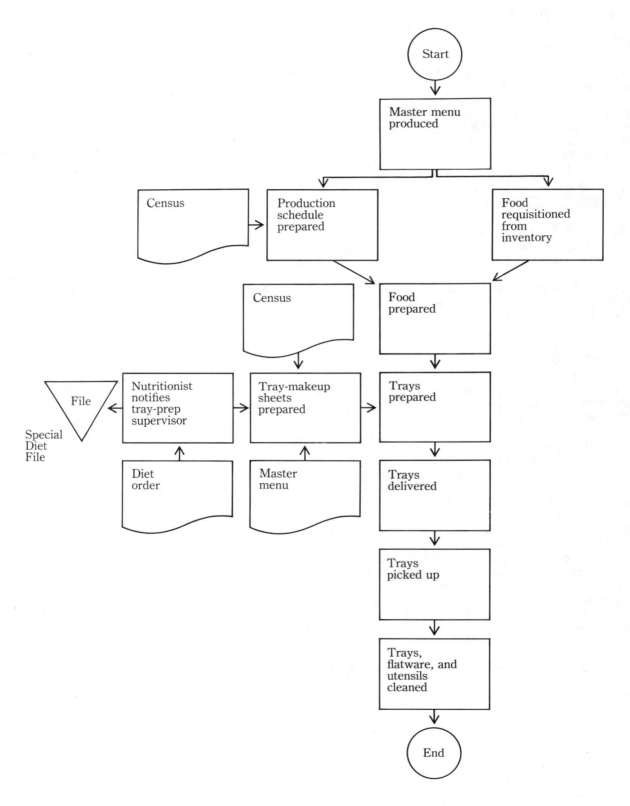

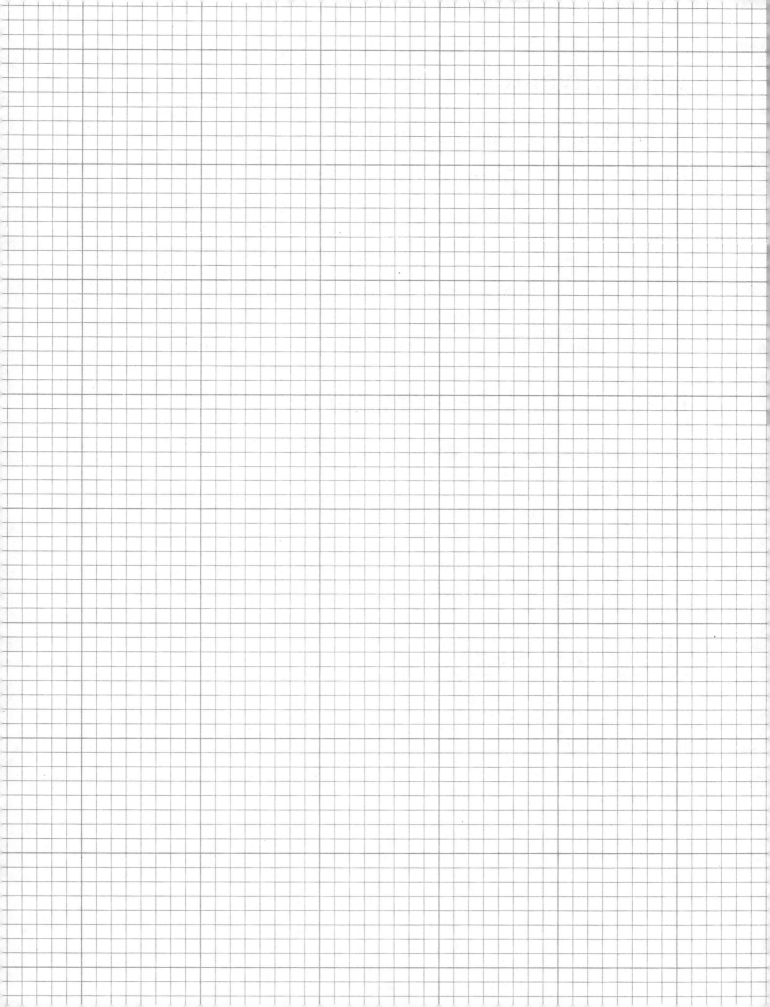

Input Inventory 1.4.1

A. Food Service Department Head

your document title
↓

1. Diet-Change notification from Nursing Station. A B C ☐ ☐ ☐ _____

2. Food requisition from Food Preparation Supervisor. ☐ ☐ ☐ _____

3. Patient menus. ☐ ☐ ☐ _____

4. Admission/discharge/transfer notification. ☐ ☐ ☐ _____

USE INPUT DOCUMENT ANALYSIS FORM

A = same document title   B = minor variations   C = significant differences

Master File Inventory 1.4.1

A. Food Service Supervisor

Notes
↓

A B C

1. Master Menu. ☐ ☐ ☐ _____

2. Nutritionist's patient file. ☐ ☐ ☐ _____

3. Census master sheet. ☐ ☐ ☐ _____

USE MASTER FILE ANALYSIS FORM

A = essentially similar   B = minor variations   C = significant differences

Report Inventory 1.4.1

A. Food Service Supervisor

your document title
↓

A B C

1. Production schedule. ☐ ☐ ☐ _____

2. Tray preparation sheets. ☐ ☐ ☐ _____

3. Monthly activity report. ☐ ☐ ☐ _____

USE REPORT ANALYSIS FORM

A = essentially similar   B = minor variations   C = significant differences

System Performance Standards 1.4.1

	Units	A	B
1. How often are meals delivered after a patient has been transferred or discharged?	times monthly _____	☐	☐
2. How long does it take from the time a physician writes a dietary order until the order is carried out?	hours_____	☐	☐
3. How often is a dietary order not carried out or improperly carried out?	times per month _____	☐	☐
4. How many patients with special diets are seen by a Nutritionist?	using one given time, number of patients seen divided by number of patients with special orders _____	☐	☐
5. How long does it take to prepare a tray?	seconds_____	☐	☐
6. How long does it take to deliver a completed tray?	minutes_____	☐	☐

USE PERFORMANCE STANDARDS ANALYSIS FORM

A = we have a standard   B = we do not have a standard

System Cost Factors 1.4.1

1. What is the cost of special equipment used to notify Food Service of admissions, discharges, and transfers? $ _____

2. How much food is wasted because of bad census information? $ _____

3. How much food is wasted because of inaccuracies in the production schedule or tray-preparation sheets? $ _____

4. What is the size of the food inventory? $ _____

5. How much Nursing time is spent serving food? $ _____

USE SYSTEM COST ANALYSIS FORM *(also see Instructions, p. 15)*

System 1.4.2: Linen/Laundry

Description 1.4.2

Notes
↓

The bulk of the Laundry's activity involves cleaning and supplying sheets, pillowcases and bedclothes for inpatient use. In addition, the department keeps the Operating Room, the Emergency Department, and other treatment areas supplied with surgical drapes, scrub suits, and other needed linen.

A B C
□ □ □ _____

Preparing the Bed

The inpatient cycle begins when a physician writes a discharge order or a patient is transferred. In addition to notifying Admitting of the discharge or transfer, the Nursing Station also informs Housekeeping, either by telephoning or by sending a copy of the discharge/transfer notice to that department. In response, Housekeeping dispatches a maid to prepare the now-empty bed for a new patient.

□ □ □ _____

As part of that task, the maid removes the dirty linen from the bed and places it in the Nursing Station's soiled-linen area. This can be a small closet, a hamper, or a laundry chute. The maid then takes clean linen from the Nursing Station's linen closet and makes the bed. It should be noted that in some hospitals, nursing personnel are responsible for stripping and making beds.

□ □ □ _____

Periodically, Laundry technicians pick up the dirty laundry from the soiled-laundry areas or from a centralized pickup point. They bring the soiled linen to the Laundry, where it is sorted and then washed. Some hospitals log the receipt of dirty linen to assure that Laundry has received all the linen it sent out. The receipt log may record batches of linen received, weight of linen received, or item counts of linen received.

□ □ □ _____

After washing, the linen is weighed. Pounds-of-linen-washed is the traditional measure of productivity for the Laundry.

□ □ □ _____

After weighing, the linen is inspected for tears. Those items that need mending are set aside. Items that cannot be mended are taken out of circulation. The rest of the items are ironed, folded, and stored.

□ □ □ _____

A = essentially similar   B = minor variations   C = significant differences

The Laundry usually restocks Nursing Stations and other linen users on a daily basis. Laundry technicians pack a cart with needed linen and take it to each Nursing Station. Each linen closet has a predetermined stocking level for each item. The Laundry technicians, who have copies of these stocking lists, bring each closet up to its proper inventory level. The technicians also record on their own logs how much of each item went into each closet. These logs are filed in Laundry.

A B C
□ □ □ _____

There are other approaches to resupplying. Some hospitals prefer the exchange-cart approach. As with the linen-closet method outlined above, each Nursing Station has a pre-set inventory level for each linen item. Two supply carts are assigned to each Nursing Station. Periodically – usually daily – Laundry Technicians fill one cart with a complete supply of linen, deliver it to the Nursing Station, and bring the second cart back to Laundry. They then restock this cart to the proper level, recording on their logs how much of each item was needed. The next day the process is repeated, with the second cart exchanged for the first.

□ □ □ _____

Another approach for preparing a bed for a new patient is to supply Housekeeping with discharge packs – sets that contain all the linen needed to prepare a room for a new patient. When Housekeeping is notified of a discharge or transfer, a maid takes one pack to the room that is to be prepared. This approach reduces the amount of linen that must be stored at each Nursing Station.

□ □ □ _____

Some hospitals restock only on the basis of a requisition. Periodically, the Head Nurse or Supervisor reviews the linen inventory, completes a requisition, and sends it to Laundry.

□ □ □ _____

Finally, some hospitals use an informal approach to restocking. When the linen level appears low, the Nursing Station telephones a request for more linen.

□ □ □ _____

Nursing Stations need linen supplies for uses other than preparing beds for new patients. On a daily basis, each patient receives fresh towels, with the soiled ones being placed in the soiled-linen area or in a laundry chute.

□ □ □ _____

Once a patient has been admitted, Housekeeping or Nursing changes the bedclothes periodically. If Nursing is responsible for the change, the Head Nurse keeps track of which patients need fresh sheets on a particular day. If the respon-

---

A = essentially similar   B = minor variations   C = significant differences

sibility is Housekeeping's, that department either reviews the census daily and monitors the length-of-stay figure, or keeps a tally sheet showing which patients are due for a bed change. There must also be a tally sheet listing those patients who need frequent sheet changes (e.g., patients with open sores or bowel-control problems).

A B C
☐ ☐ ☐ _____

Finally, patients in isolation often have special needs in the area of linen supply. Accomodating those needs involves three units — Nursing, the hospital's Infection Control Committee, and Housekeeping. These units work together to establish procedures for handling isolation cases.

☐ ☐ ☐ _____

Surgery

In most other treatment areas that need sheets or other linen, the cleaning-restocking cycle is identical to that described for the Nursing Station. In the Operating Room, however, there are additional considerations.

☐ ☐ ☐ _____

Nonsterile linen items are processed in the same manner as Nursing Station linen. Some hospitals may control the dispensing of scrub suits and other uniforms by insisting on a one-for-one exchange. But, basically, Laundry's procedure is to pick up the soiled linen, then bring the linen supply area back up to proper inventory levels.

☐ ☐ ☐ _____

When dealing with linen that must be sterile, there are additional processes followed by Laundry. If Central Service is responsible for supplying all sterile items to the Operating Room, Laundry simply washes all Operating Room linen and sends to Central Service those items that must be sterilized.

☐ ☐ ☐ _____

If Laundry is responsible for sterilizing, the department has a special section that makes up the surgical linen packs, sterilizes them, stocks them, and then resupplies the Operating Room.

☐ ☐ ☐ _____

Uniforms

In some hospitals, the Laundry washes, irons, and stores uniforms for certain employees and physicians. Typically, the uniforms are delivered to the Laundry in batches and are kept separate from bedclothes and other linen. The uniforms, which are marked with the user's name, are returned after they are laundered.

☐ ☐ ☐ _____

A = essentially similar   B = minor variations   C = significant differences

Outside Laundries

Some hospitals have done away with their
Laundry Department. They either contract with
a private firm to handle the hospital's linen, join
with other hospitals in operating a shared
laundry, or contract with a linen-supply
company.

A B C

☐ ☐ ☐ _____

With an outside or shared-laundry system, it
becomes very important to keep an accurate
accounting of the amount of laundry leaving the
institution and returning to it. One control
technique is to have both the hospital and the
outside laundry log the number of batches sent
to the laundry and the number received from it
each day. A comparison of the two logs will
validate that all linen leaving the institution is
returned.

☐ ☐ ☐ _____

A = essentially similar   B = minor variations   C = significant differences

Flow Chart 1.4.2

Linen Flow at Nursing Station

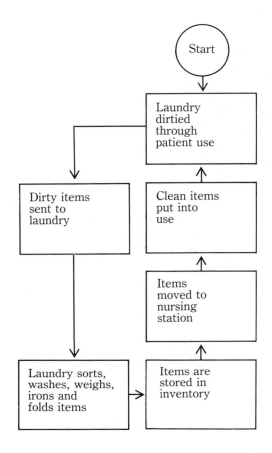

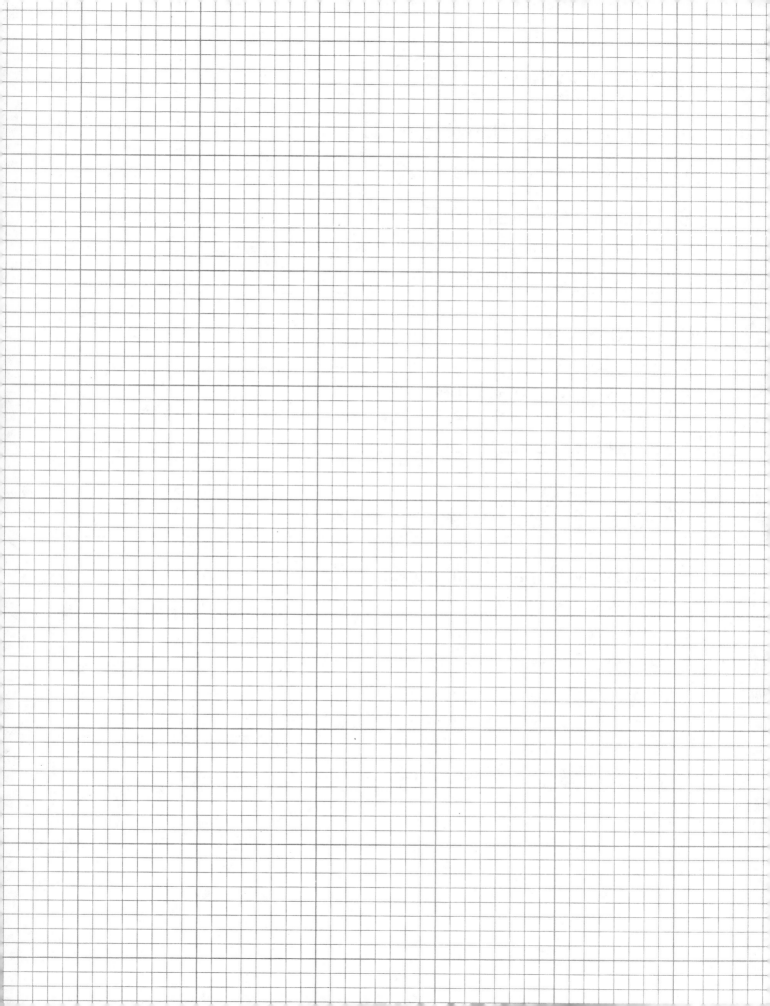

Input Inventory 1.4.2

your document title
↓

A. Housekeeping Department Head

	A	B	C	
Discharge/transfer notice sent to Housekeeping.	☐	☐	☐	_____

B. Laundry Department Head

	A	B	C	
1. Stocking lists for linen closets or carts.	☐	☐	☐	_____
2. Restocking logs used by technicians in restocking closets or carts.	☐	☐	☐	_____

C. Head Nurse

	A	B	C	
1. Laundry requisition.	☐	☐	☐	_____
2. Notification of isolation patient or other special case.	☐	☐	☐	_____

USE INPUT DOCUMENT ANALYSIS FORM

A = same document title	B = minor variations	C = significant differences

Master File Inventory 1.4.2

Notes
↓

A. Laundry Department Head

	A	B	C	
1. Log for receipt of soiled linen.	☐	☐	☐	_____
2. Log of weight of cleaned linen.	☐	☐	☐	_____
3. Log of linen items disposed.	☐	☐	☐	_____
4. Current inventory.	☐	☐	☐	_____
5. Listing of isolation patients and other special cases.	☐	☐	☐	_____

USE MASTER FILE ANALYSIS FORM

A = essentially similar	B = minor variations	C = significant differences

Report Inventory 1.4.2

A. Laundry Department Head

your document title
↓

                                           A B C
1. Monthly department productivity report.   □ □ □   _____

2. Linen usage by Nursing Station and
   department.   □ □ □   _____

USE REPORT ANALYSIS FORM

A = essentially similar   B = minor variations   C = significant differences

System Performance Standards 1.4.2

	Units	A	B
1. How many pounds of linen does the Laundry process?	pounds per month divided by average number of beds occupied in that month _____	□	□
2. Is there an established level for each Nursing Station and department?	yes or no _____	□	□
3. What is the linen turnover?	estimated value of linen inventory divided by amount spent for linen in last 12 months _____	□	□
4. How often does a Nursing Station run out of a linen item?	number of times per week ____	□	□
5. How often does surgery run out of a linen item?	number of times per month __	□	□
6. How long does linen last?	mean age of items being thrown away _____	□	□
7. How much of the hospital's linen is disposable?	annual cost of disposable linen divided by sum of numerator and annual budget for reusable linen and Laundry labor _____	□	□

USE PERFORMANCE STANDARDS ANALYSIS FORM

A = we have a standard   B = we do not have a standard

System Cost Factors 1.4.2

1. What is the dollar value of extra linen stored at the Nursing Stations? $ _____

2. How much nursing time is spent requisitioning linen and assuring the proper
   stock levels are maintained? $ _____

3. What is the dollar value of linen stolen every year? $ _____

USE SYSTEM COST ANALYSIS FORM *(also see Instructions, p. 15)*

System 1.4.3: Patient Transportation

Description 1.4.3

Notes

There are four approaches to the problem of moving patients from one location to another. Hospitals may elect to use one of these or a combination of several. The approaches:

                                                      A B C

1. To centralize transportation by forming an independent department. ☐ ☐ ☐ _____

2. To assign transporters to individual departments, such as ancillary departments and the Operating Room. ☐ ☐ ☐ _____

3. To give Nursing the responsibility for moving patients. ☐ ☐ ☐ _____

4. To rely on volunteers. ☐ ☐ ☐ _____

Centralized Transportation

The process begins when the Transportation Department is notified that a patient must be moved. This can take place in several ways. The ancillary department requesting the patient may telephone or send a requisition to Transportation, or the ancillary department may call the Nursing Station, requesting the patient but giving Nursing the responsibility for contacting Transportation. ☐ ☐ ☐ _____

Another approach is for the Nursing Station to send requisitions to both the ancillary department and Transportation. Transportation then contacts the appropriate department to determine when the patient should be picked up. ☐ ☐ ☐ _____

Finally, each ancillary department may put out a daily list showing when patients are scheduled to undergo treatment or diagnostic testing. From this list, the transportation supervisor prepares daily work schedules. ☐ ☐ ☐ _____

Regardless of the approach, Transportation must be given the following information: the patient's name, hospital number and room and bed number, the department to which the patient is to be taken, the time the patient should arrive, and the desired method of transportation (wheelchair, stretcher, etc.). ☐ ☐ ☐ _____

A = essentially similar   B = minor variations   C = significant differences

Once Transportation is notified of the need to move a patient, the Transportation Supervisor logs the information listed above and prepares a dispatch ticket. At the appropriate time, the supervisor gives the ticket to a transporter, sends the transporter to the Nursing Station, and logs the transporter out of the department.

A B C
□ □ □ _____

The transporter reports to the Nursing Station, notifies the Charge Nurse that the patient is about to be picked up, and records the pickup on the Nursing Station log. The transporter's entry should include the patient's name, room, and bed number; the destination; the time of pickup; and the transporter's initials. The Nursing Station should then supply the transporter with any written clinical information that will be needed by the ancillary department. Such information usually includes the patient's history and physical examination results, medications being taken and indications for the requested procedure. In some hospitals, the full medical record accompanies the patient.

□ □ □ _____

When the patient arrives at the ancillary department, the accompanying transporter gives the dispatch ticket and the clinical information forms to the department's receptionist. The transporter then returns to the Transportation Department and is logged back in by the supervisor.

□ □ □ _____

When the ancillary department finishes with the patient, it notifies Transportation that the patient is ready to be returned to the Nursing Station. The ancillary department must give Transportation the same information that Transportation received when picking up the patient at the Nursing Station – name, room, and bed number, etc. The Transportation Supervisor logs the call and dispatches a transporter to pick up and deliver the patient to the appropriate Nursing Station. The transporter logs the patient back into the Nursing Station, then returns to Transportation, where he or she is then logged in.

□ □ □ _____

Departmental Transporters

At the beginning of the work day, a supervisor prepares a work schedule for the department. This schedule lists the patients who are to be seen, their room and bed numbers, and, occasionally, the time tests are to be performed. Working from this schedule, the supervisor dispatches transporters to pick up the scheduled patients. Usually, the transporter is given a copy of the requisition form as a dispatch ticket.

□ □ □ _____

A = essentially similar   B = minor variations   C = significant differences

In Surgery, a scheduling secretary, working from the day's surgery schedule, completes dispatch tickets and sends transporters to the Nursing Stations. As patients arrive, the clerk logs their names and times of arrival.

A B C
☐ ☐ ☐

At the Nursing Station, the transporter logs the pickup and takes the patient to the appropriate department.

☐ ☐ ☐

When the department finishes with the patient, a supervisor instructs a transporter to return the patient.

☐ ☐ ☐

Other Approaches

When Nursing handles its own transportation, the process is usually informal. When a patient is to be moved, the Charge Nurse tells those responsible – usually attendants or orderlies – where to take the particular patient. When a department finishes with a patient, the Nursing Station is contacted. Nursing then dispatches the personnel responsible for transporting.

☐ ☐ ☐

When volunteers are used, the process is much the same, with direction coming from the Director of Volunteers and the supervisors of the departments to which the volunteers are assigned. Typically, volunteers are assigned to Admitting and Nursing.

☐ ☐ ☐

A = essentially similar   B = minor variations   C = significant differences

Flow Chart 1.4.3a

Centralized Transportation

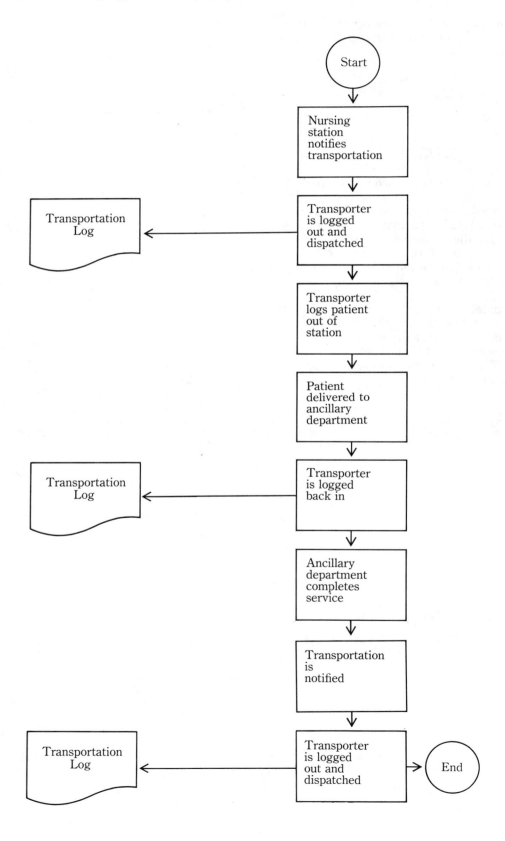

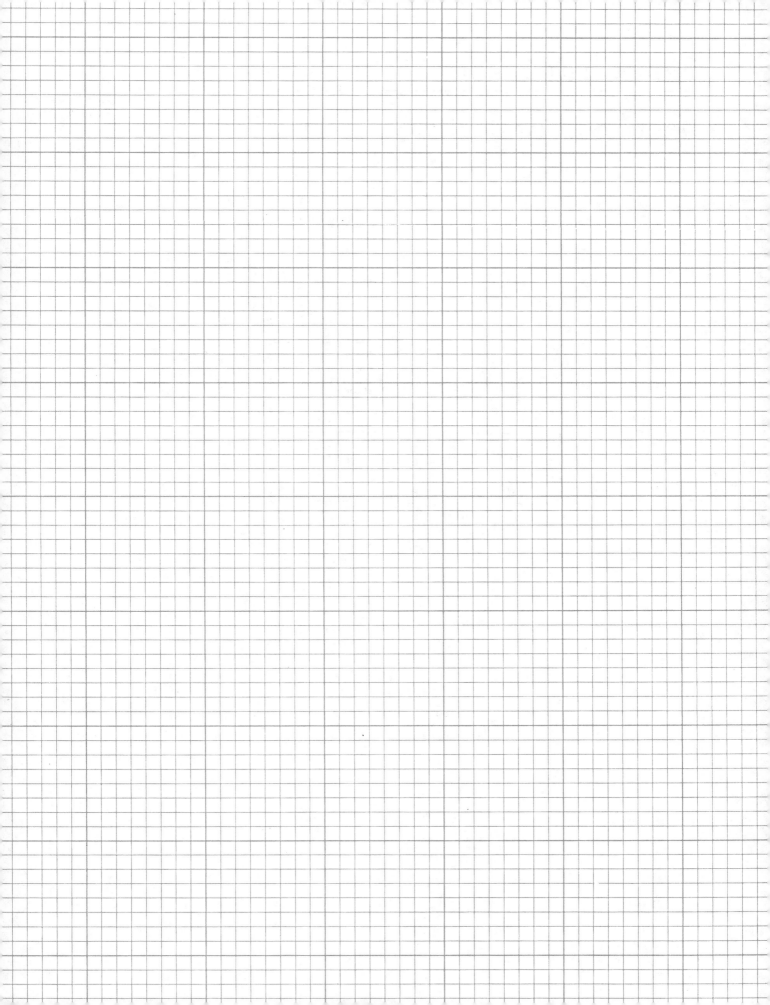

Flow Chart 1.4.3b

Departmental Transportation

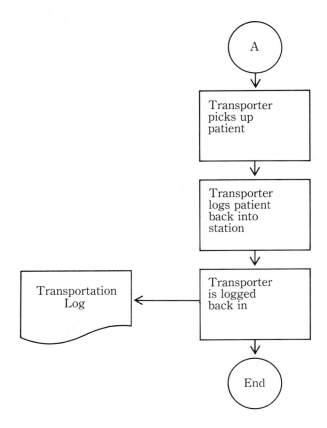

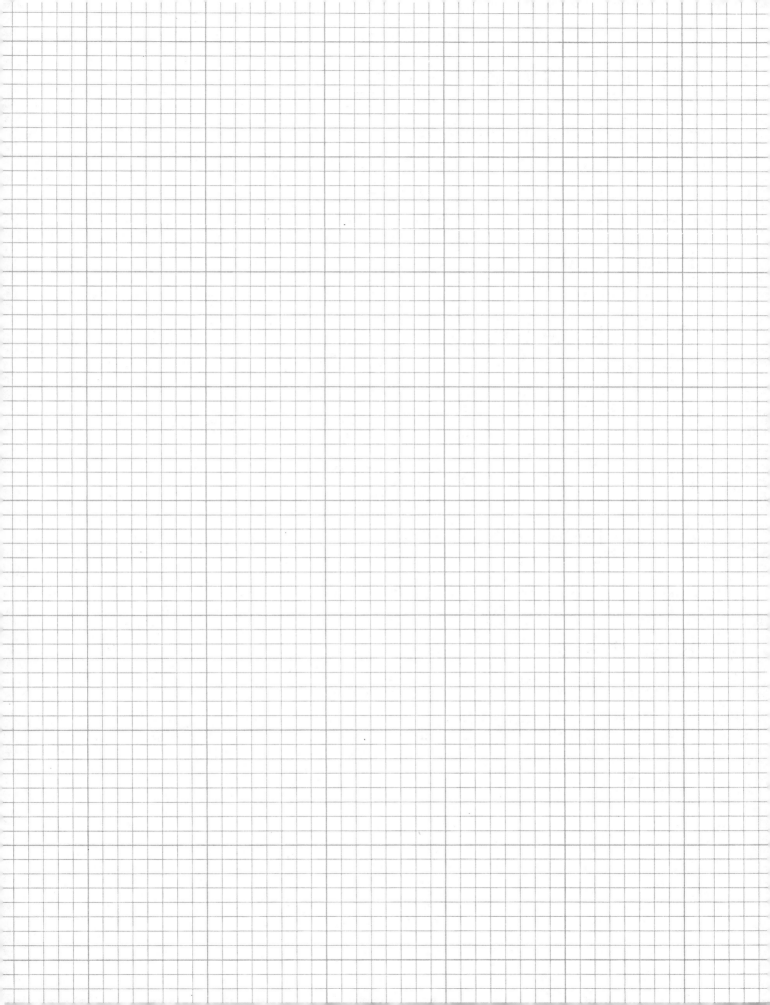

Input Inventory 1.4.3

A. Transportation Supervisor

your document title
↓

          A B C

1. Dispatch ticket.   ☐ ☐ ☐   _____

2. Requisition for service.   ☐ ☐ ☐   _____

3. Work schedules from ancillary departments.   ☐ ☐ ☐   _____

B. Head Nurse

Clinical information sheets.   ☐ ☐ ☐   _____

C. Head Nurse, Surgery

Surgery dispatch ticket.   ☐ ☐ ☐   _____

USE INPUT DOCUMENT ANALYSIS FORM

A = same document title	B = minor variations	C = significant differences

Master File Inventory 1.4.3

A. Transportation Supervisor

Notes
↓

          A B C

1. Transportation Log.   ☐ ☐ ☐   _____

2. Inventory records on Transportation's equipment (wheelchairs, stretchers, etc.).   ☐ ☐ ☐   _____

B. Head Nurse

Log of patient's whereabouts.   ☐ ☐ ☐   _____

USE MASTER FILE ANALYSIS FORM

A = essentially similar	B = minor variations	C = significant differences

Report Inventory 1.4.3

A. Transportation Supervisor

your document title
↓

	A	B	C	
1. Productivity report.	□	□	□	_____
2. Transportation Department's work schedule.	□	□	□	_____

USE REPORT ANALYSIS FORM

A = essentially similar	B = minor variations	C = significant differences

System Performance Standards 1.4.3

	Units		A	B
1. What is the average time it takes for a dispatched transporter to reach a Nursing Station?	minutes_____		□	□
2. What is the average time a transporter spends at a Nursing Station?	minutes_____		□	□
3. What is the average time it takes a transporter to move a patient from a Nursing Station to an ancillary department?	minutes_____		□	□
4. Are transporters required to examine a patient's identification (ID) bracelet before they move the patient?	yes or no _____		□	□
5. How often does a transporter pick up the wrong patient?	number of times per month __		□	□
6. How often does a transporter arrive at a Nursing Station and find the patient is not there?	number of times per month __		□	□
7. How often are patients scheduled to be in two different ancillary departments at the same time?	number of times per month __		□	□
8. What is the average waiting time in Radiology between the time a test is completed and the time a patient is back in bed?	minutes_____		□	□
9. How often is Surgery delayed or cancelled because of delays in delivering a patient?	number of times per month __		□	□
10. What is the average time between the completion of the admitting process and the arrival of the patient at the Nursing Station?	minutes_____		□	□

USE PERFORMANCE STANDARDS ANALYSIS FORM

A = we have a standard	B = we do not have a standard

System Cost Factors 1.4.3

1. How many wheelchairs and stretchers does the hospital have? $ _____

2. How much time do transporters spend waiting between assignments? $ _____

3. Is special communication equipment used to connect the Transportation
   Department with Nursing Stations and ancillary departments? $ _____

4. If the patient's medical record accompanies the patient to an ancillary
   department, how often does a physician miss seeing the chart because the
   patient is undergoing diagnosis or treatment? $ _____

USE SYSTEM COST ANALYSIS FORM *(also see Instructions, p. 15)*

System 1.4.4: Housekeeping
Description 1.4.4

Housekeeping's major responsibilities are to prepare patient rooms after discharges and transfers, follow specialized cleaning procedures for the rooms of isolation patients, clean all areas of the hospital on a rotating basis, respond to emergency calls, and remove trash.

A B C
□ □ □

Preparing the Bed

The inpatient cycle begins when a physician writes a discharge order or when a patient is transferred. In addition to notifying Admitting of the discharge or transfer, the Nursing Station also informs Housekeeping, either by telephoning or sending a copy of the discharge/transfer notice. In response Housekeeping dispatches a maid to prepare the now-empty bed for a new patient.

□ □ □

The maid performs predetermined assignments, which include stripping and washing the bed, putting on clean linen, washing the area around the bed, and cleaning the bathroom. When the bed is ready for use, the maid notifies Admitting either by telephoning or sending a room-ready notification.

□ □ □

The maid who prepares the bed may either be assigned directly to the Nursing Station, in which case he or she has full responsibility for cleaning the unit; or the maid may be assigned to the Housekeeping Office, which dispatches him or her specifically to prepare rooms for incoming patients.

□ □ □

Other Duties

Housekeeping maintains a master production schedule, which shows when each area of the hospital is to be cleaned, how often it is to be cleaned, and who is responsible for the cleaning.

□ □ □

As emergencies arise (a patient vomiting, a major spill, etc.), the supervisor in that area calls Housekeeping, which dispatches personnel to clean the area in question. Logs are kept of these emergency calls.

□ □ □

A = essentially similar   B = minor variations   C = significant differences

Another log is kept, listing all patients who have been placed in isolation. Housekeeping is responsible for following special cleaning procedures required by each type of isolation.

Notes ↓

A B C
☐ ☐ ☐ _____

Housekeepers may be permanently assigned to areas with an ongoing need for cleanup, such as the Operating Room and the ED.

☐ ☐ ☐ _____

Outside Contracts

Some hospitals contract with housekeeping firms who then take responsibility for cleaning the institution. These contracts come in two forms: the outside firm has complete responsibility, including hiring all employees and supplying equipment; or the outside firm simply provides management services.

☐ ☐ ☐ _____

A = essentially similar   B = minor variations   C = significant differences

Flow Chart 1.4.4

Preparing the Patient Room

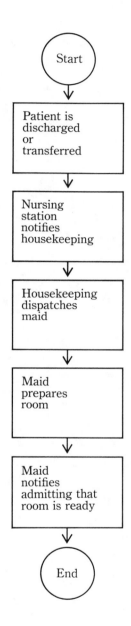

Start

Patient is discharged or transferred

Nursing station notifies housekeeping

Housekeeping dispatches maid

Maid prepares room

Maid notifies admitting that room is ready

End

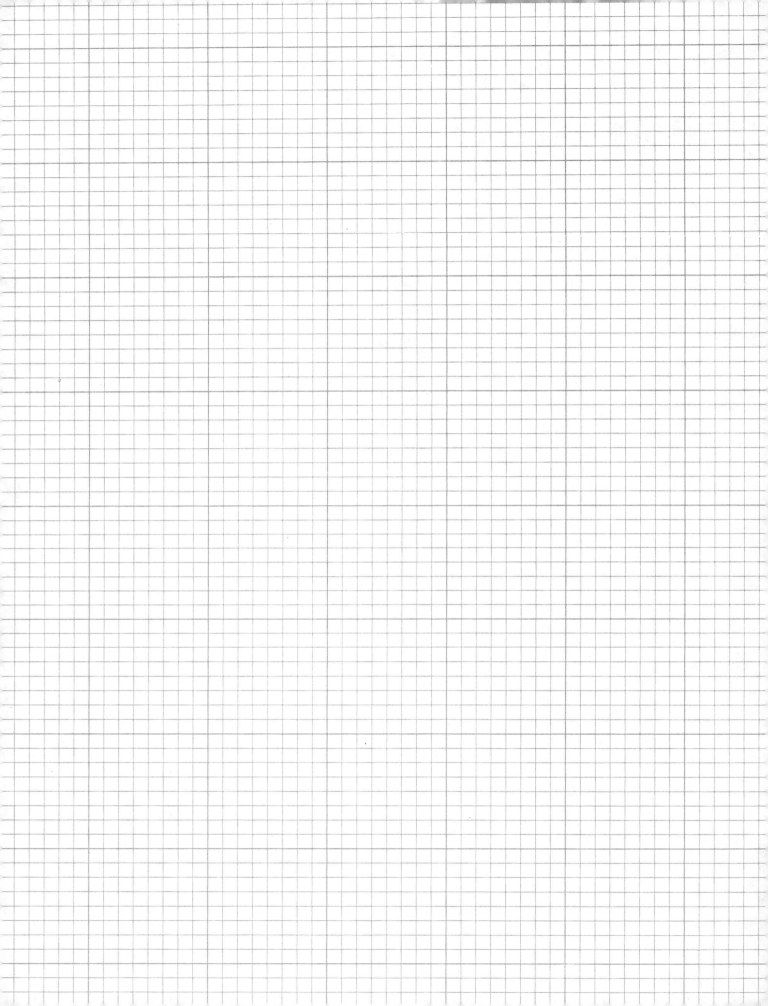

Input Inventory 1.4.4

A. Housekeeping Supervisor

your document title
↓

	A	B	C	
1. Room-ready notification.	□	□	□	_____
2. Isolation patient notification.	□	□	□	_____
3. Request for special services.	□	□	□	_____

USE INPUT DOCUMENT ANALYSIS FORM

A = same document title   B = minor variations   C = significant differences

Master File Inventory 1.4.4

A. Housekeeping Supervisor

Notes
↓

	A	B	C	
1. Daily census.	□	□	□	_____
2. Log of emergency calls.	□	□	□	_____
3. Log of special-service calls.	□	□	□	_____
4. Listing of isolation patients.	□	□	□	_____
5. Production schedule.	□	□	□	_____

USE MASTER FILE ANALYSIS FORM

A = essentially similar   B = minor variations   C = significant differences

Report Inventory 1.4.4

A. Housekeeping Supervisor

your document title
↓

	A	B	C	
Productivity report.	□	□	□	_____

USE REPORT ANALYSIS FORM

A = essentially similar   B = minor variations   C = significant differences

System Performance Standards 1.4.4

		Units	A	B
1.	How long does it take a maid to clean and prepare a newly vacated bed?	minutes_____	☐	☐
2.	How often does a maid arrive at a room and find that the discharged patient has not yet left?	times per month _____	☐	☐
3.	How long does it take Housekeeping to notify Admitting that a room is ready?	minutes_____	☐	☐
4.	How often does Admitting have to call the Nursing Station to determine if a bed is ready for use?	times per week _____	☐	☐
5.	How long does it take to clean an occupied room?	minutes_____	☐	☐
6.	How many emergency calls does Housekeeping receive?	number per week _____	☐	☐
7.	What is the Housekeeping Department's staffing ratio?	number of Housekeeping employees divided by the number of square feet in the hospital_____	☐	☐

USE PERFORMANCE STANDARDS ANALYSIS FORM

A = we have a standard   B = we do not have a standard

System Cost Factors 1.4.4

1. What is the cost for forms or communication equipment the Nursing Stations use to notify Housekeeping that a patient has been transferred or discharged? $ _____

2. How many workhours are lost because Housekeeping personnel have no way of logging when assignments begin and end? $ _____

3. How many Housekeeping-oriented functions do nursing personnel perform? $ _____

USE SYSTEM COST ANALYSIS FORM *(also see Instructions, p. 15)*

System 1.4.5:
Social Services

Description 1.4.5

Social Service is either an independent department or part of Nursing. Its major responsibility is to serve as an interface between the patient and agencies outside the hospital.

A B C
☐ ☐ ☐ _____

Its most common activities are:

1. To bring the patient in contact with community agencies that will help the patient cope with medical problems. Examples of such organizations are United Fund agencies, Alcoholics Anonymous, diabetic-training groups, and visiting-nurse associations.

☐ ☐ ☐ _____

2. To assist patients and their families in arranging transfers to nursing homes.

☐ ☐ ☐ _____

3. To coordinate or insure that patients are trained in the special procedures, diet selection, and other skills needed to handle certain medical problems after discharge.

☐ ☐ ☐ _____

4. To assist the Financial Counselor in helping a patient enroll in Medicaid, municipal welfare, and other financial-assistance programs.

☐ ☐ ☐ _____

Social Service workers become involved with patients in several different ways. The attending physician may order Social Service assistance. The Utilization Review Coordinator also may involve Social Service, either by direct order or by suggesting Social Service involvement to the admitting physician. Standing admission orders for certain types of patients, such as stroke victims, may trigger Social Service involvement. The Social Service worker may study the daily census, looking for likely candidates for assistance. Finally, informal contacts from Nursing may bring a worker in contact with a patient.

☐ ☐ ☐ _____

Once involved, the worker visits the patient and takes appropriate action. The worker records such action on the patient's medical record. In some hospitals, nurses note Social Service involvement on their nursing notes.

☐ ☐ ☐ _____

A = essentially similar   B = minor variations   C = significant differences

The Social Worker also records the action taken in the patient's Social Service file, which is kept in the department.

A B C
☐ ☐ ☐

A = essentially similar   B = minor variations   C = significant differences

Flow Chart 1.4.5

Social Service Involvement

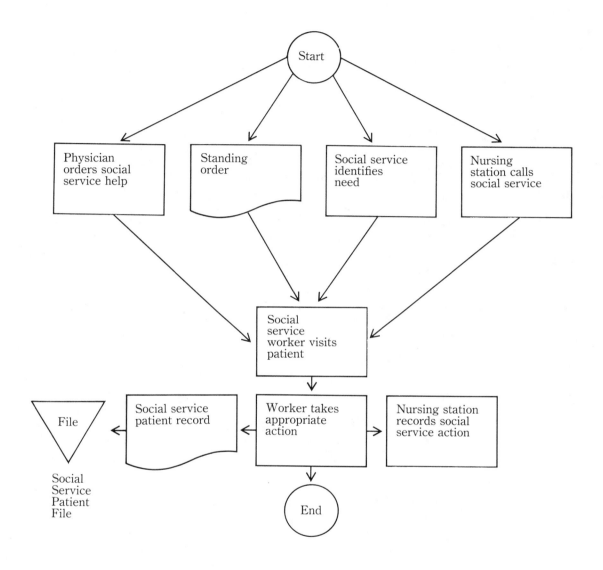

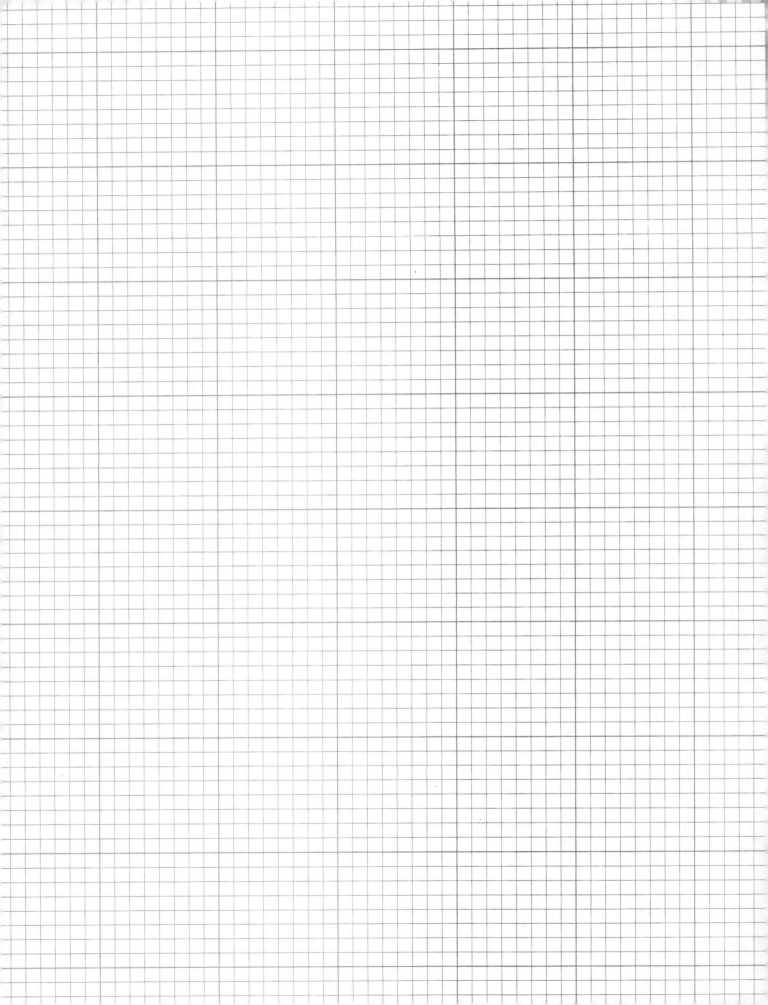

Input Inventory 1.4.5

A. Social Service Supervisor

your document title
↓

	A	B	C	
1. Departmental progress note.	☐	☐	☐	_____
2. Nursing Home transfer form.	☐	☐	☐	_____

USE INPUT DOCUMENT ANALYSIS FORM

A = same document title   B = minor variations   C = significant differences

Master File Inventory 1.4.5

A. Social Service Supervisor

Notes
↓

	A	B	C	
1. Patient file.	☐	☐	☐	_____
2. Listing of current patients being assisted.	☐	☐	☐	_____
3. Follow-up file to remind worker to check progress of discharged patients.	☐	☐	☐	_____

USE MASTER FILE ANALYSIS FORM

A = essentially similar   B = minor variations   C = significant differences

Report Inventory 1.4.5

A. Social Service Supervisor

your document title
↓

	A	B	C	
Periodic report on number of patients seen.	☐	☐	☐	_____

USE REPORT ANALYSIS FORM

A = essentially similar   B = minor variations   C = significant differences

System Performance Standards 1.4.5

Units

		A	B
1. What percentage of patients are seen by the Social Service Department?	number of patients seen divided by total number of patients discharged _____	☐	☐
2. How often are patients kept in the hospital because nursing home openings cannot be located?	times per month _____	☐	☐

3. What percentage of patients are seen as a result of standing orders?

number of patients seen
because of standing orders
divided by total number of
patients seen _____   A   B
                               ☐   ☐

USE PERFORMANCE STANDARDS ANALYSIS FORM

A = we have a standard   B = we do not have a standard

System Cost Factors 1.4.5

(none)

System 1.4.6:
Patient Information Services
Description 1.4.6

The Information Desk and the Switchboard share responsibility for interacting with the public to provide general information about patients. In some hospitals these two areas are combined, but the more common practice is to have separate units.

A B C
□ □ □

During the hours when the Information Desk is staffed, the desk conducts several major activities. The receptionist greets visitors and directs them to patient rooms. If the hospital has a pass system to control visitors, the receptionist issues the passes. The receptionist also: serves telephone callers, checking whether a person has been admitted and giving condition reports; helps clergymen locate members of their congregations, and may provide physicians with financial information about patients to assist them in their billing. This last service is particularly valuable to specialists seeking information about patients who were referred to them after admission.

□ □ □

Information Flow

The flow of information to the Information Desk begins when the patient is admitted. Admitting sends an admission notification to the Information Desk. Usually this notification is a copy of the Admitting Form, which also serves as the source for billing information given to physicians.

□ □ □

The receptionist files the form or extracts from it the information most often needed by the desk (patient name, age, sex, address, physician, religion, room and bed number, and hospital number), writing this information on an index card. This document is filed in alphabetical order and serves as a quick reference for handling visitor questions.

□ □ □

The receptionist then writes the patient's name next to the appropriate room and bed number on the census, which was sent to the Information Desk the previous night. Finally, the receptionist files the Admitting Form in alphabetical order.

□ □ □

A = essentially similar   B = minor variations   C = significant differences

During the evening the Information Desk receives two reports. The first is the daily census from Admitting. Once this census has been received, the receptionist throws away the previous day's, and then cross-checks the new census with the quick-reference file. If the two do not agree, the receptionist calls Admitting.

A B C

☐ ☐ ☐ _____

The other report is the Condition Report. Each Nursing Station sends the Information Desk a list of all patients and their conditions (i.e., good, fair, critical). The receptionist enters this information on the quick-reference cards. In part of the Condition Report, the Nursing Stations may also indicate if there are any visitor restrictions.

☐ ☐ ☐ _____

The desk also receives the Surgery Schedule. Normally, the receptionist will enter surgery dates on the quick-reference cards.

☐ ☐ ☐ _____

As patients are transferred, the Nursing Station sends a copy of the transfer notification. This is either sent directly or through Admitting. The receptionist then updates the desk files and census. When a patient expires, the Nursing Station notifies the desk by telephone.

☐ ☐ ☐ _____

When a patient is discharged, the Nursing Station sends the desk a copy of the discharge notification. Again, this is either sent directly or through Admitting. The receptionist lines out the patient's name on the census, pulls the patient's card from the quick-reference file, and pulls the Admitting Form from its file.

☐ ☐ ☐ _____

Other Services

The Information Desk may be responsible for preparing a census for each physician, listing only his or her patients and their room and bed numbers. Physicians pick up these censuses before making rounds.

☐ ☐ ☐ _____

Switchboard

In addition to operating the switchboard and the hospital's paging system, switchboard operators normally are responsible for monitoring alarm and security systems.

☐ ☐ ☐ _____

Hospitals have a variety of systems to guard against fire, provide security, and check the status of critical equipment. The alarm portions of these systems are usually found in the switchboard room. Among the systems so located are smoke and fire alarms, closed-circuit monitors, and the temperature gauge/alarm for the Blood Bank refrigerator.

☐ ☐ ☐ _____

A = essentially similar   B = minor variations   C = significant differences

96

Flow Chart 1.4.6

Information Desk

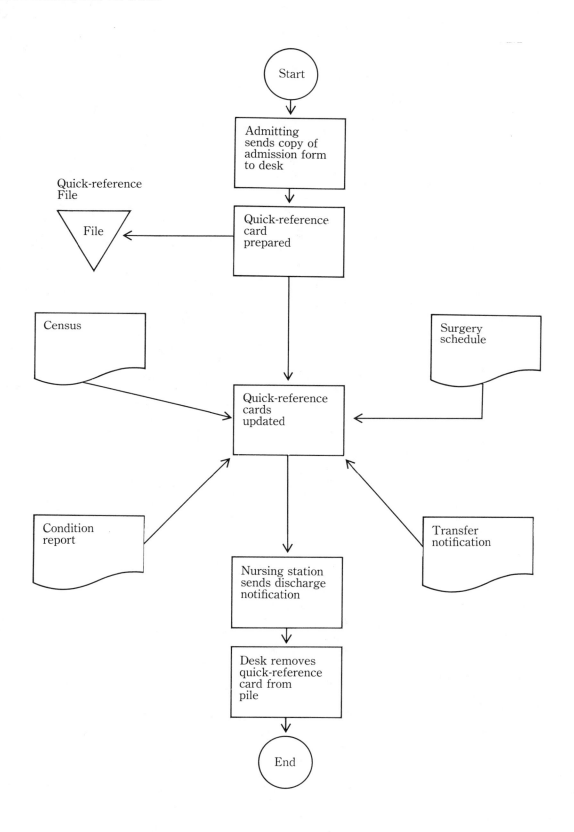

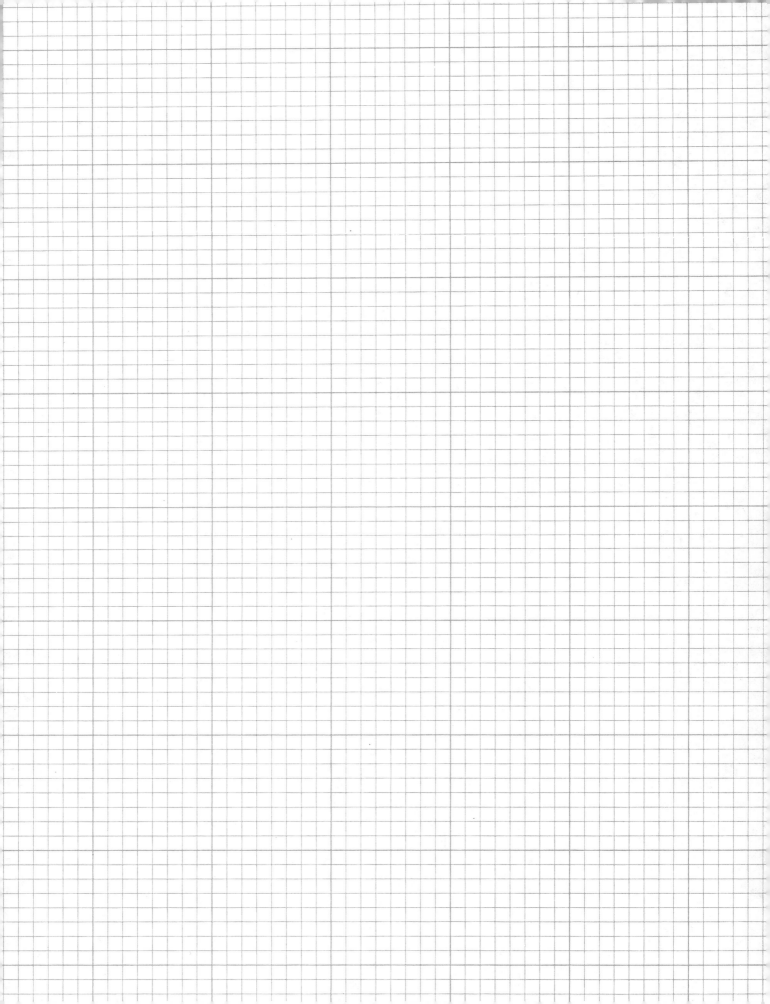

Input Inventory 1.4.6

A. Information Desk Supervisor

your document title
↓

	A	B	C	
1. Condition Report.	☐	☐	☐	_____
2. Admission notification (if Admitting Form is not used).	☐	☐	☐	_____
3. Transfer and discharge notifications.	☐	☐	☐	_____
4. Quick-reference card.	☐	☐	☐	_____

USE INPUT DOCUMENT ANALYSIS FORM

A = same document title   B = minor variations   C = significant differences

Master File Inventory 1.4.6

A. Information Desk Supervisor

Notes
↓

	A	B	C	
1. Admitting Forms.	☐	☐	☐	_____
2. Quick-reference file.	☐	☐	☐	_____
3. Census.	☐	☐	☐	_____
4. Employee listing.	☐	☐	☐	_____
5. Physician listing.	☐	☐	☐	_____

USE MASTER FILE ANALYSIS FORM

A = essentially similar   B = minor variations   C = significant differences

Report Inventory 1.4.6

A. Information Desk Supervisor

your document title
↓

	A	B	C	
Physician's census.	☐	☐	☐	_____

USE REPORT ANALYSIS FORM

A = essentially similar   B = minor variations   C = significant differences

System Performance Standards 1.4.6

		Units	A	B
1.	What is the accuracy of the quick-reference file?	ratio of incorrect bed and room information to total number of patients in hospital_____	☐	☐
2.	How long does it take for the Information Desk to answer the telephone?	seconds_____	☐	☐
3.	How long does it take for the switchboard operator to answer the telephone?	seconds_____	☐	☐
4.	How much nursing time is spent preparing the Condition Report?	minutes_____	☐	☐
5.	How much time does the Information Desk spend transferring information from one report to another?	minutes daily _____	☐	☐

USE PERFORMANCE STANDARDS ANALYSIS FORM

A = we have a standard   B = we do not have a standard

System Cost Factors 1.4.6

(none)

Ambulatory Care
Services Systems

System 2.1:
Emergency Services
Description 2.1

The typical Emergency Department (ED) deals not only with life-or-death situations but also with routine medical problems. At least 75 percent of all patients coming to an ED have nonurgent conditions. The contemporary ED is actually two facilities in one – a trauma center and a walk-in physician's office.

A B C
☐ ☐ ☐

Registration

When a patient arrives for service, the ED Clerk fills out an ED Form. This multicopy document contains the patient's reason for seeking ED services (complaint), demographic information (name, age, sex, address, etc.), financial information (type of insurance, employer, etc.), and an ED number. The form also has blank spaces for physician orders, physician treatment notes, and nursing notes.

☐ ☐ ☐

After the clerk completes the form, he or she obtains the patient's signature on both a consent-for-treatment statement and an assignment statement (which allows the hospital to bill the patient's insurance company). Normally, these statements are printed on the ED Form.

☐ ☐ ☐

The clerk also obtains the patient's signature on any appropriate insurance forms. The clerk then asks the patient for identification. If the ED has a copying machine, the clerk copies the ID cards as well as any insurance cards. All of this additional paperwork is clipped together and filed alphabetically.

☐ ☐ ☐

Finally, the clerk prepares an identification bracelet and puts it on the patient's wrist.

☐ ☐ ☐

In some hospitals, the first person a patient encounters is not the clerk but a Triage Nurse. The Triage Nurse's responsibility is to evaluate the patient's condition and determine if the patient should be treated immediately. In cases where the patient does bypass the ED Clerk, the clerk visits the patient in the treatment area at a convenient time in order to gather the necessary information and signatures for the ED Form.

☐ ☐ ☐

A = essentially similar   B = minor variations   C = significant differences

Treatment Begins

The ED Clerk directs the patient to the waiting area and takes the ED Form to the treatment area. After reviewing the form, an ED Nurse brings the patient to the treatment area and assigns him or her a room. The nurse then writes the room number on the top of the form.

A B C
☐ ☐ ☐ _____

The next step is the patient's evaluation by a physician. Hospitals use two approaches to ensure that physicians identify the patient with the correct room. The ED Nursing Station may use a chart rack with a room designation over each slot. The second approach is to have a blackboard with each room number permanently written down the left-hand side. The ED Nurse then writes the present patient's name and problem next to the appropriate room number.

☐ ☐ ☐ _____

The physician taking a particular case picks up the ED Form and examines the patient. After evaluating the situation, the physician writes orders on the form and gives it to the nurse. These orders delineate procedures the physician will carry out (e.g., suturing), procedures the nurse will carry out, requests for consultations and assistance from specialists, and requests for services from ancillary departments.

☐ ☐ ☐ _____

Requisitions

1. Radiology—The nurse completes a Radiology requisition form and telephones that department. Depending on the procedure requested, Radiology either dispatches a transporter to pick up the patient or sends a technician with a mobile x-ray unit.

☐ ☐ ☐ _____

   Once the mobile x-ray is completed, the ED physician makes a preliminary reading. The film then goes to the radiologist for final interpretation. If the patient is still in the ED, the radiologist will telephone his or her report to the ED physician before dictating it.

☐ ☐ ☐ _____

   In cases where the x-ray is taken in the Radiology Department where a radiologist is on duty, the film goes directly to the radiologist.

☐ ☐ ☐ _____

   When a radiologist is not available, the film is returned to the ED, where the ED physician makes a reading. The film is then returned to Radiology to await interpretation by a radiologist.

☐ ☐ ☐ _____

A = essentially similar   B = minor variations   C = significant differences

104

Notes

Once the x-ray film has been developed, it is interpreted by the radiologist, who telephones his report to the ED before dictating it.

A B C
□ □ □ _____

2. Laboratory—The nurse completes the appropriate Laboratory requisitions and telephones that department. A phlebotomist is dispatched to obtain the necessary samples and pick up the requisitions. Once the tests are complete, the department telephones the results to the ED.

□ □ □ _____

3. EKG—The nurse completes an EKG requisition and telephones the department, which dispatches a technician. After the technician has taken an EKG, the ED physician reviews it. The technician then takes the strip, along with the requisition, back to the department, where a cardiologist provides the final interpretation.

□ □ □ _____

4. Respiratory Therapy—The nurse completes the appropriate requisition and telephones the department. A technician is dispatched to render the required service. Normally, the technician will record that service on the ED Form. The technician then returns to the department with the requisition.

□ □ □ _____

5. Medications—The ED normally has a large stock of drugs. When a physician orders a drug, the nurse takes that drug from the stocking area, administers it, and records the administration.

□ □ □ _____

If the ED does not have a needed drug, a courier is dispatched to the Pharmacy with a requisition.

□ □ □ _____

6. Supplies—ED supplies range from dressings to surgical trays to casts. As supplies are needed, the nurse takes them from the stocking area, uses them, and records their use on the patient's ED Form.

□ □ □ _____

Dismissal

After a patient has received all necessary treatment, the physician writes a dismissal order on the ED Form. The physician also notes all necessary instructions for the patient. The nurse reviews these instructions with the patient, gives the patient a copy, and asks the patient to sign a statement acknowledging that the instructions were given.

□ □ □ _____

The nurse then escorts the patient to the ED Desk and returns the form to the ED Clerk.

□ □ □ _____

A = essentially similar B = minor variations C = significant differences

At this point, some hospitals make an effort to collect the patient's bill. Normally, the clerk will not have all of the information needed to prepare a completely accurate bill. Instead, the clerk prepares an estimated bill, which contains a note stating that a supplementary billing may be necessary.

A B C
☐ ☐ ☐ _____

To generate a bill, the ED Clerk estimates charges as follows:

1. The fee for use of the ED facilities is usually a flat rate plus an hourly charge. The clerk can compute this fee by noting the arrival and dismissal times.

☐ ☐ ☐ _____

2. For the services of ancillary departments, the clerk reviews the tests and services performed, looks up the prices in a price book, and itemizes those charges.

☐ ☐ ☐ _____

3. The cost for supplies and medication is also obtained by reviewing the ED Form and looking up the prices on supplies and medication used.

☐ ☐ ☐ _____

4. If the hospital includes the charge for physician services in its bill, the clerk includes that fee. Physician charges are usually based on the type of services rendered or time spent.

☐ ☐ ☐ _____

After computing all estimated charges, the ED Clerk types a bill and presents it to the patient. In some hospitals, the ED Registration Desk has its own cashiering station, where the clerk collects any payment the patient may make. In other hospitals, the patient is directed to the Centralized Cashiering Station. In either case, if a payment is made, it is deducted from the patient's bill, and the patient receives a receipt.

☐ ☐ ☐ _____

Billing

Periodically (usually daily) each ancillary department segregates all requisitions received from the ED. The charge copies are returned to the ED Desk with the appropriate prices written on them.

☐ ☐ ☐ _____

As these copies return, the ED Clerk attaches them to the Business Office copy of the ED Form. The clerk normally holds the Business Office copy for a fixed number of days to ensure that charge copies for all requisitions have been received. The clerk then sends the copy, the requisitions, and the insurance paperwork to the Business Office, where an accurate, detailed bill

---

is prepared. Once the bill has been mailed, the billing material is placed in the Accounts Receivable file.

A B C
□ □ □

_____

Charting

Written clinical results are gathered and filed in much the same manner as billing information. Each ancillary department, for example, sends the ED Clerk a copy of the test results for each patient.

□ □ □ _____

For Radiology and EKG, results are contained in a written and signed report. For the Laboratory, results are written on a copy of the requisition form.

□ □ □ _____

The clerk attaches all results to the Medical Records copy of the ED Form and files the copy either in the ED or in Medical Records.

□ □ □ _____

Distribution

The typical ED Form has more than half-a-dozen copies, with the distribution varying from hospital to hospital. The following distribution is common:

1. Medical Records copy is stored in the ED or Medical Records.

   □ □ □ _____

2. Attending copy is sent to the patient's physician.

   □ □ □ _____

3. ED copy is given to the physician.

   □ □ □ _____

4. Business Office copy becomes part of the patient's account file.

   □ □ □ _____

5. Billing copy accompanies the Business Office copy to the billing section, then is mailed with the insurance company bill.

   □ □ □ _____

Another copy usually goes to Radiology with the requisition. The clinical information it contains assists the radiologist in interpreting the film.

□ □ □ _____

Some forms include a checklist of ED-stocked supplies and medications. After a patient's treatment has been completed, the nurse notes the items used, then gives the checklist to the clerk for use in preparing the estimated bill.

□ □ □ _____

A = essentially similar   B = minor variations   C = significant differences

Log

The ED Clerk keeps a log listing all patients who receive service. The log, which lists patients by time of arrival, contains the patient's name, address, sex, age, and complaint. In addition, there is space for the clerk to write the final resolution of the case (e.g., referred to Dr. Smith, dismissed, admitted to 240C).

A B C
☐ ☐ ☐ _____

The Admitted Patient

If the physician decides to admit a patient, the ED Nurse contacts Admitting, which dispatches an Admitting Clerk to complete an Admitting Form.

☐ ☐ ☐ _____

In cases where the patient is going to Surgery after being stabilized in the department, the Admitting Clerk gathers as much information as possible. An ED Nurse prepares a medical record for the patient, which includes the Admitting Form, and sends the record to Surgery with the patient.

☐ ☐ ☐ _____

Once a room and bed have been assigned, that information, along with the patient's new, inpatient hospital number, is written on any additional requisitions sent out by the ED. This ensures that ancillary departments will send test results to the Nursing Station and charge copies of the requisitions to the Business Office.

☐ ☐ ☐ _____

For requisitions that had been sent before the admission, the ED Clerk must write the appropriate room and bed number and the new patient number on all results and charge copies and send them to both the Nursing Station and Business Office.

☐ ☐ ☐ _____

Billing for physician services can be handled in one of four ways:

1. If the physician is salaried, a physician-services fee is included in the final bill. The fee is simply another general-revenue item, like drugs and lab tests.

   ☐ ☐ ☐ _____

2. The physician may handle his or her own billing.

   ☐ ☐ ☐ _____

3. The physician may contract with the hospital to handle his or her billing. The hospital then prints separate bills for the physician's services.

   ☐ ☐ ☐ _____

A = essentially similar   B = minor variations   C = significant differences

4. The hospital may include the physician's
   fee as part of the ED bill. It then passes on
   to the physician the amount of physician
   fees billed minus a service charge and a
   bad-debt allowance.

A B C
☐ ☐ ☐ _____

_____

A = essentially similar   B = minor variations   C = significant differences

Flow Chart 2.1

Processing the Emergency Room Patient

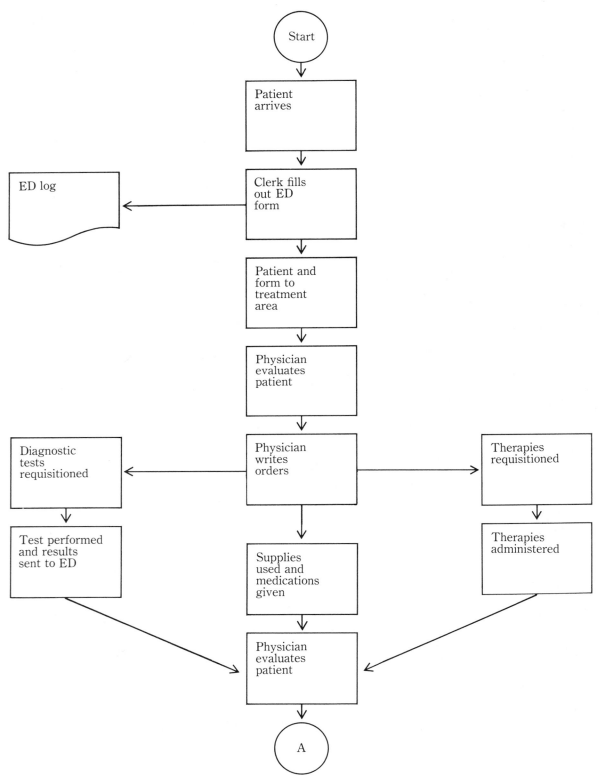

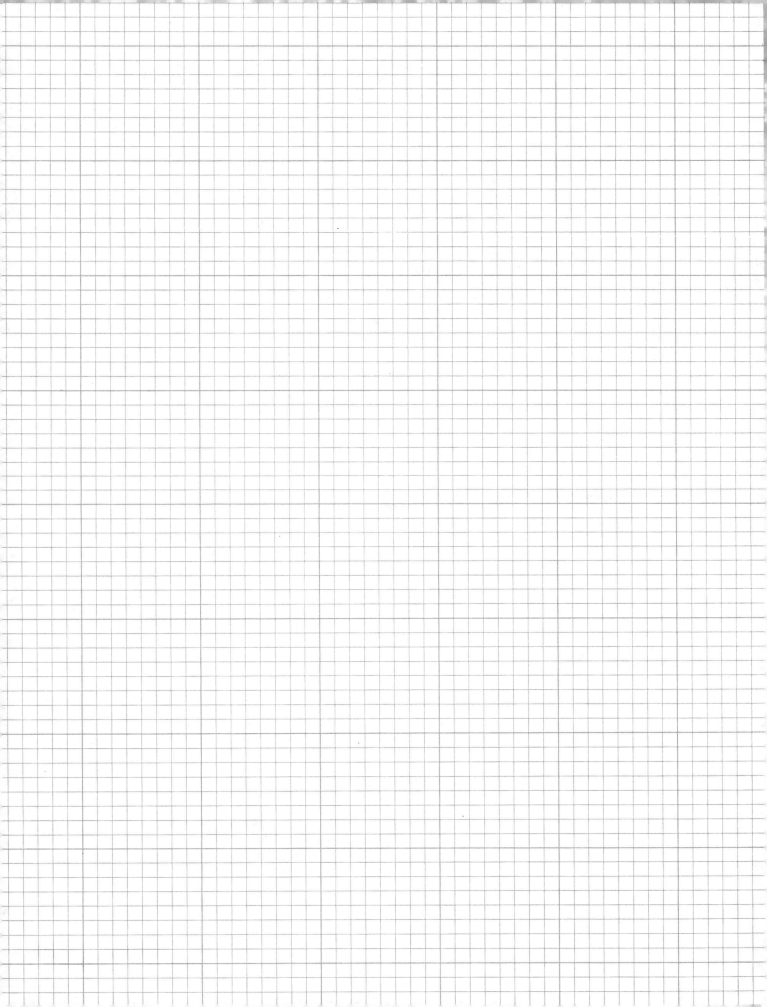

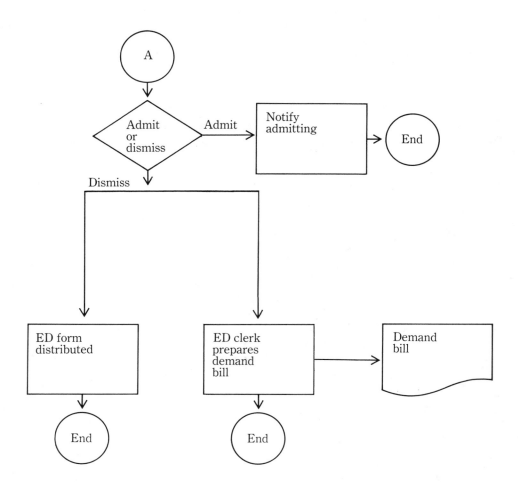

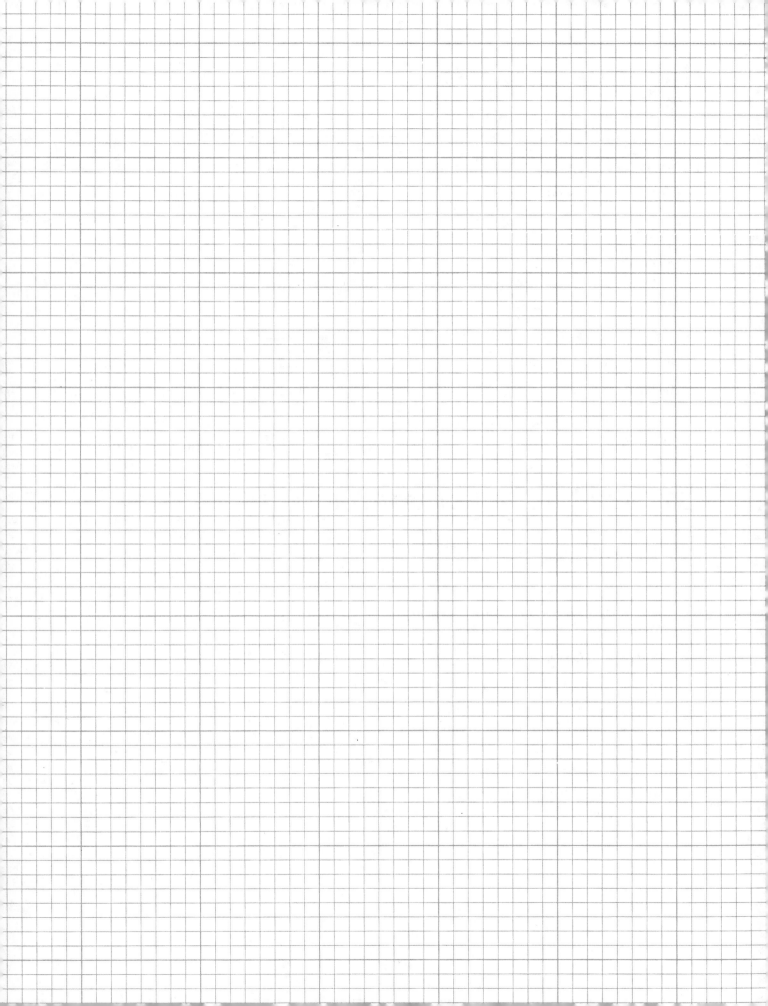

Input Inventory 2.1

A. Head Nurse, ED

your document title
↓

	A	B	C	
1. ED Form.	□	□	□	_____

2. Requisitions for services, treatment, or supplies.

- Radiology
- Laboratory
- Respiratory Therapy
- EKG
- Supplies

	A	B	C	
• Drugs	□	□	□	_____
3. Instructions to patient.	□	□	□	_____
4. Acknowledgment of receipt of instructions.	□	□	□	_____
5. Insurance forms.	□	□	□	_____

USE INPUT DOCUMENT ANALYSIS FORM

A = same document title	B = minor variations	C = significant differences

Master File Inventory 2.1

A. Head Nurse, ED

Notes
↓

	A	B	C	
1. ED Log.	□	□	□	_____
2. File of medical record copy of ED Form for past patients.	□	□	□	_____
3. Call roster of physicians.	□	□	□	_____
4. Suspense file of completed insurance forms.	□	□	□	_____
5. Business Office copies of ED Form being held until charge copies of requisitions arrive.	□	□	□	_____
6. Price book.	□	□	□	_____

USE MASTER FILE ANALYSIS FORM

A = essentially similar	B = minor variations	C = significant differences

Report Inventory 2.1

A. Head Nurse, ED

your document title
↓

A B C

Monthly activity report.   □ □ □   _____

B. ED Clerk

1. Estimated bills.   □ □ □   _____

2. Receipt.   □ □ □   _____

USE REPORT ANALYSIS FORM

| A = essentially similar | B = minor variations | C = significant differences |

System Performance Standards 2.1

Units

A B

1. How much time is spent matching charge tickets to ED Forms?   hours per week _____   □ □

2. How much time is spent matching printed results to ED Forms?   hours per week _____   □ □

3. How long does it take to register a patient?   minutes_____   □ □

4. How much cash does the ED Clerk collect?   cash collected yearly in the ED divided by yearly ED revenue_____   □ □

5. How long does it take to produce an estimated bill?   minutes_____   □ □

6. How many ED Forms have incorrect billing information (incorrect insurance numbers, wrong addresses, etc.)?   number of forms yearly with incorrect information divided by annual number of patients seen in ED _____   □ □

7. How many charge copies of requisitions for admitted patients come back to ED instead of going to the Business Office?   number per week _____   □ □

8. How long does a registered patient wait before being taken to the treatment area?   minutes_____   □ □

9. How long does it take to retrieve the record of a past ED patient?   minutes_____   □ □

USE PERFORMANCE STANDARDS ANALYSIS FORM

| A = we have a standard | B = we do not have a standard |

System Cost Factors 2.1

1. What is the estimated loss of revenue due to ED Nurses' failure to chart all medications given and supplies used? $ _____

2. What is the value of the drug and supply inventories maintained in the ED? $ _____

3. How much nursing time is spent writing requisitions? How legible are they? $ _____

4. How many requisitions do not get to the Business Office for billing because they cannot be matched with ED Forms? $ _____

USE SYSTEM COST ANALYSIS FORM *(also see Instructions, p. 15)*

System 2.2:
Referred Outpatient Services
Description 2.2

A referred outpatient is a patient sent to the hospital by his private physician for outpatient treatment or diagnostic services. In effect, the physician is using the hospital's sophisticated equipment and personnel as part of an overall treatment plan while maintaining primary responsibility for treating the patient.

A B C
☐ ☐ ☐ _____

There are two types of referred outpatients: the episodic, who come for one service or one battery of services, and the recurring, who come on a periodic, scheduled basis for ongoing therapeutic treatment.

☐ ☐ ☐ _____

Diagnostic radiology, laboratory tests, and nuclear-medicine procedures are examples of outpatient services normally rendered on an episodic basis. Physical, respiratory, and x-ray therapy are examples of services normally rendered on a recurring basis.

☐ ☐ ☐ _____

The Flow

The rendering of services to a referred outpatient begins when the patient's physician schedules the service. In most cases the physician's secretary calls the clinical department. The department's receptionist then enters the service in the Schedule Book. In some cases, such as the formulation of a radiation therapy program, the patient's physician will discuss the case with the physicians in the hospital department.

☐ ☐ ☐ _____

After the service has been scheduled, the physician gives the patient a prescription for the service. The prescription blanks may be supplied by the hospital, in which case they provide a space where the physician writes the patient's name, the service to be rendered, the scheduled date and time, a signature, and printed directions telling the patient how to get to the proper registration point.

☐ ☐ ☐ _____

In some cases, the physician will simply write a prescription, give it to the patient, and leave the scheduling responsibility to the patient.

☐ ☐ ☐ _____

A = essentially similar   B = minor variations   C = significant differences

On the scheduled day, the patient goes to the Outpatient Registration Desk, where a clerk completes the Outpatient Form. This document, which usually has three copies, contains demographic information, financial information for billing purposes, the name of the department to which the patient is going, and spaces for entering services rendered and their prices at a later date. Also on the form are sections pertaining to consent-for-treatment and assignment-of-benefits. The clerk first obtains the patient's signature for these sections and for any appropriate insurance forms, then makes copies of the patient's ID and insurance cards.

A B C
☐ ☐ ☐ _____

Next, the clerk removes one copy of the form, attaches the insurance forms and copies of the ID and insurance cards, and files the material alphabetically in a suspense file.

☐ ☐ ☐ _____

The clerk gives the remaining two copies to the patient and directs him or her to the appropriate department. After the patient leaves, the clerk enters the patient's name, the patient's physician, the department involved, and the date in an Outpatient Log.

☐ ☐ ☐ _____

When the patient arrives at the department, the receptionist logs him or her in, prepares the appropriate intradepartmental paperwork, attaches both copies of the Outpatient Form to this paperwork, and takes the patient and the form to the area where service is to be rendered.

☐ ☐ ☐ _____

After treatment has been completed, a technician records all services rendered on both copies of the Outpatient Form and returns the patient and the form to the receptionist. The receptionist enters the appropriate charges, removes one copy, gives it to the patient, directs the patient to the Outpatient Desk, and files the remaining copy alphabetically.

☐ ☐ ☐ _____

When the patient returns to the desk, a clerk takes the second copy and uses it to prepare a bill. If the patient wishes to pay, the clerk accepts payment and gives the patient a receipt. In hospitals with centralized cashiering functions, the clerk gives the patient the bill to take to the cashier.

☐ ☐ ☐ _____

In some hospitals, the Outpatient Form may have four copies, with one serving as the bill that is presented to the patient at the time of treatment. In other hospitals, this bill is a separate form.

☐ ☐ ☐ _____

While the patient is at the desk, the clerk also removes the suspense copy of the Outpatient Form, detaches it from the other paperwork,

A = essentially similar　　　　B = minor variations　　　　C = significant differences

and files it alphabetically. The copy returned by the patient is attached to the insurance paper-work, along with a copy of the receipt if the patient has paid. This is sent to the Business Office for final posting and billing.

A B C

☐ ☐ ☐

At the end of the day, the clerk reviews all forms remaining in the suspense file and then contacts the departments involved to determine what services were rendered and what charges must be made. The clerk enters this information on the form, makes a copy for the alphabetical Outpatient files, and sends the copy and the insurance papers to the Business Office.

☐ ☐ ☐

The suspense file, therefore, assures that a bill will be prepared even if a patient fails to return to the desk.

☐ ☐ ☐

Decentralized Method

Some hospitals do not have a separate Out-patient Desk. Instead, each department is responsible for processing its own outpatients.

☐ ☐ ☐

The flow begins when the test is scheduled by the patient's physician. When the patient arrives at the hospital, he or she goes to the department's Reception Desk, where the receptionist completes an Outpatient Form and logs the patient into the department. Some hospitals have a standard three-copy form that is used by all clinical departments. In others, each department has its own Outpatient Form. This form usually has more than three copies, with the additional ones serving intradepartmental needs (e.g., envelope label, results copy for the patient's physician, billing copy for physicians in the department).

☐ ☐ ☐

The receptionist completes the form, obtains the necessary signatures, then takes the patient and the form to the treatment area. After service is complete, the technician records the services performed and returns the patient and the form to the receptionist. The receptionist enters the appropriate charges, gives one copy to the patient, and directs the patient to the cashier. The receptionist then attaches the insurance forms to another copy and sends it to the Business Office. The remaining copy is filed alpha-betically in the department.

☐ ☐ ☐

Recurring Patients

The key to processing recurring patients is the fact that both the Outpatient Desk and the department keep copies of the Outpatient Forms

Notes
↓

A = essentially similar   B = minor variations   C = significant differences

119

for these patients in a separate, active file.
Periodically, the forms are taken from the file,
and billing information is sent to the Business
Office.

A B C

□ □ □

The first time a recurring patient arrives, he or
she is processed in the same manner as an
episodic patient, with the following exceptions:

1. "Recurring" is written or stamped on all
copies of the form.

□ □ □

2. The desk and the department put their
copies of the Outpatient Form into the
recurring file. Nothing is sent to the
Business Office.

□ □ □

On subsequent visits, the patient goes directly to
the department. The receptionist takes the two
copies of the patient's form from the recurring
file and sends them with the patient to the treatment area. The technician writes the services
performed and the date and sends the copies
back to the receptionist. The receptionist enters
the charge and places the forms back in the
recurring file.

□ □ □

Periodically (usually monthly), the receptionist
removes the forms, sends one copy to the Outpatient Desk and places the second back in the
recurring file.

□ □ □

The Outpatient Clerk totals the charges, takes
the copy of the form from the suspense file,
records the date the copy was received from the
receptionist, then sends the copy with the
charges to the Business Office. Next the Outpatient Clerk prepares a new Outpatient Form
for the patient and sends it to the department
for use in noting charges for subsequent visits.
The receptionist places this new form in the
suspense file along with the remaining copy of
the original.

□ □ □

Reports/Termination Order

The end point of the flow of a referred outpatient through the system is the sending of a
report to the patient's physician, or, for
recurring outpatients, the cancellation of the
service by the patient's physician.

□ □ □

Notes
↓

Flow Chart 2.2a

Referred Outpatient/Centralized Registration

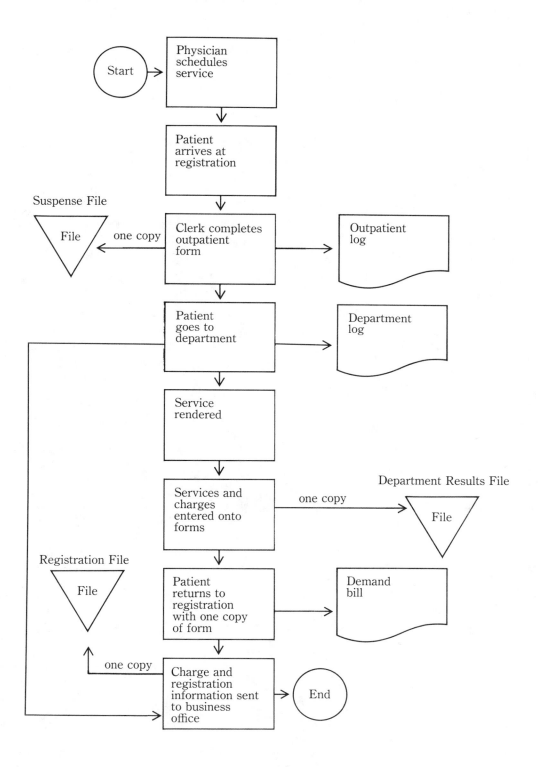

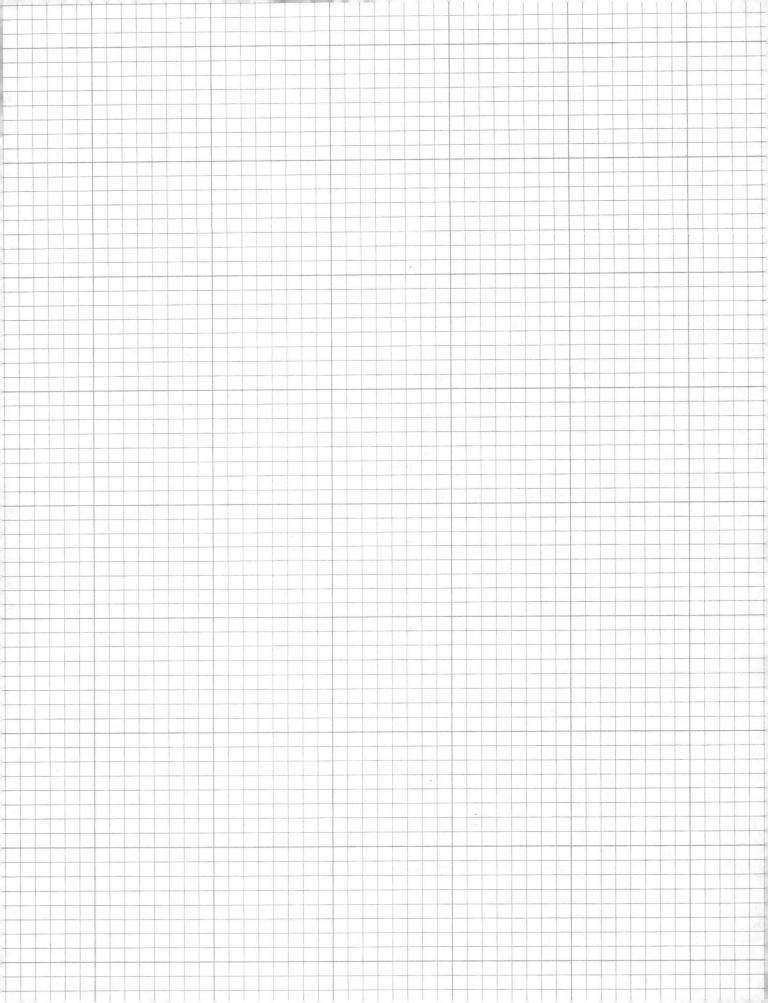

Flow Chart 2.2b

Referred Outpatient/Decentralized Registration

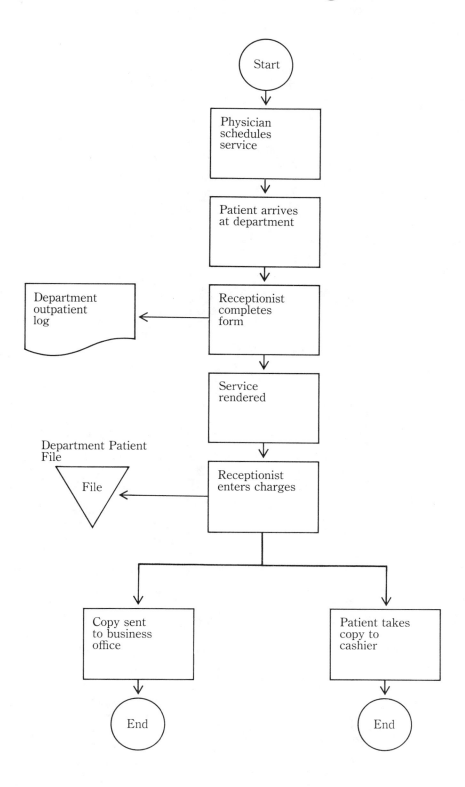

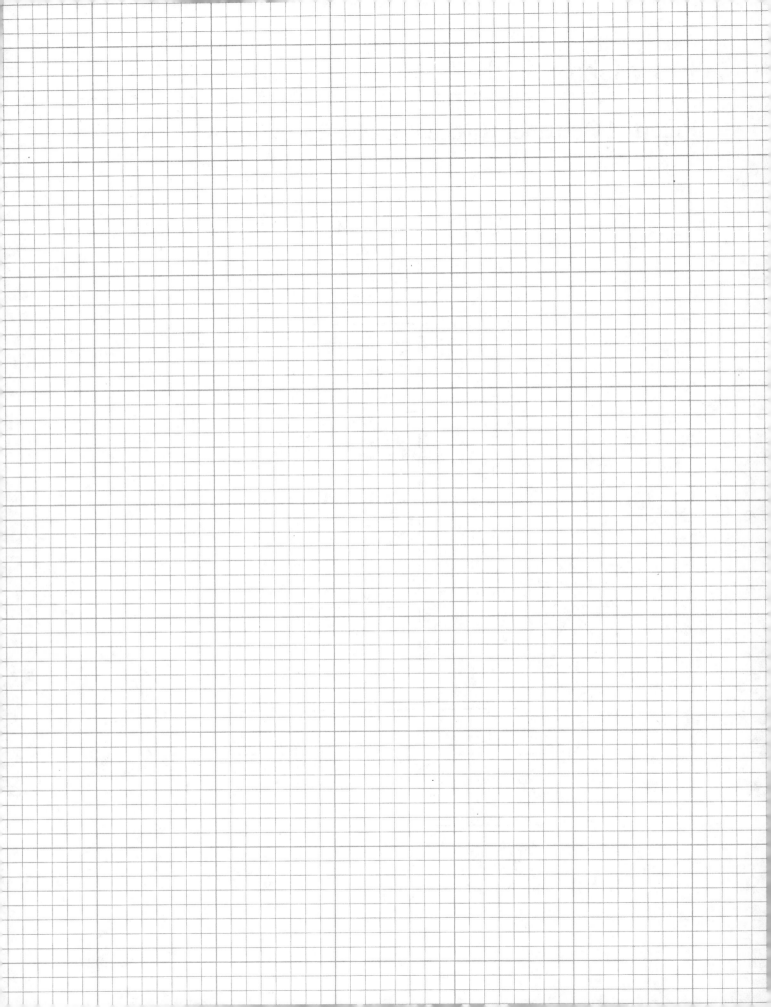

Flow Chart 2.2c

Billing Recurring Outpatient/Centralized Registration

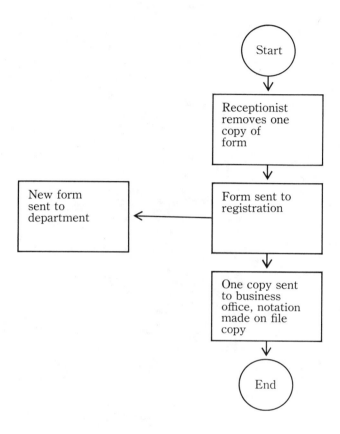

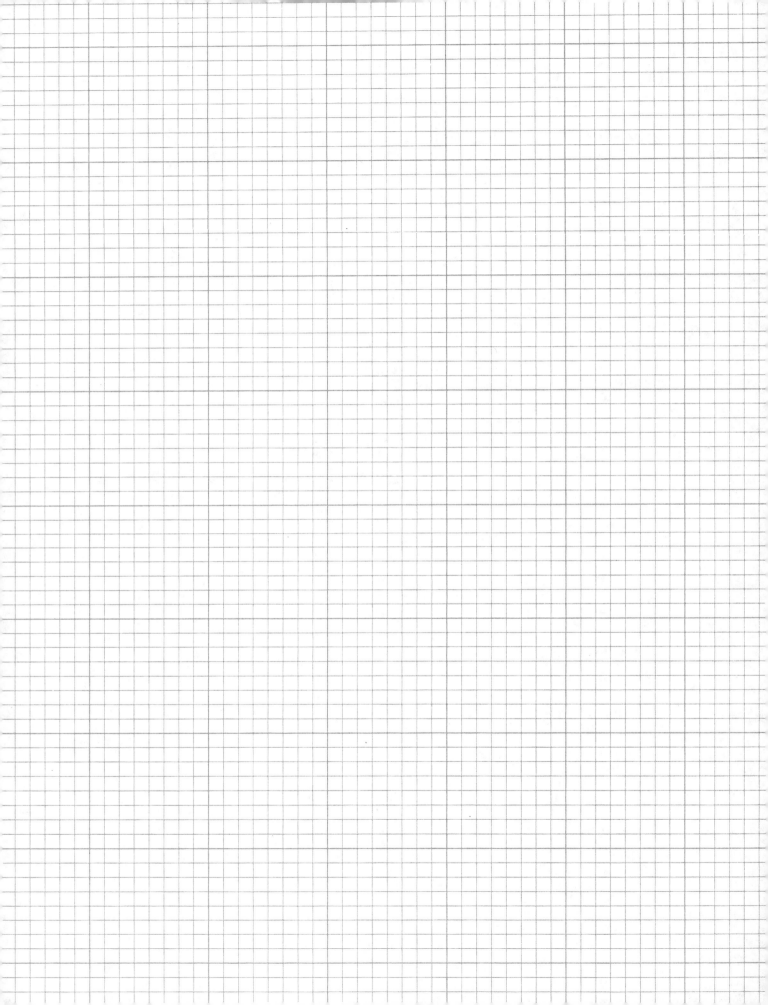

Input Inventory 2.2

A. Registration Supervisor

your document title
↓

	A	B	C	
1. Outpatient Form.	☐	☐	☐	_____
2. Prescription.	☐	☐	☐	_____
3. Insurance Forms.	☐	☐	☐	_____
4. Receipt.	☐	☐	☐	_____

B. Clinical Department Supervisor

| 1. Departmental Outpatient Form. | ☐ | ☐ | ☐ | _____ |
| 2. Scheduling Pad. | ☐ | ☐ | ☐ | _____ |

USE INPUT DOCUMENT ANALYSIS FORM

A = same document title   B = minor variations   C = significant differences

Master File Inventory 2.2

A. Registration Supervisor

Notes
↓

	A	B	C	
1. Suspense file.	☐	☐	☐	_____
2. Recurring patients.	☐	☐	☐	_____
3. Log.	☐	☐	☐	_____
4. Patient file.	☐	☐	☐	_____

B. Clinical Department Supervisors

1. Log.	☐	☐	☐	_____
2. Recurring patients.	☐	☐	☐	_____
3. Old schedules.	☐	☐	☐	_____

USE MASTER FILE ANALYSIS FORM

A = essentially similar   B = minor variations   C = significant differences

Report Inventory 2.2

A. Registration Supervisor

your document title ↓

A B C

1. Bill. ☐ ☐ ☐ _____

2. Report on number of patients registered by department. ☐ ☐ ☐ _____

USE REPORT ANALYSIS FORM

A = essentially similar   B = minor variations   C = significant differences

System Performance Standards 2.2

	Units	A	B
1. How long does it take to register a patient?	minutes_____	☐	☐
2. How much cash is collected from outpatients at the time of service?	cash collected yearly divided by yearly referred-outpatient revenue_____	☐	☐
3. How often are tests cancelled because of scheduling errors?	times per month _____	☐	☐
4. How many Registration Forms contain incomplete or incorrect information, thereby delaying billing?	number per month _____	☐	☐
5. How often are recurring patients billed?	times per quarter_____	☐	☐

USE PERFORMANCE STANDARDS ANALYSIS FORM

A = we have a standard   B = we do not have a standard

System Cost Factors 2.2

1. How much time is spent logging patients in Registration and in the departments? $ _____

2. How often are patients "lost" (i.e., they register but end up with no records on file at the department)? $ _____

3. How often must credits be issued because the wrong tests were conducted due to mistakes made in filling out the prescription or because no prescription was written? $ _____

4. Is the clerk able to review Accounts Receivable records before registering the patient? $ _____

USE SYSTEM COST ANALYSIS FORM *(also see Instructions, p. 15)*

System 2.3:
Clinics

Description 2.3

Notes

A hospital clinic is a section that either renders ongoing primary care (i.e., serves as a patient's family physician) or renders highly specialized care in an outpatient setting. The number of clinics a hospital may have can range from zero to fifty or more, with the higher numbers considered standard at large teaching hospitals.

A B C
☐ ☐ ☐

The existence of clinics is normally associated with one of two conditions – the need to provide primary care to a medically indigent population or the need to provide a training environment for residents.

☐ ☐ ☐

In hospitals with few clinics, each clinic is treated, from the point of view of patient flow, as another clinical department rendering outpatient care. The patient is registered as a recurring outpatient, and the flow of information and forms follows much the same course as outlined in Section 2.2.

☐ ☐ ☐

When a patient first comes to a clinic the staff will initiate a medical record, which the clinic will then store. This record contains order sheets, progress notes for the use of the clinic's physicians and nurses, a history and physical, and the results of any tests run by the ancillary clinical departments.

☐ ☐ ☐

When a physician in a clinic orders tests or treatments from clinical departments, he or she writes an order on the patient's clinic chart. A clinic nurse then completes a requisition.

☐ ☐ ☐

In some hospitals the requisition is sent directly to the department. In others, the patient is required to reregister as a referred outpatient for any services the clinic itself cannot provide.

☐ ☐ ☐

In cases where the requisition goes directly to the department, the receptionist processes it in much the same manner an outpatient requisition is processed. After the test is performed or the service is rendered, the patient is sent back to the clinic. Both the results copy of the requisition, if there is one, and the charge copy are also returned to the clinic. Printed results are placed in the patient's file. The charge copy is

---

A = essentially similar   B = minor variations   C = significant differences

attached to the copy of the Outpatient Form that will be sent to Outpatient Registration for billing purposes.

A B C
☐ ☐ ☐

Centralized Clinic Office

In hospitals with a large number of clinics, a special department may exist to handle some or all of the administrative tasks associated with clinic operation. Such tasks include registering, scheduling, and storing medical records. The last activity is particularly important in hospitals where a patient may be enrolled in more than one clinic. In such situations, the hospital normally wants to keep only one outpatient record – a unit or unitized record – for the patient, thereby establishing the need for a central records-storage area.

☐ ☐ ☐

With the centralized approach, a new patient first goes to the Clinic Registration Desk. There the patient is interviewed, and a Clinic Registration Form is completed. This form contains demographic information, billing information, and the reasons why the patient is seeking treatment.

☐ ☐ ☐

After the interview is completed, the patient is sent home and told to contact the Clinic Office on a certain day. The Clinic Form is sent to the office. One copy is sent to the clinic to which the patient is assigned. The remaining copies are placed in the patient's file in the Clinic Office.

☐ ☐ ☐

When the patient calls, a Scheduling Clerk reviews the schedule for the particular clinic and sets a date and time for the patient's visit.

☐ ☐ ☐

Each day, the clinic schedules for the following day are reviewed by a Scheduling Clerk, who then prepares the next day's daily schedule for each clinic. One copy goes to the clinic, another goes to the Clinic Registration Desk, and a third goes to the medical-records section of the Clinic Office. A Medical Records Technician pulls the files for all patients scheduled to be seen the next day. These files are then delivered to the appropriate clinics.

☐ ☐ ☐

When the patient arrives, he or she goes to the Clinic Registration Desk and signs in. The patient then goes to the appropriate clinic, where clinical personnel make the needed entries into the patient's record. After treatment, the patient is dismissed.

☐ ☐ ☐

A = essentially similar   B = minor variations   C = significant differences

Finally, the clinic nurse sends the record back to the central records area, after printed test results received from clinical departments have been added.

A B C
☐ ☐ ☐ _____

If there is a fixed fee for each clinic visit, the clinic takes no further steps. If the clinic fee is variable – depending on services rendered and supplies used – a clinic Unit Secretary completes a charge document and sends it to the Clinic Office.

☐ ☐ ☐ _____

A Clinic Office Billing Secretary then prepares a list of services rendered and the appropriate charges and forwards it to the Business Office for billing. For the first billing, a copy of the patient's Clinic Registration Form accompanies the list of services. The Billing Secretary obtains information about services from the following sources:

☐ ☐ ☐ _____

1. If there is a fixed clinic fee, that fee is written on the charge document.

☐ ☐ ☐ _____

2. If there is a variable fee, the fee indicated on the charge document that comes from the clinic is recorded.

☐ ☐ ☐ _____

3. Charge copies of requisition forms are sent by the clinical departments to the Billing Secretary.

☐ ☐ ☐ _____

A = essentially similar   B = minor variations   C = significant differences

Flow Chart 2.3

Centralized Clinic Department

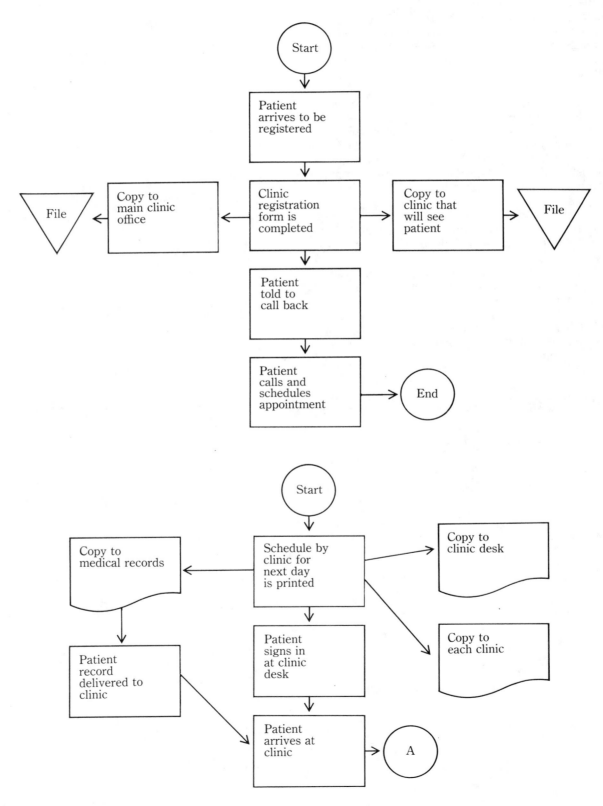

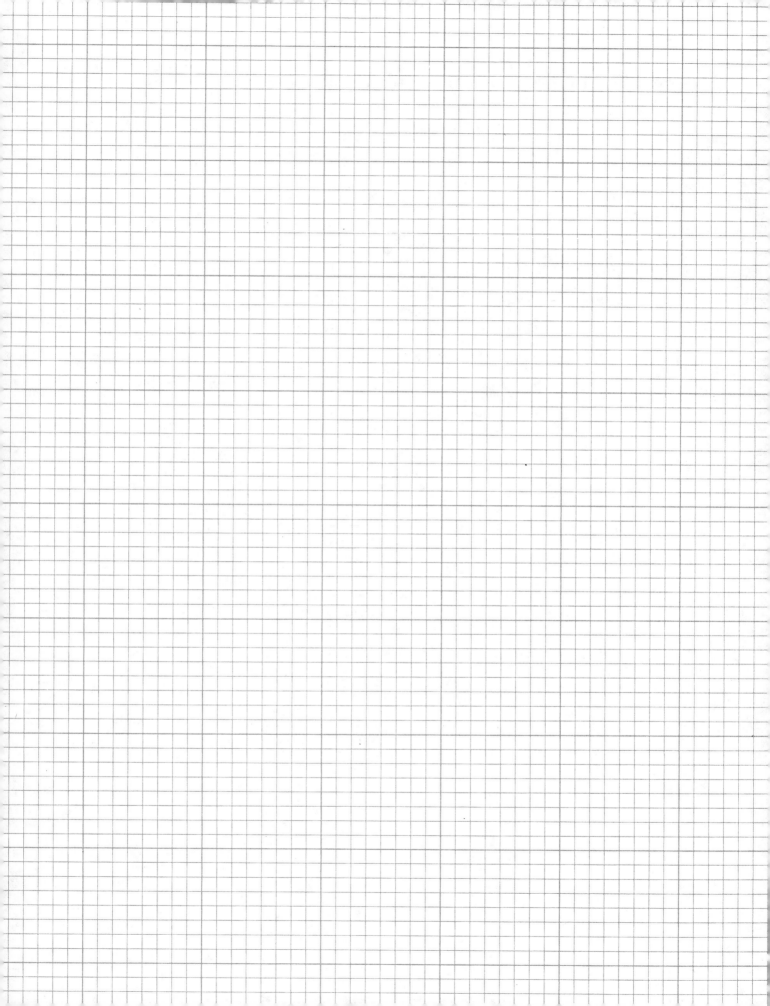

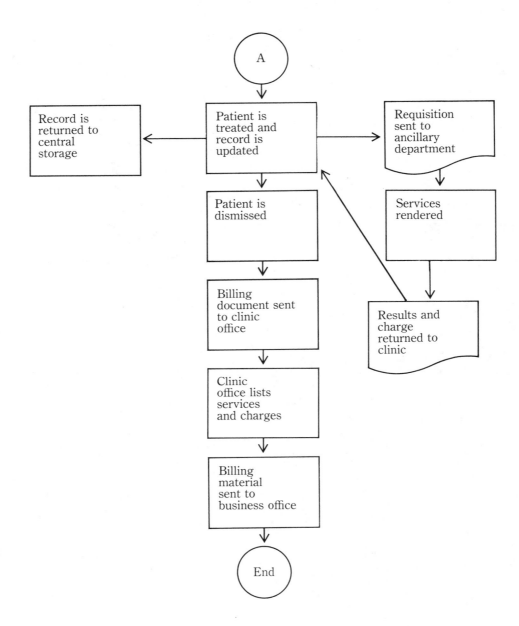

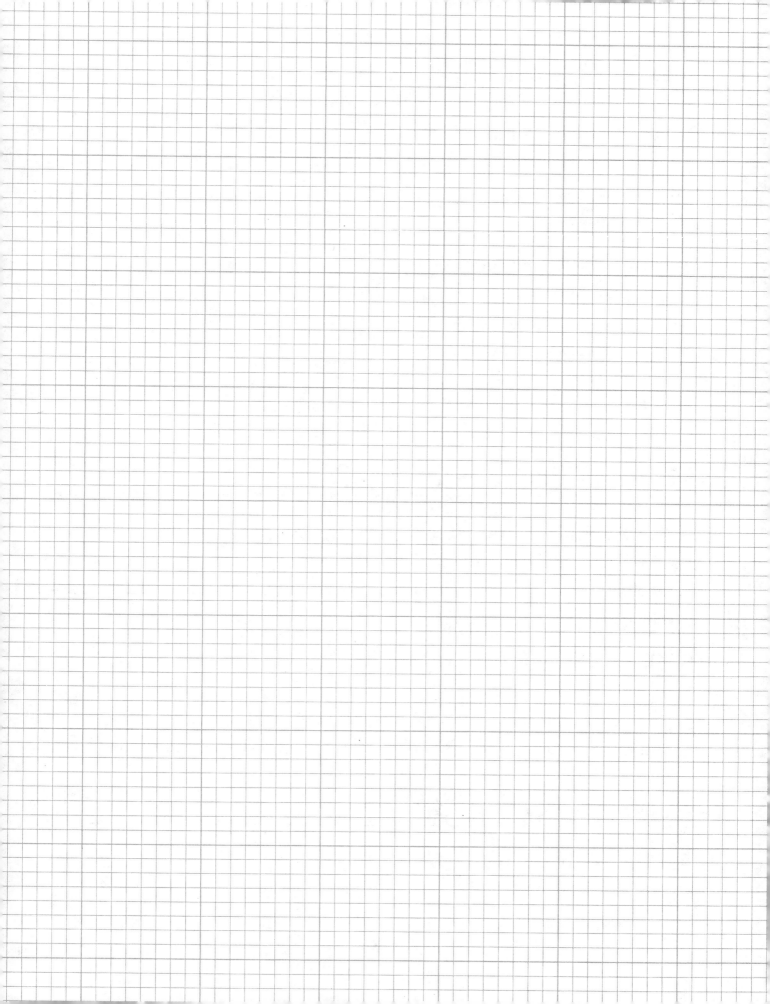

Input Inventory 2.3

A. Clinic Office Supervisor

your document title
↓

A B C

1. Clinic registration form. ☐ ☐ ☐ _____

2. Fee listing for Business Office. ☐ ☐ ☐ _____

3. Patient interview form. ☐ ☐ ☐ _____

B. Head Nurse, Clinic

1. Forms for Medical Record. ☐ ☐ ☐ _____

2. Charge document sent to Clinic Office. ☐ ☐ ☐ _____

3. Requisition for services from ancillary departments. ☐ ☐ ☐ _____

USE INPUT DOCUMENT ANALYSIS FORM

A = same document title   B = minor variations   C = significant differences

Master File Inventory 2.3

A. Clinic Office Supervisor

Notes
↓

A B C

1. Sign-in sheet. ☐ ☐ ☐ _____

2. Patient file. ☐ ☐ ☐ _____

3. Schedule book. ☐ ☐ ☐ _____

B. Head Nurse, Clinic

Patient file (medical). ☐ ☐ ☐ _____

USE MASTER FILE ANALYSIS FORM

A = essentially similar   B = minor variations   C = significant differences

Report Inventory 2.3

A. Clinic Office Supervisor

your document title
↓

A B C

1. Monthly activity report. ☐ ☐ ☐ _____

2. Daily schedules by clinic. ☐ ☐ ☐ _____

3. Reports to private physicians.

A B C
☐ ☐ ☐

USE REPORT ANALYSIS FORM

| A = essentially similar | B = minor variations | C = significant differences |

System Performance Standards 2.3

	Units	A	B
1. How long does it take to register a clinic patient?	minutes_____	☐	☐
2. How long does it take to get an appointment at a clinic?	mean time for all clinics in days _____	☐	☐
3. How often is a physician not at a clinic at the scheduled starting time?	number of times per week____	☐	☐
4. How often does a patient arrive at a clinic without his or her records on file?	times per week _____	☐	☐
5. How many records are lost?	number per month _____	☐	☐
6. How much is lost in revenue because charge tickets cannot be matched with patient visits?	dollars _____	☐	☐
7. How many scheduled patients do not show up for an appointment?	number per week _____	☐	☐
8. What is the waiting time for service once a scheduled patient arrives at a clinic?	minutes_____	☐	☐

USE PERFORMANCE STANDARDS ANALYSIS FORM

| A = we have a standard | B = we do not have a standard |

System Cost Factors 2.3

How many workhours are involved in moving the records of clinic patients? $ _____

USE SYSTEM COST ANALYSIS FORM (also see Instructions, p. 15)

General Patient
Services Systems

System 3.1.1: Laboratory

Description 3.1.1

Notes
↓

The Laboratory is made up of five basic areas, each of which is involved in performing diagnostic tests on various types of specimens.

A B C
☐ ☐ ☐ _____

These sections are:

- Chemistry
- Cytology
- Hematology
- Histology
- Microbiology

☐ ☐ ☐ _____

Also associated with the Clinical Laboratory is the Blood Bank, which will be analyzed separately in this section.

☐ ☐ ☐ _____

Larger laboratories may further divide these clinical areas into subunits specializing in coagulation studies, immunology, serology, steroid analysis, toxicology, urinalysis, and virology.

☐ ☐ ☐ _____

Most laboratory activity involves running tests on specimens from patients. But this department may also play a role in employee physicals, nosocomial infection control, and testing specimens sent by other hospitals.

☐ ☐ ☐ _____

Ordering the Service

Laboratory information flow begins when a physician orders a specific laboratory test. This order may be either for one test to be done once or a test to be repeated daily until cancelled by the physician. The Nursing Station prepares a requisition for the desired test.

☐ ☐ ☐ _____

If the test is to run STAT or requires special handling (e.g., time specimens, isolation, etc.), the text slip is marked accordingly. The request for these procedures is called to the Laboratory. Upon receiving a STAT or special handling order, the Laboratory Clerk notifies a phlebotomist, who immediately proceeds to the Nursing Station. The phlebotomist obtains the requisition and proceeds to the patient's room. After checking the patient's identification with the name on the request slip, the phlebotomist obtains the required amount of blood and enters

---

the time and initials the requisition. The blood-sample tubes are labeled with the patient's name and hospital number, and the sample and request slip are hand-carried to the lab and delivered to the appropriate testing section.

A B C
☐ ☐ ☐ _____

For non-STAT procedures that require a phlebotomist, the requsition is delivered to the Laboratory receiving area. Typically these requisitions are delivered in the evening and are sorted according to Nursing Station. Specimens are then obtained the following morning during the scheduled pick-up rounds. In many hospitals, however, specimen pick-up rounds are made during the day.

☐ ☐ ☐ _____

The phlebotomist takes the requisition to the patient's room. From this point, the procedure is the same as described previously for STAT procedures.

☐ ☐ ☐ _____

Many specimens (e.g., urine, sputum, etc.) do not require the service of a phlebotomist. For these cases, a requisition is still prepared. The specimen is then collected, labeled by the Nursing Station, and hand-carried to the Laboratory with the requisition. Usually the specimen is delivered to the appropriate Laboratory section. All sections provide a log book to note the patient's name, room number, specimen type, time, and the deliverer's name.

☐ ☐ ☐ _____

Processing the Sample

Chemistry

Most specimens analyzed by Chemistry are blood samples. Once received by Chemistry, the sample is allowed to clot. The serum is then separated off and put into a tube with the patient's name on it. The requisition is checked by the technologist to determine what procedures will be required. The patient's name, room number, and physician are written in the Chemistry procedure log book. Each ordered test is also marked in the log book.

☐ ☐ ☐ _____

The requisition, along with the serum sample, is delivered to the procedural area. The technologist receiving the requisition and sample writes the patient's name in a notebook or sheet designed for the procedure area. This notebook or sheet aids in test sequencing when more than one sample is being tested. A check is made to insure that the name on the serum sample tube matches the name on the test slip.

☐ ☐ ☐ _____

Notes
↓

A = essentially similar   B = minor variations   C = significant differences

142

The technologist runs the required procedure. STAT procedures are given first priority. Automated procedures result in some type of graphic or digital printout, which is interpreted and checked against standards for validity. Manual results are similarly read, interpreted, and checked. Valid results are recorded on the patient's requisition while questionable results are referred to the supervisor and retested. The technologist signs each requisition and records the test results in the Chemistry procedures log book. STAT results are phoned to the floor or physician. The requisition is then sent to the Clerical Area.

A B C
☐ ☐ ☐ _____

Cytology

Cytology is concerned with the cell structure of a large variety of biological specimens. When a specimen is delivered to Cytology, a staffer records the patient's name, room number, specimen type, the time delivered, and the signature of the deliverer in the Cytology specimen log book.

☐ ☐ ☐ _____

After matching the specimen label with the request slip, the technician assigns a sequential number to the specimen and writes it onto the requisition. The technician then prepares slides of the specimen, which are then examined. The results are recorded on the requisition. Abnormal results are reviewed by the supervisor and the pathologist.

☐ ☐ ☐ _____

The completed requisition is signed and dated and sent to the Clerical Area.

☐ ☐ ☐ _____

Hematology

Hematology concentrates on the study of anti-coagulated blood samples.

☐ ☐ ☐ _____

Once received by Hematology, blood samples and requisitions are matched according to the patient's name. Both sample tube and test slip are numbered sequentially. STAT procedures receive priority as to positioning in the test run sequence. A peripheral smear of the patient's blood is made on a slide. The patient's name and the assigned sample number are written on the slide. This slide is stained for differential and descriptive purposes.

☐ ☐ ☐ _____

The technologist runs the blood sample through the machine, and the blood count is printed out on the test slip. The results are checked for validity. Samples giving questionable results are repeated. STAT procedure results are phoned to the floor, emergency room, or physician.

☐ ☐ ☐ _____

A = essentially similar   B = minor variations   C = significant differences

The blood smear is examined microscopically with differential and descriptive results written onto the requisition. Abnormal findings are referred to the supervisor. If the results appear normal, the technologist signs the lab slip and writes the date and time. These results are recorded in the Hematology procedures log book following the above-mentioned numerical sequencing.

A B C
□ □ □ _____

Completed requisitions are sent to the Clerical Area.

□ □ □ _____

Histology

Histology involves the pathologist rather than the technologist. The major portion of the workload is the preparation and examination of surgically removed tissues and organs.

□ □ □ _____

Upon arrival from Surgery, each specimen is recorded in the specimen log book. A technician numbers each specimen and prepares slides. The pathologist examines each specimen and all slides, then dictates findings. This dictation is typed onto a Histology report form and returned to the pathologist for approval and signature.

□ □ □ _____

Copies of the completed Histology report form go to the patient's chart, to the patient's physicians, and to the Histology file. The requisition is sent to the Clerical Area.

□ □ □ _____

Microbiology

Microbiology receives the largest variety of biological specimens of any of the Clinical Laboratory sections. It is responsible for the proper handling, setting up, growth, identification, and drug-sensitivity testing of all microbial cultures. Work centers around identification and sensitivity testing of bacteria. Due to the incubation time necessary for bacterial growth, results are not available for 24 to 72 hours. When a specimen arrives at Microbiology, the person delivering the specimen writes the patient's name, room number, specimen type, delivery time, and deliverer's name in the daily Microbiology specimen log sheet. All specimens are assigned a sequential number, which is placed on the requisition, on all subsequent cultures, and on all subsequent tubes and plates.

□ □ □ _____

After all test procedures have been completed, the technologist records the results on the requisition and sends it to the Clerical Area.

□ □ □ _____

Results Reporting

Some hospitals have decentralized files in their Laboratories. Each section keeps one copy of the requisition for its result file.

A B C
☐ ☐ ☐ _____

In other hospitals, there is only one file, with all results going into that file.

☐ ☐ ☐ _____

In the Clerical Area, a clerk separates each requisition. One copy goes to the patient's chart; another may be sent to the patient's physician. If the Laboratory's file is centralized, a copy is placed in the file. On the fourth copy, the clerk enters a charge, then sends the copy to the Business Office.

☐ ☐ ☐ _____

The Histology requisition typically has only one copy, which goes to the Business Office.

☐ ☐ ☐ _____

Blood Bank

The Blood Bank is responsible for obtaining and storing blood and providing blood to patients.

☐ ☐ ☐ _____

The blood is obtained from donors, community blood banks, and commercial sources.

☐ ☐ ☐ _____

Each unit is typed and labeled, then stored in a refrigerator. The Blood Bank keeps a log called the Blood-Unit Record File, which shows the following information for each stored unit – date drawn, source, type, identification number, and expiration date. A Blood Bank technician reviews this log daily to assure that blood is available and that no out-of-date units remain in storage.

☐ ☐ ☐ _____

The Flow

When a physician orders a transfusion, a Blood Bank requisition is completed, and the Blood Bank is notified by telephone. A phlebotomist is dispatched, who draws a blood sample and places bands labeled with a Blood Bank number on the patient's wrist and ankle. The number is also placed on the sample tube and on all units that are cross-matched for the patient.

☐ ☐ ☐ _____

When the patient's blood sample is delivered with a transfusion requisition, the sample and slip are checked for matching identification. The blood sample is allowed to clot and then is centrifuged. The patient's serum is separated into another tube, which is then labeled with all relevant patient information. The patient's blood

---

A = essentially similar   B = minor variations   C = significant differences

is typed, and an antibody screen is set up. Possible compatible units of blood to be cross-matched are checked in the blood unit record file.

A B C
□ □ □ _____

After obtaining the units to be cross-matched from storage, a technician sets up a cross-match for each unit. The Blood Bank numbers and blood types of all units being cross-matched are recorded on the transfusion requisition. A Blood Bank worksheet is also completed. On this work-sheet are recorded: the date of the cross-match, the patient's name and hospital number, the ordering physician, the patient's ABO and Rh types, the reactions to the antibody screen, the Blood Bank numbers for the units cross-matched with the results for each cross-match, the time the process began and finished, and the tech-nologist's initials. Blood Bank tags with the patient's name, room number, physician, blood type, the Blood Bank unit number, the unit type, the unit outdating date, the date of cross-match, the Blood Bank number and the technologist's initials are clipped to the unit of blood, and the unit is returned to the storage shelf.

□ □ □ _____

After completing the cross-match, the technician notifies the using station or department that the needed units are available for transfusion. A cross-match slip with the patient's name, room number, physician, blood type, Blood Bank band number, and the Blood Bank unit number is filed with the unit record in the Blood Bank unit record file. This insures that the unit is not recross-matched for another patient. These slips remain with the unit record for the amount of time required by Laboratory policy.

□ □ □ _____

The transfusion requisition is sent to the Clerical Area. One copy is placed on the patient's chart; another is filed. A clerk enters charges onto the third and sends it to the Business Office.

□ □ □ _____

Another important document is the blood sign-out sheet. When a unit of blood is to be trans-fused, a staff person from the floor or ED comes to the Blood Bank with a request for a blood slip. This slip has the patient's name, room number, hospital number, and Blood Bank number recorded on it. The type of blood (whole blood or packed cells) is also written on the slip. This information is duplicated on the sign-out sheet, along with the blood unit number, unit type, the patient's blood type, the time the unit is taken, and the initials of both the staff person taking the unit of blood and the technologist who issues the unit.

□ □ □ _____

A = essentially similar   B = minor variations   C = significant differences

Other pertinent information collected and stored by the Blood Bank includes: an antibody file (containing patient name and antibody identified in a previously completed cross-match procedure) and a donor file (containing information concerning past voluntary donors).

A B C
☐ ☐ ☐ _____

_____

A = essentially similar   B = minor variations   C = significant differences

Flow Chart 3.1.1a

Requisition Flow/Non STAT

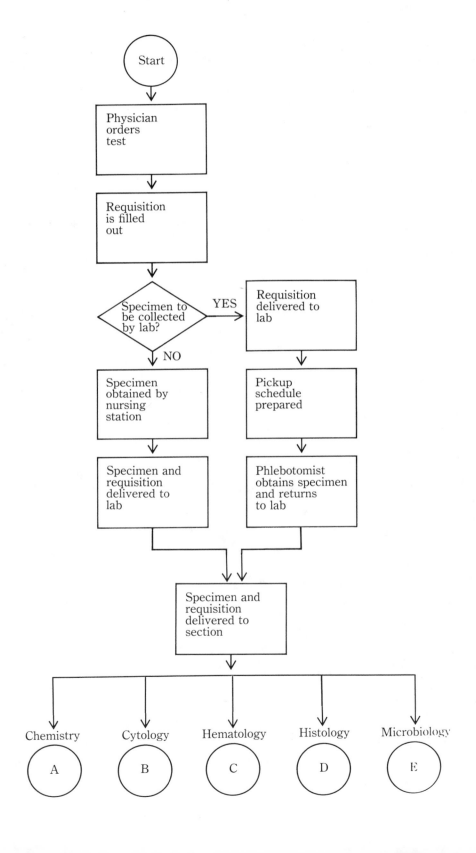

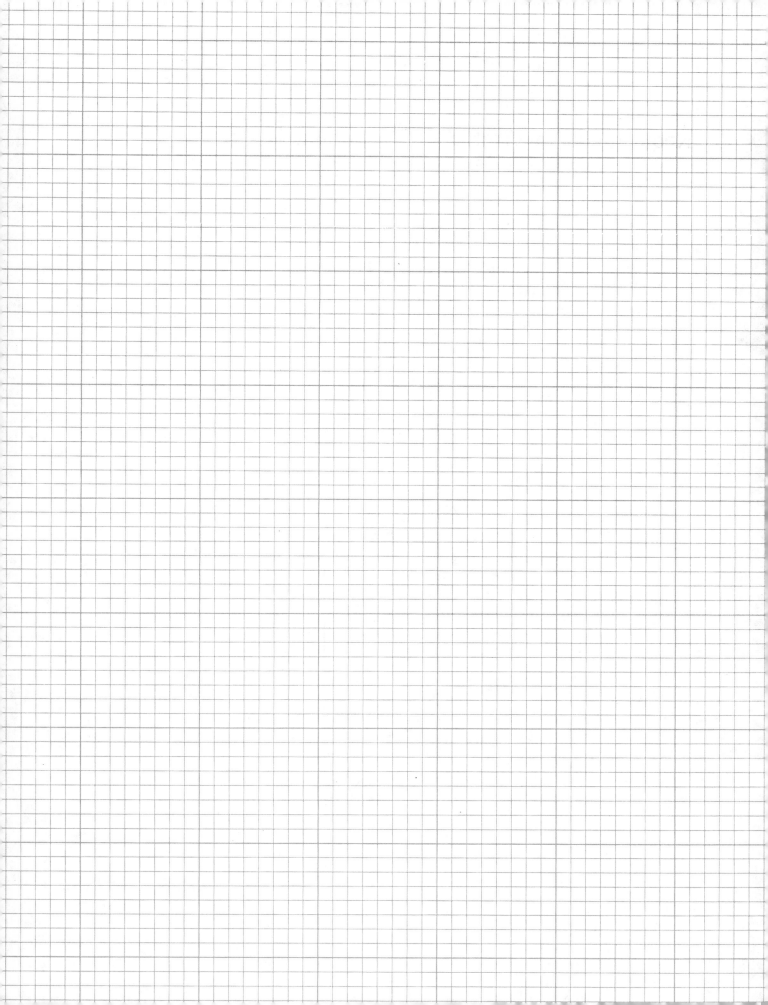

Requisition Flow/Non STAT, continued

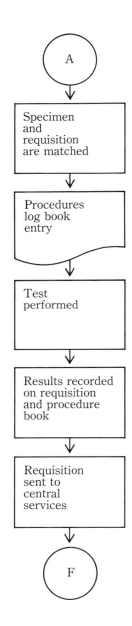

A

Specimen
and
requisition
are matched

Procedures
log book
entry

Test
performed

Results recorded
on requisition
and procedure
book

Requisition
sent to
central
services

F

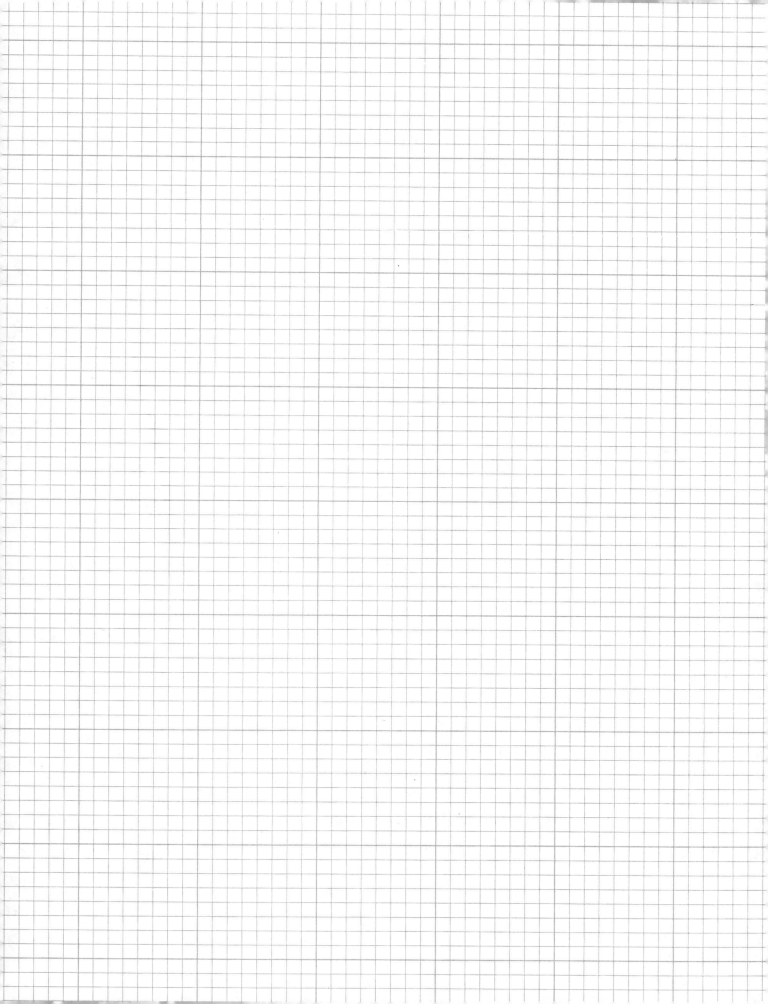

Requisition Flow/Non STAT, continued

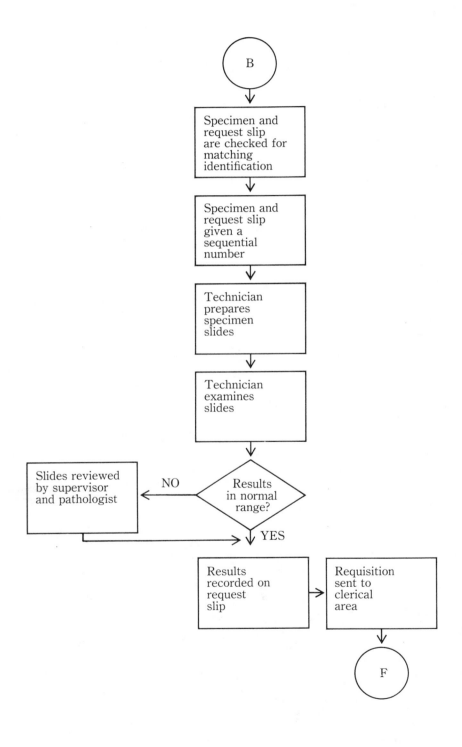

Requisition Flow/Non STAT, continued

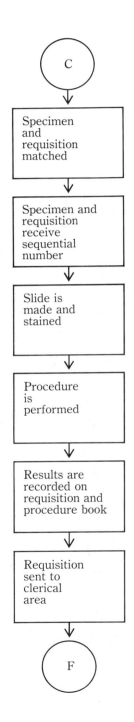

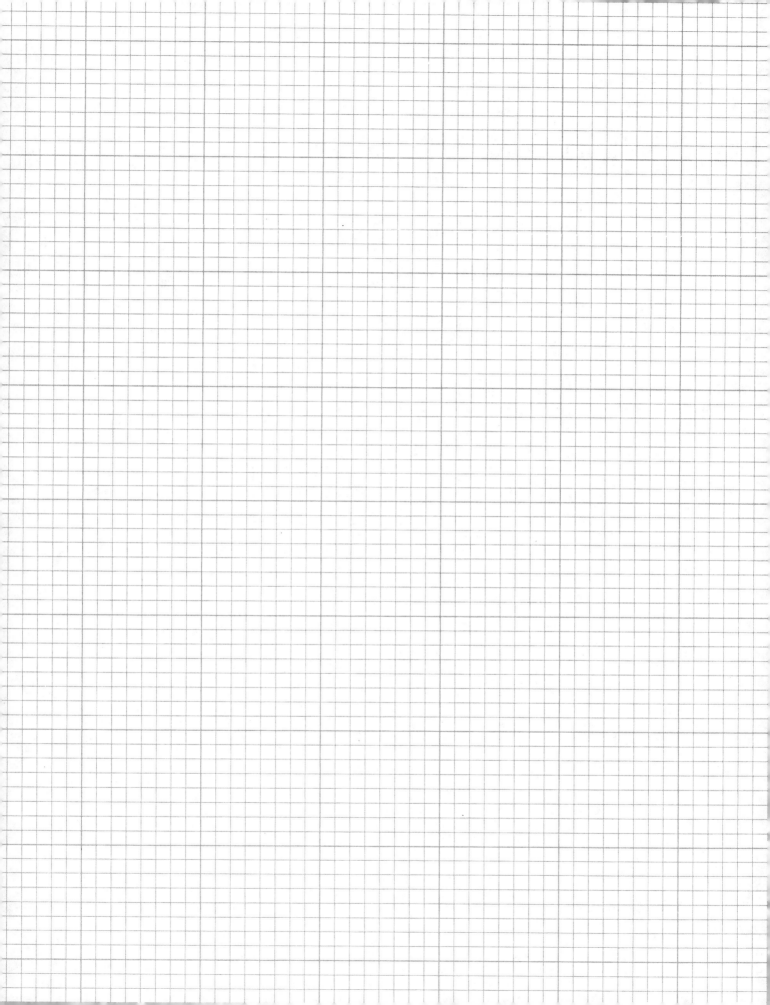

Requisition Flow/Non STAT, continued

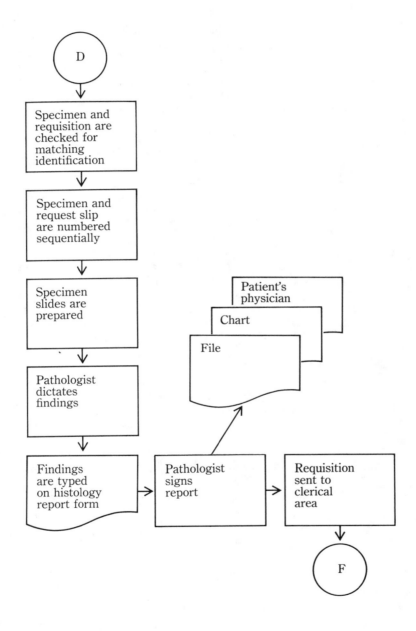

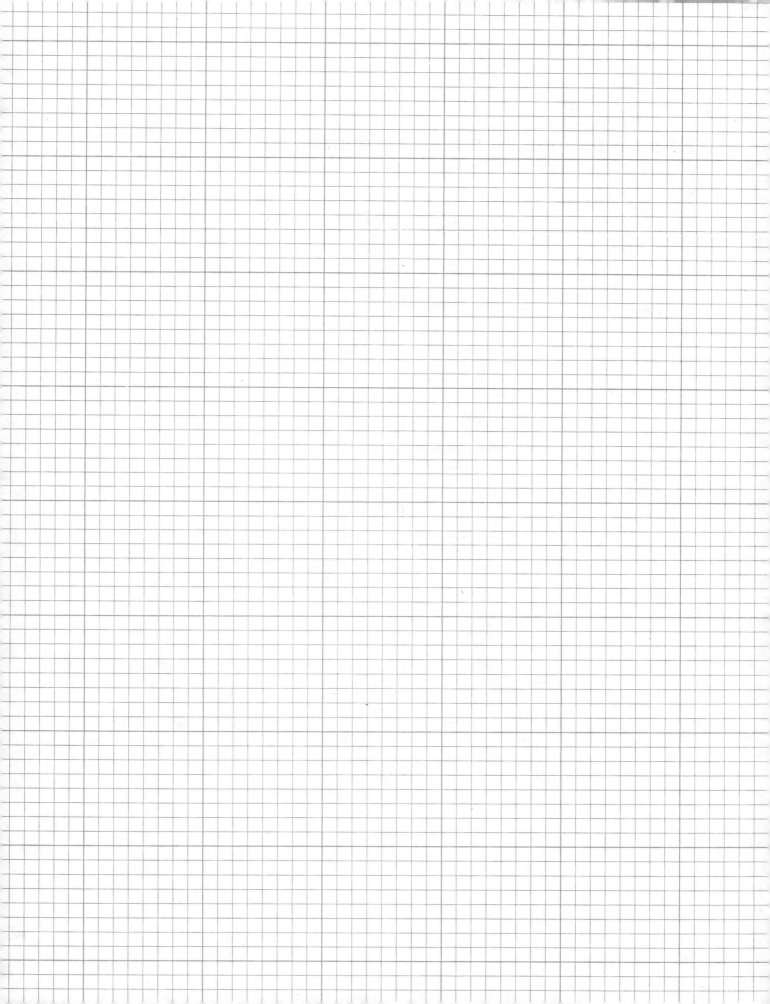

Requisition Flow/Non STAT, continued

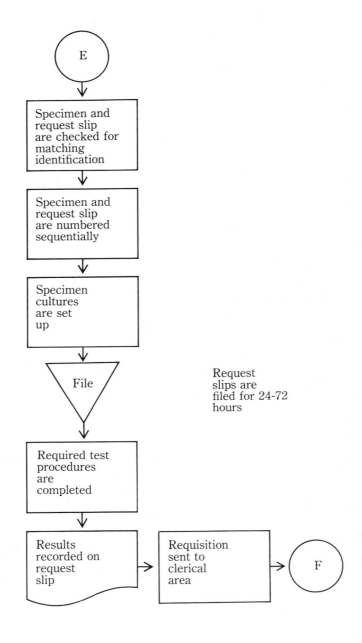

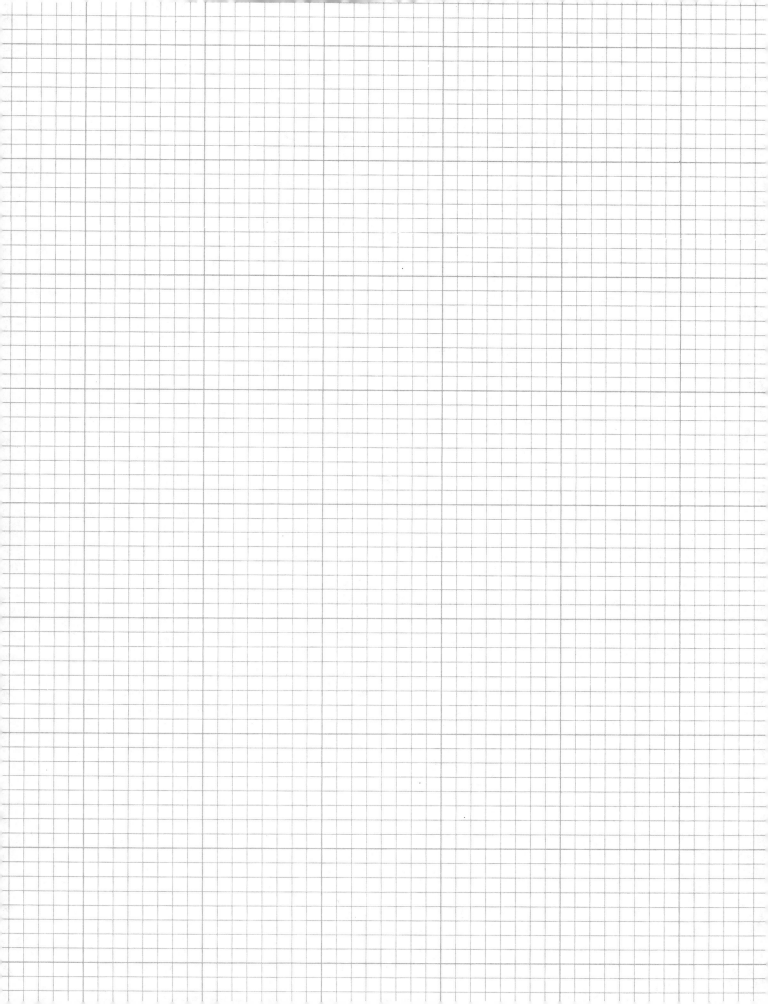

Requisition Flow/Non STAT, continued

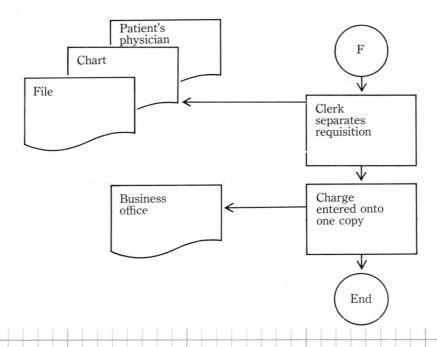

Flow Chart 3.1.1b

Blood Bank

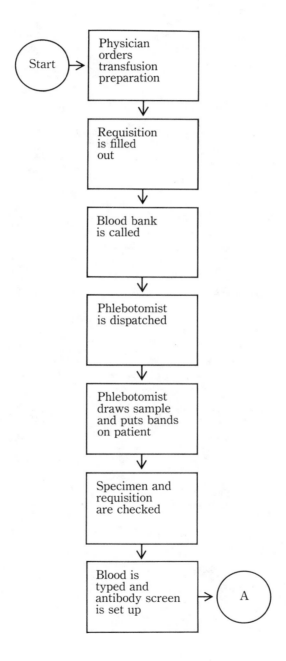

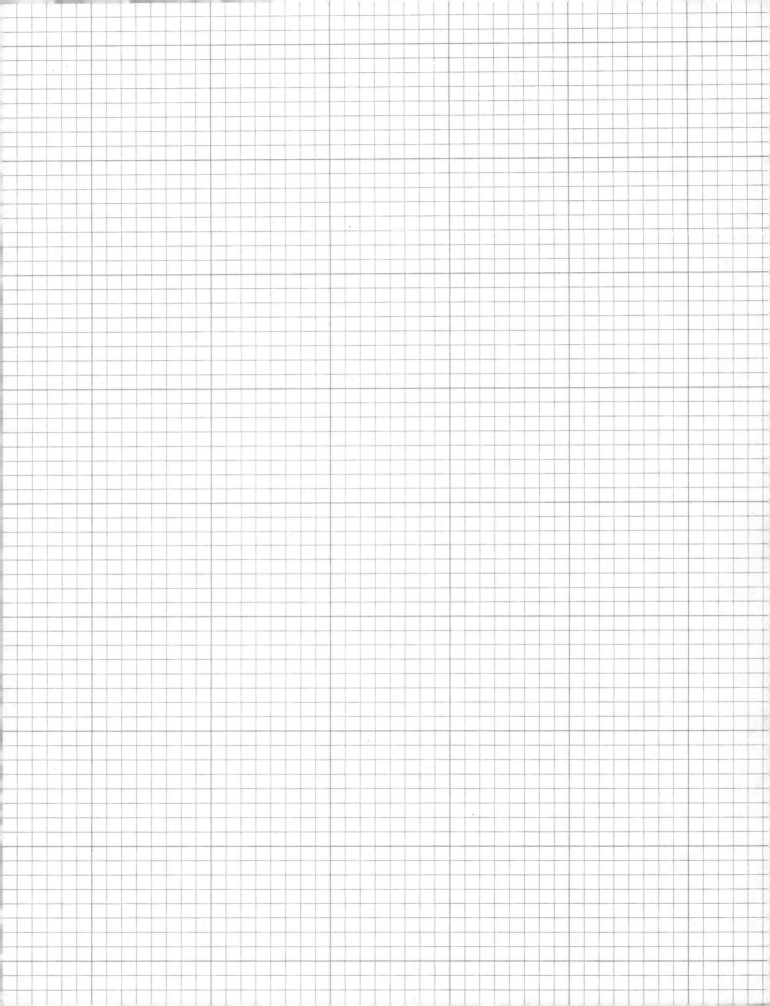

Blood Bank, continued

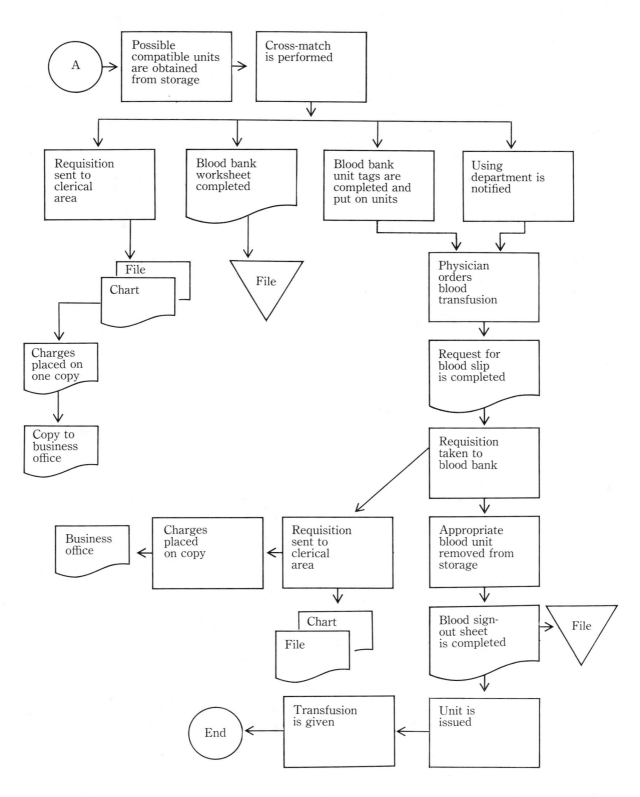

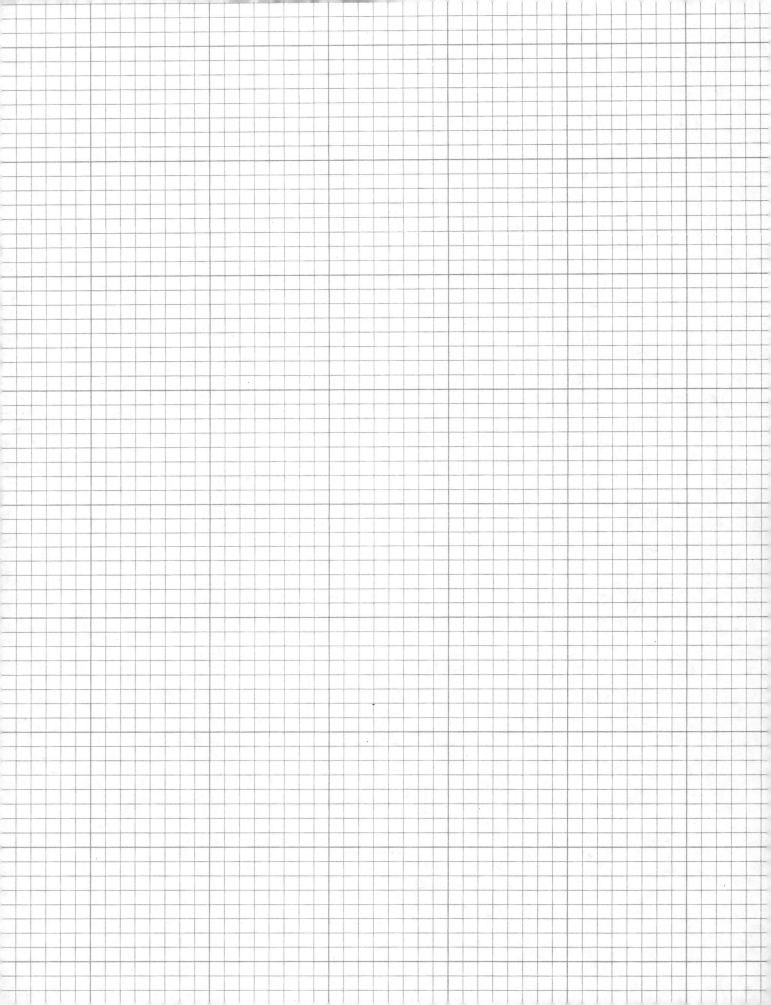

Input Inventory 3.1.1
Laboratory

A. Head Nurse

your document title
↓

A B C

1. Laboratory requisitions.

   a. Automated Chemistry request slips (e.g., SMA–12, SMA–6, etc.). ☐ ☐ ☐ _____

   b. Manual Chemistry request slip. ☐ ☐ ☐ _____

   c. Miscellaneous Chemistry request slip. ☐ ☐ ☐ _____

   d. Cytology request slip. ☐ ☐ ☐ _____

   e. Hematology request slip (e.g., CBC). ☐ ☐ ☐ _____

   f. Special Hematology request slip (e.g., phase platelet count, hemosiderin). ☐ ☐ ☐ _____

   g. Microbiology request slip. ☐ ☐ ☐ _____

   h. Other request slips.

- Coagulation
- Immunology
- Serology
- Steroid analysis
- Toxicology
- Urinalysis
- Virology ☐ ☐ ☐ _____

   i. Miscellaneous lab request slip. ☐ ☐ ☐ _____

2. STAT and Special Handling tags. ☐ ☐ ☐ _____

USE INPUT DOCUMENT ANALYSIS FORM

A = same document title	B = minor variations	C = significant differences

Blood Bank

A. Head Nurse

your document title
↓

A B C

1. Transfusion requisition. ☐ ☐ ☐ _____

2. Request for blood slip. ☐ ☐ ☐ _____

B. Blood Bank Supervisor

A B C

1. Unit Record Form.   □ □ □   _____

2. Blood Bank unit tags.   □ □ □   _____

3. Unit sign-out sheets.   □ □ □   _____

USE INPUT DOCUMENT ANALYSIS FORM

A = same document title   B = minor variations   C = significant differences

Master File Inventory 3.1.1
Laboratory

Notes
↓

A. Head Nurse

A B C

List of all procedures laboratory is able to perform.   □ □ □   _____

B. Laboratory Section Supervisor

1. Hematology

    a. Procedures log book.   □ □ □   _____

    b. Daily reagent control logs.   □ □ □   _____

    c. Bone marrow report forms.   □ □ □   _____

    d. Daily instrument control logs.   □ □ □   _____

2. Chemistry

    a. Procedures log book.   □ □ □   _____

    b. Daily reagent control logs.   □ □ □   _____

    c. Daily instrument control logs.   □ □ □   _____

C. Clerical Area

Results.   □ □ □   _____

USE MASTER FILE ANALYSIS FORM

A = essentially similar   B = minor variations   C = significant differences

Blood Bank

A. Blood Bank Supervisor

A B C

1. Voluntary donor file.　　　□ □ □　　_____

2. Patient antibody file.　　　□ □ □　　_____

3. Blood Bank worksheet.　　　□ □ □　　_____

4. Daily reagent control logs.　□ □ □　　_____

5. Requisition file.　　　　　　□ □ □　　_____

USE MASTER FILE ANALYSIS FORM

A = essentially similar	B = minor variations	C = significant differences

Report Inventory 3.1.1
Laboratory

A. Laboratory Clerical Area

your document title
↓

Statistical report listing the number of tests　A B C
performed per desired time period.　　　　　□ □ □　_____

USE REPORT ANALYSIS FORM

A = essentially similar	B = minor variations	C = significant differences

Blood Bank

A. Blood Bank Supervisor

your document title
↓

A B C

Monthly Activity Report.　　　□ □ □　_____

USE REPORT ANALYSIS FORM

A = essentially similar	B = minor variations	C = significant differences

System Performance Standards 3.1.1
Laboratory

	Units	A	B
1. Once a specimen arrives in the Laboratory, how much time elapses before it is logged in the proper section?	minutes_____	☐	☐
2. Once a test is completed, how much time elapses before it is posted on the patient's chart?	minutes_____	☐	☐
3. How much time is spent transposing results from requisitions to log books?	hours daily _____	☐	☐
4. How much time is spent telephoning results?	hours per day _____	☐	☐
5. How many telephone calls come into the Laboratory?	number received each day____	☐	☐
6. How many requisitions are STAT?	number of STAT calls received in a week divided by the total number of requisitions received in a week __	☐	☐
7. How many abnormal results are reported?	mean number per day _____	☐	☐
8. How much time is spent in the Clerical Area separating, filing, and charging?	hours per day _____	☐	☐
9. How often is a sample taken from the wrong patient?	number of times per week____	☐	☐

USE PERFORMANCE STANDARDS ANALYSIS FORM

A = we have a standard   B = we do not have a standard

Blood Bank

	Units	A	B
1. From the time a blood request is received, how long does it take to have the cross-matching performed?	minutes_____	☐	☐
2. How much blood is lost because it is not used before its expiration date?	number of units per month __	☐	☐
3. How often must blood be obtained on an emergency basis from outside the hospital?	number of times per year ____	☐	☐

USE PERFORMANCE STANDARDS ANALYSIS FORM

A = we have a standard   B = we do not have a standard

System Cost Factors 3.1.1
Laboratory

1. How much is spent annually on log books? $ _____

2. How much phlebotomist and technologist time is wasted because of short-comings in scheduling the pickup of specimens and the performing of tests? $ _____

3. Are results formatted in a way that permits the physician to read and compare results quickly? $ _____

USE SYSTEM COST ANALYSIS FORM *(also see Instructions, p. 15)*

Blood Bank

How many clerical people are employed in the Blood Bank? $ _____

USE SYSTEM COST ANALYSIS FORM *(also see Instructions, p. 15)*

System 3.1.2:
Diagnostic Radiology
Description 3.1.2

The Radiology Department's two major functions are performing diagnostic radiological procedures and administering radiation therapy. In some hospitals, the use of radioactive materials in diagnostic procedures (e.g., Nuclear Medicine) also is the responsibility of the department.

A B C
□ □ □ _____

The Flow

Pursuant to a physician's order, Radiology receives a copy of a requisition from the Nursing Station. The document states what procedures are to be done and gives the patient's name, hospital number, room and bed number, attending and consulting physicians, and the admitting diagnosis. It may also contain additional clinical information, such as the reason for the requested procedures.

□ □ □ _____

The requisition goes to a radiology clerk, who enters information from it into the Radiology Log. The radiology clerk then reviews an index card file, which contains one card for every patient the department has seen. The cards are in alphabetical order, with a patient number assigned by Radiology as well as a listing of the dates of service.

□ □ □ _____

If the clerk finds that the patient has been to the department before, the patient's Radiology number is written on the requisition and in the Log. If the patient has not been to the department before, the clerk assigns the next available number, makes up a new index card for the patient, files it, and writes the Radiology number on the requisition and Log. The clerk also prepares a label that will be placed on the envelope used to hold the patient's x-ray films and prepares a Radiology Form, which will be used in transcribing the radiologist's report.

□ □ □ _____

The requisition, the label, and the form are given to a scheduling technician, who schedules the procedures requested. Normally, the tests or therapy will be performed that day or the next.

□ □ □ _____

The requisition and form then go to a file clerk. If the patient has been to the department before, the clerk uses the patient's Radiology number to locate the envelope containing x-rays and reports from previous visits. These envelopes are filed in numerical order. If the requisition and form are accompanied by a label, the file clerk knows this material is for a new patient. In this case, the file clerk places the label on a new envelope.

A B C
☐ ☐ ☐ _____

The requisition, form, and envelope are clipped together and placed in a suspense file to await the arrival of the patient. Normally, all the material for patients who are expected the next day is filed alphabetically near the Reception Desk.

☐ ☐ ☐ _____

In the evening, a scheduling secretary types the schedule for the following day. This schedule details the day's activity by radiology room, listing in chronological order the names of the patients and the procedures for each room.

☐ ☐ ☐ _____

When the patient arrives, a receptionist enters the arrival time in the Log next to the patient's name. If necessary, the patient is taken to a dressing room, then to a waiting area.

☐ ☐ ☐ _____

When it is time for the patient to receive the test or treatment, a technician picks up the envelope and other material from the suspense file, reviews the requisition, and brings the patient to the proper radiology room.

☐ ☐ ☐ _____

After the procedure has been completed, the patient returns to the waiting area. While the exposed film is being developed, the envelope and other material are placed in a second suspense file near the developing area. After the films are developed, the technician examines them to make sure that they are readable. If they are not, the procedure may be performed again. If they are readable, the patient is sent back to his room or, in the case of outpatients, to the Outpatient Registration Desk, where a receptionist logs the departure time.

☐ ☐ ☐ _____

Meanwhile, a technician places the film in the envelope and delivers it and the associated material to a reading room where a radiologist reads the film. For recurring patients, the radiologist has the old films and reports available in the envelope. The radiologist then dictates a report. In many cases, the radiologist will also telephone a report to the Nursing Station or attending physician or handwrite an abbreviated report, which is sent immediately to the Nursing Station. The radiologist then reviews the requisition for completeness and accuracy and initials it to show the report has been dictated.

☐ ☐ ☐ _____

A = essentially similar   B = minor variations   C = significant differences

A clerk then sorts the material. The requisition is taken to a receptionist, who enters charges on the form, records the total charge in the Log, notes the date of the service on the patient's index card, and sends the requisition to the Business Office.

A B C
☐ ☐ ☐ _____

The requisition usually has two copies. One goes to the Business Office; the other stays with the Radiology Form and is filed in the patient's envelope.

☐ ☐ ☐ _____

The Radiology Form goes to a transcriber, who may or may not be in Radiology. Some hospitals centralize transcription while others staff each clinical department with its own transcribers.

☐ ☐ ☐ _____

The envelope is then returned to the file clerk, who puts it in a suspense file.

☐ ☐ ☐ _____

When the transcribed report is returned to the department, the radiologist reviews and signs it. Next, a clerk sends one copy to the Nursing Station for the patient's record, one copy to a file clerk, who places it in the appropriate envelope for filing, and the remaining copies to the patient's physicians.

☐ ☐ ☐ _____

Other Paths

The flow of outpatient and ED patients is almost identical to the flow described for inpatients.

☐ ☐ ☐ _____

Even when Radiology has satellites, such as a room in the ED area, the procedures remain similar. The technician in the ED keeps a Log, which is sent periodically to Radiology's clerical supervisor. The films, requisitions, and Radiology Forms are all sent to the main department, where they are processed in the manner described above.

☐ ☐ ☐ _____

When mobile x-ray units are used, the technician performs the requested procedures, then returns the requisition and exposed film to a Radiology Clerk who reviews the index file, puts the proper Radiology number on the requisition and Radiology Form, finds the proper envelope, logs the request, and delivers the material to the radiologist for review.

☐ ☐ ☐ _____

Physician Billing

The hospital may use one of three ways to provide compensation for radiologists. They may be salaried; they may receive a percentage of the department's revenue; or they may bill patients themselves for their services.

☐ ☐ ☐ _____

A = essentially similar   B = minor variations   C = significant differences

172

Flow Chart 3.1.2

Radiology

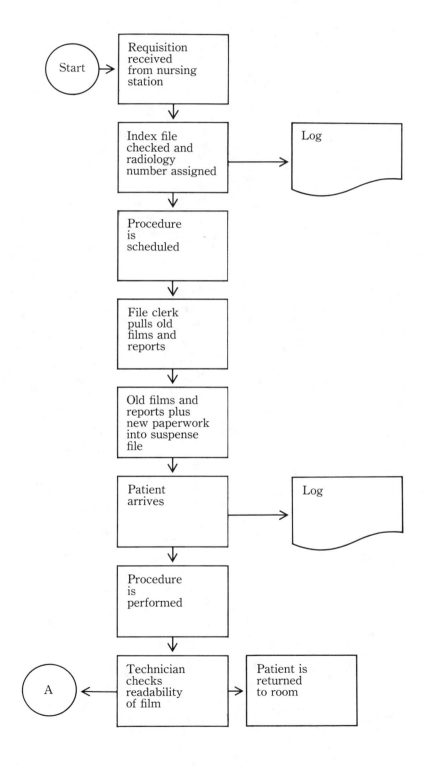

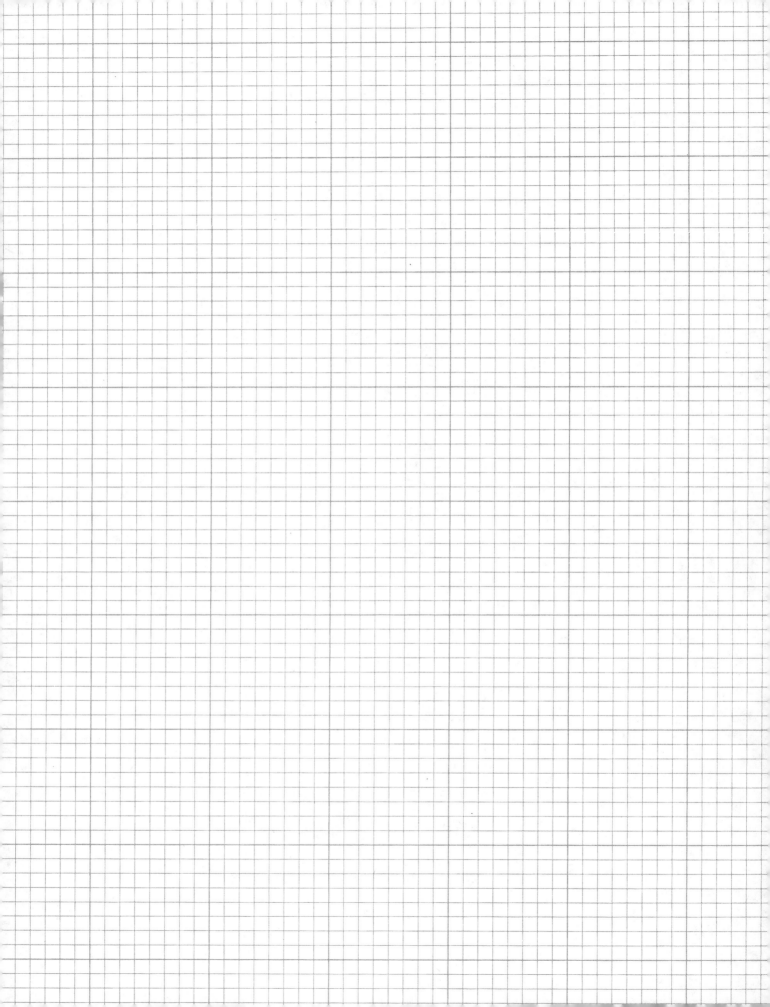

Radiology, continued

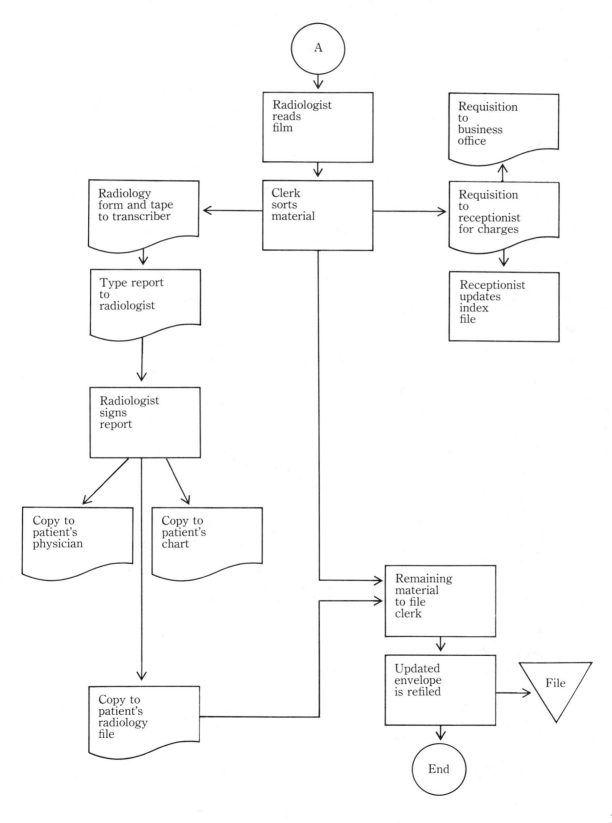

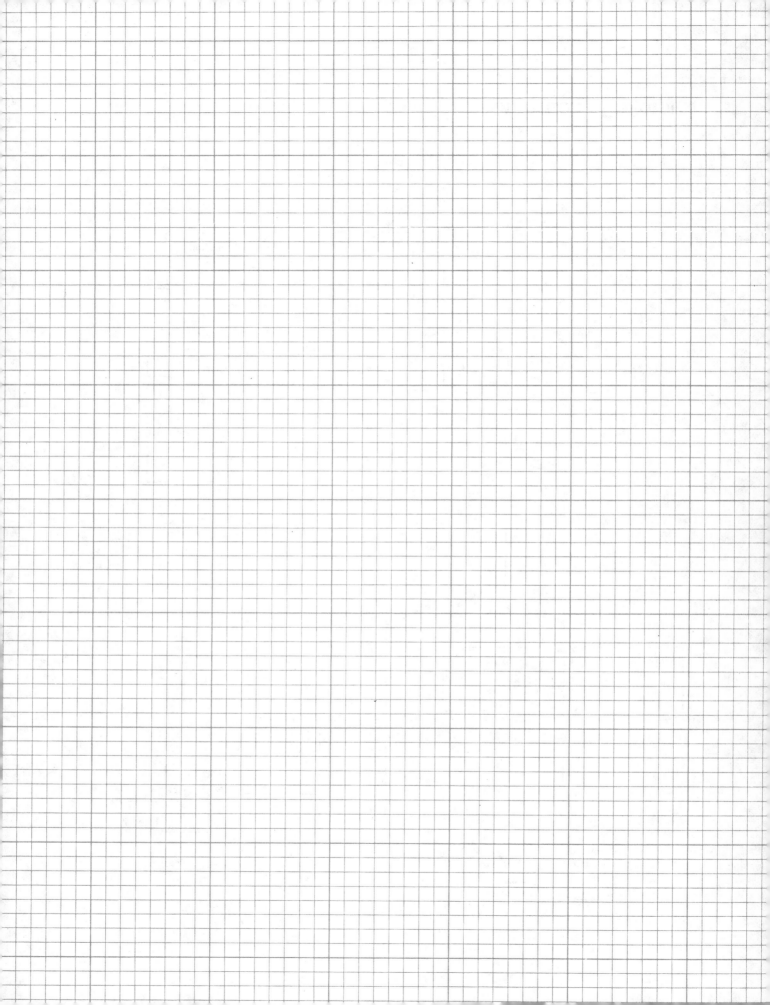

Input Inventory 3.1.2

A. Chief Technician

your document title
↓

	A	B	C	
1. Envelope for films and reports.	☐	☐	☐	_____
2. Index card.	☐	☐	☐	_____
3. Radiology (report) form.	☐	☐	☐	_____
4. Label.	☐	☐	☐	_____

USE INPUT DOCUMENT ANALYSIS FORM

A = same document title   B = minor variations   C = significant differences

Master File Inventory 3.1.2

A. Chief Technician

Notes
↓

	A	B	C	
1. Listing of scheduled services.	☐	☐	☐	_____
2. Film/report file.	☐	☐	☐	_____
3. Index card file.	☐	☐	☐	_____
4. Suspense file (patients due to arrive).	☐	☐	☐	_____
5. Radiology Log.	☐	☐	☐	_____
6. Suspense file (reports to be signed).	☐	☐	☐	_____

USE MASTER FILE ANALYSIS FORM

A = essentially similar   B = minor variations   C = significant differences

Report Inventory 3.1.2

A. Chief Technician

your document title
↓

	A	B	C	
1. Monthly productivity report.	☐	☐	☐	_____
2. Signed report from radiologist.	☐	☐	☐	_____
3. Quick report.	☐	☐	☐	_____
4. Daily schedule.	☐	☐	☐	_____

USE REPORT ANALYSIS FORM

A = essentially similar   B = minor variations   C = significant differences

System Performance Standards 3.1.2

Units

		A	B
1. How many clerical staffers does the department employ?	number of full-time equivalent divided by number of procedures performed yearly	☐	☐
2. How much film is wasted by the department?	dollars per month _____	☐	☐
3. How many procedures are not billed because requisitions do not reach the Business Office?	number per month _____	☐	☐
4. How long does a patient wait from the time of arrival in the department until the time the procedure begins?	mean time in minutes_____	☐	☐
5. From the time a procedure is completed, how long does it take to generate a signed report?	minutes_____	☐	☐
6. How long does it take for a signed report to reach the patient's chart?	minutes_____	☐	☐
7. How often are films misplaced?	times per month when file clerk cannot locate envelopes immediately_____	☐	☐
8. What is the utilization rate of each radiology room?	mean hours of use daily divided by 24 hours _____	☐	☐

USE PERFORMANCE STANDARDS ANALYSIS FORM

A = we have a standard   B = we do not have a standard

System Cost Factors 3.1.2

1. What is the yearly postage charge for sending reports to physicians? $ _____

2. How much time is spent looking for old reports in files? $ _____

3. How often does the radiologist have to wait because there is a backlog in developing film or moving patients from rooms? $ _____

4. What is the cost of special equipment used in filing and retrieving? $ _____

5. What practices are followed to ensure that the right procedure is being done on the right patient? $ _____

USE SYSTEM COST ANALYSIS FORM *(also see Instructions, p. 15)*

System 3.1.3: Therapeutic Radiology

Description 3.1.3

Notes
↓

In most cases, a patient begins receiving radiation therapy when he is an inpatient, with treatments continuing on an outpatient basis after dismissal.

A B C
☐ ☐ ☐ _____

Flow

After consultation with physicians in the Radiology Department and other specialists, the patient's attending physician completes an order for radiation therapy.

☐ ☐ ☐ _____

A nurse completes a requisition form and sends it to the department. A clerk then logs the requisition and sends it to the supervisor of Radiation Therapy.

☐ ☐ ☐ _____

A file is opened for the patient. Initially this file contains a copy of the treatment plan agreed upon by the attending physician who will be rendering the therapy. Normally, the file also contains a consent form, signed by the patient and witnessed by the attending physician or the physician supervising the therapy.

☐ ☐ ☐ _____

Whenever therapy is to be rendered, the patient is taken to the Therapy Section, where he is logged in by a section clerk. The therapy is rendered, and the patient is logged out of the department and returned to the Nursing Station.

☐ ☐ ☐ _____

The physician rendering the therapy notes the date and other important data in the patient's file. Normally, the Nursing Station is responsible for recording in the medical record the fact that the patient was taken to therapy.

☐ ☐ ☐ _____

Periodically, the physician rendering therapy dictates a progress report. This is transcribed, with one copy going to the patient's file, one copy to the patient's medical record if he or she is still an inpatient, and one copy to the patient's physician.

☐ ☐ ☐ _____

Working from the log book, a clerk completes a charge ticket and sends it to the Business Office.

☐ ☐ ☐ _____

A = essentially similar   B = minor variations   C = significant differences

Before the patient is discharged, the Therapy
Section informs him or her of the times
scheduled for further treatments after dismissal.
Once dismissed, the patient becomes a recurring
outpatient.

A B C
☐ ☐ ☐

A = essentially similar   B = minor variations   C = significant differences

Flow Chart 3.1.3

Therapeutic Radiology

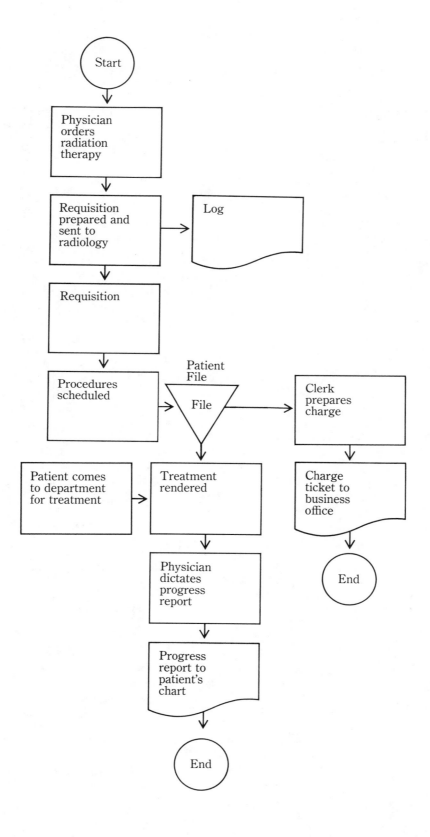

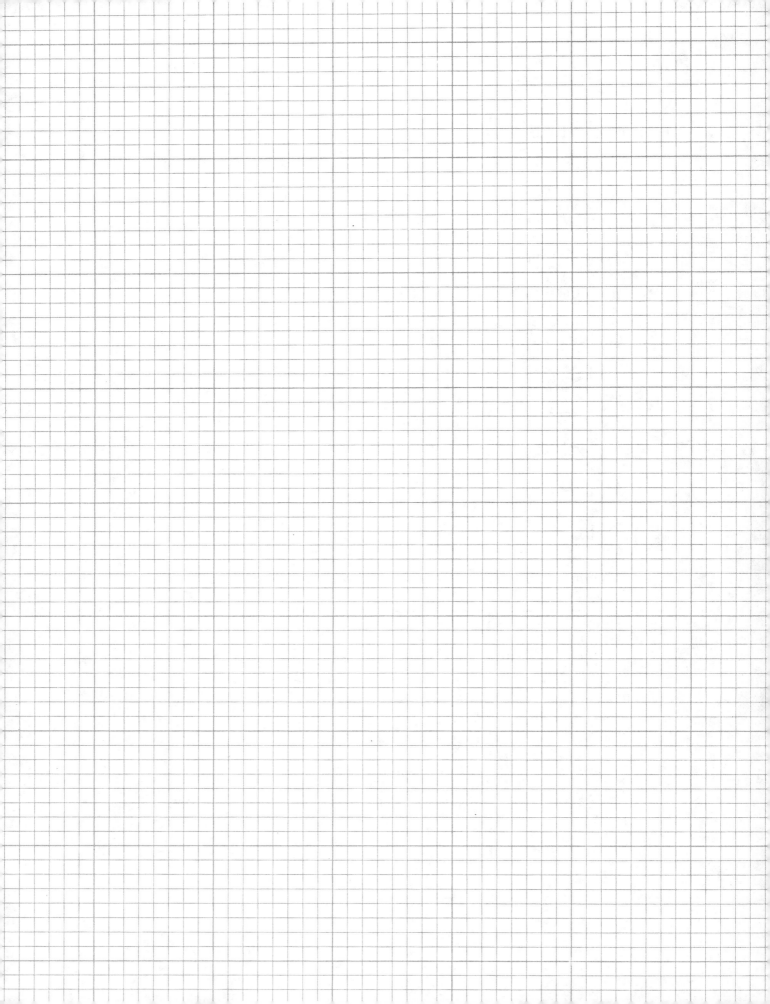

Input Inventory 3.1.3

A. Therapy Supervisor

your document title
↓

	A	B	C	
1. Requisition.	□	□	□	_____
2. Consent form.	□	□	□	_____
3. Charge ticket.	□	□	□	_____
4. Treatment record.	□	□	□	_____

USE INPUT DOCUMENT ANALYSIS FORM

A = same document title   B = minor variations   C = significant differences

Master File Inventory 3.1.3

A. Therapy Supervisor

Notes
↓

	A	B	C	
1. Section log.	□	□	□	_____
2. Schedule.	□	□	□	_____
3. Patient file.	□	□	□	_____

USE MASTER FILE ANALYSIS FORM

A = essentially similar   B = minor variations   C = significant differences

Report Inventory 3.1.3

A. Therapy Supervisor

your document title
↓

	A	B	C	
1. Monthly activity report.	□	□	□	_____
2. Treatment report.	□	□	□	_____

USE REPORT ANALYSIS FORM

A = essentially similar   B = minor variations   C = significant differences

System Performance Standards 3.1.3

	Units	A	B
1. What is the utilization of the therapy equipment?	number of hours the equipment is utilized each week divided by the product of 168 and the number of treatment rooms_____	☐	☐
2. What is the waiting time for therapy?	mean time that patients are required to wait in the department _____	☐	☐
3. How often does Nursing forget scheduled therapy?	number of times per week____	☐	☐
4. How often does a patient fail to come for therapy after dismissal?	number of patients per month _____	☐	☐

USE PERFORMANCE STANDARDS ANALYSIS FORM

A = we have a standard   B = we do not have a standard

System Cost Factors 3.1.3

(none)

System 3.1.4:
Nuclear Medicine

Description 3.1.4

The Department of Nuclear Medicine uses radioactive materials in the performance of diagnostic procedures. In some hospitals, the department is part of Radiology; in others, it is independent.

A B C
☐ ☐ ☐ _____

There are two types of Nuclear Medicine procedures – in vivo, or imaging, and in vitro. In vivo testing involves injecting radioactive material into a patient and tracing the flow of the material in the body with sensors. The specialized machine that contains the sensors is usually called a camera. Because different radioactive materials tend to concentrate in different parts of the body, Nuclear Medicine physicians can use these different materials to obtain photographic images, or scans, of different organs – liver, kidney, thyroid, etc.

☐ ☐ ☐ _____

In vitro procedures involve injecting radioactive material into blood or other samples taken from the patient and analyzing the resulting reaction.

☐ ☐ ☐ _____

The Flow

After the patient's physician orders a Nuclear Medicine procedure, the Nursing Station completes a requisition and sends it to the department. The requisition may contain clinical information, such as the admitting diagnosis and the reason for the test. If it does not, the nurse also completes a clinical-information form, which accompanies the requisition.

☐ ☐ ☐ _____

A Nuclear Medicine Clerk logs the requisition, schedules the procedure, and notifies the Nursing Station and Transportation of the time and date when the patient is expected at the department.

☐ ☐ ☐ _____

As tests are scheduled, a clerk logs each patient's scheduled procedure. This results in a complete schedule for the department for the next day.

☐ ☐ ☐ _____

A = essentially similar   B = minor variations   C = significant differences

In Vitro

For an in vitro procedure, it often is not necessary to bring the patient to the department. A technician can be dispatched to the patient's room to obtain the sample. In cases where the in vitro patient is brought to the department, a Nuclear Medicine technician takes the sample and sends the patient back to the Nursing Station.

A B C
☐ ☐ ☐

After the sample is obtained, a technician runs the appropriate tests. The technician enters the results on the report form, which usually is the requisition itself.

☐ ☐ ☐

The technician then reviews the requisition for accuracy, removes the charge copy, and gives it to a clerk, who enters the proper charges and forwards it to the Business Office.

☐ ☐ ☐

The results copies and the clinical-information form are sent to the Nuclear Medicine physician, who reviews the results and adds comments to them.

☐ ☐ ☐

One copy of the result form goes to the Nursing Station for mounting in the patient's medical record. One copy, along with the clinical-information form, goes into the patient's departmental file. The remaining copies are sent to the patient's attending physician.

☐ ☐ ☐

In Vivo

When an in vivo patient is brought to the department, a clerk logs him or her in. A technician then injects the patient with the appropriate radioactive material. After waiting for the material to concentrate, the patient is taken to a procedure room, where scans of the organ under study are made.

☐ ☐ ☐

The patient is then logged out of the department and returned to the Nursing Station. The technician reviews the requisition for accuracy and sends a copy to a clerk, who enters the appropriate charges and sends the form on to the Business Office.

☐ ☐ ☐

The output of the scanning camera is a photographic image. This image, along with the remaining copies of the requisition and the clinical-information form, is sent to the Nuclear Medicine physician, who reviews the film and dictates a report. The material is held in a suspense file while the tape containing the dictated report is sent to Transcription. When

A = essentially similar   B = minor variations   C = significant differences

the written report is returned, it is matched with the documents in the suspense file and sent to the physician, who signs the report and gives the material to a clerk. The clerk sends one copy to the Nursing Station for mounting in the patient's medical record. Another copy, together with the requisition and the clinical-information form, is placed in the patient's departmental file. The remaining copies are sent to the patient's physicians.

A B C
☐ ☐ ☐ _____

Outside Work

When the department lacks certain pieces of equipment, Nuclear Medicine sends in vitro samples to other hospitals or to independent laboratories for analysis. The flow in these cases is identical up to the point where the sample is taken.

☐ ☐ ☐ _____

A technician then prepares the sample for mailing or transporting and fills out a requisition supplied by the outside agency. The sample is then logged out of the department and sent to the agency.

☐ ☐ ☐ _____

When the results are received, they are either transcribed onto a departmental form or sent directly to the patient's record at the Nursing Station, to the patient's file, and to the patient's physicians.

☐ ☐ ☐ _____

In some hospitals, a charge ticket for the outside service is prepared and sent to the Business Office when the sample is sent out. In other hospitals, a charge document is not prepared until the results are received. In either case, the hospital treats the invoice from the outside agency as an account payable and bills the patient for the service.

☐ ☐ ☐ _____

In some cases, a physician at the outside agency submits a bill in addition to the agency's bill. Often, the physician will bill the patient directly. When that is the case, the hospital must supply the agency's physician with demographic and financial information about the patient to enable the physician to submit his bill.

☐ ☐ ☐ _____

Storage

Film is not the only medium available for storing the results of imaging. Microfilm is another approach. A third available medium is magnetic tape or discs. Nuclear Medicine cameras convert electromagnetic waves into electrical signals, which can be stored in a magnetic medium. When this approach is used, a Log is needed to show what material is on what tape.

A B C
☐ ☐ ☐ _____

Outpatients

The Nuclear Medicine Department is doing an increasing number of procedures for outpatients. The flow is basically the same as it is for inpatients. (Charging follows the flow detailed for the outpatient department.)

☐ ☐ ☐ _____

Scheduling

Scheduling is particularly crucial for many Nuclear Medicine tests. The material that is injected into the patient may have a very short shelf life. For tests involving these materials, the scheduling of patients must be coordinated with the delivery of the radioactive material. Otherwise, material will be wasted or the department will be unable to perform scheduled tests.

☐ ☐ ☐ _____

Accounting for Radioactive Material

For most radioactive materials used, the department must account for each dose. Therefore assay sheets are kept for each supply of each material delivered. The assay sheet identifies the material and contains spaces for logging the name and number of the patient receiving a dose and the date the dose was rendered. These are filed alphabetically.

☐ ☐ ☐ _____

Flow Chart 3.1.4a

In Vitro

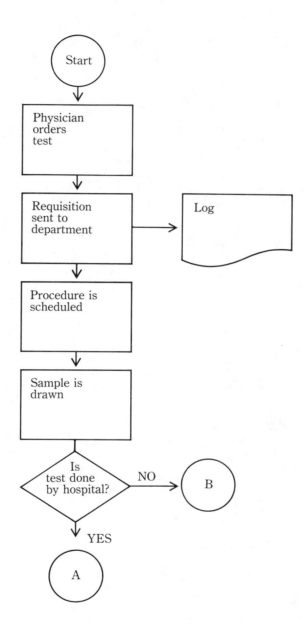

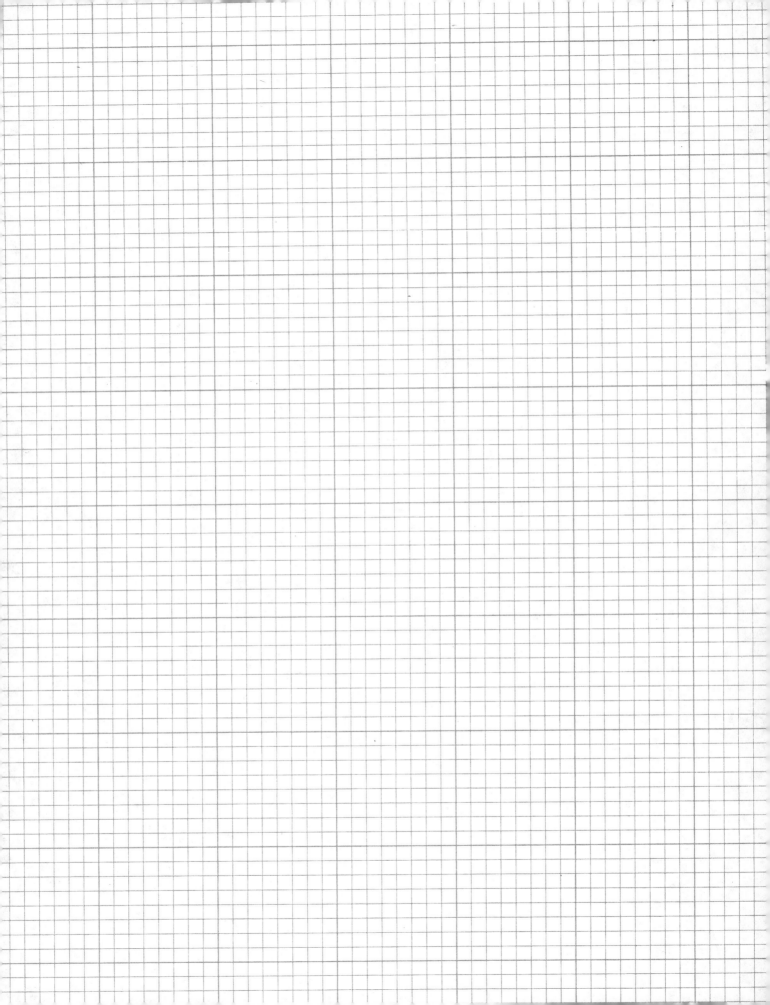

In Vitro, continued

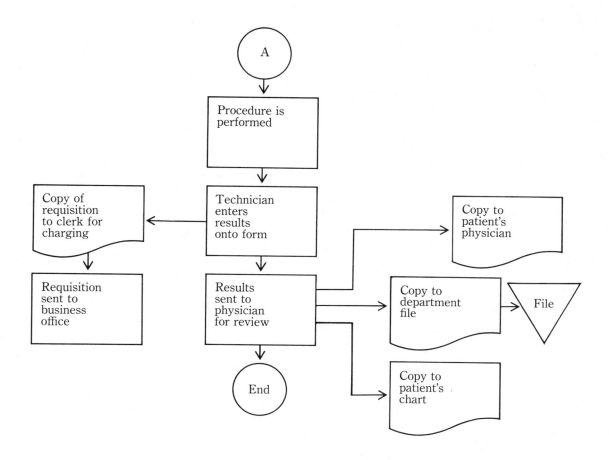

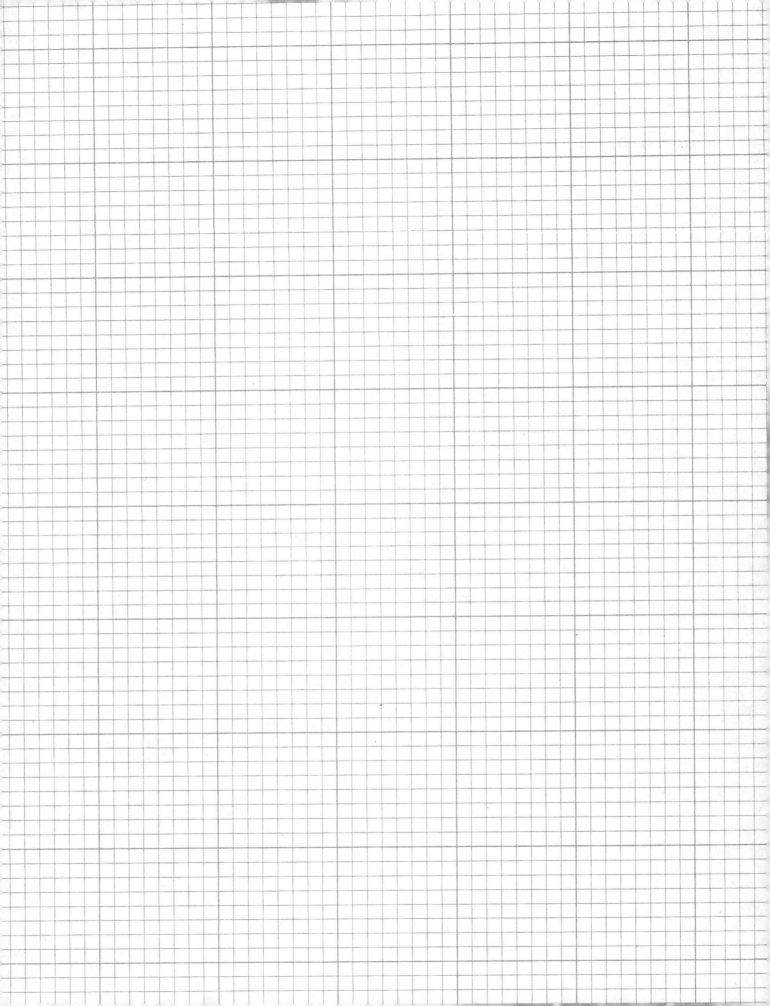

In Vitro, continued

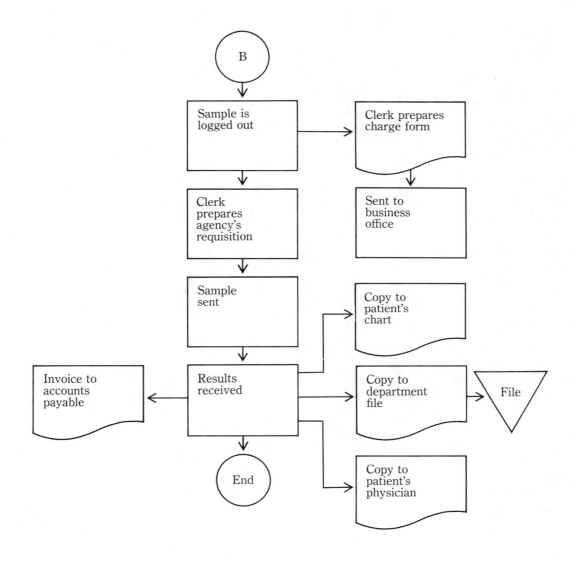

Flow Chart 3.1.4b

In Vivo

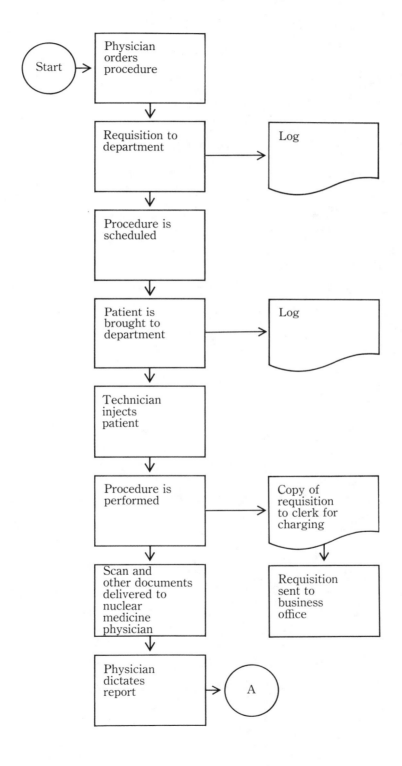

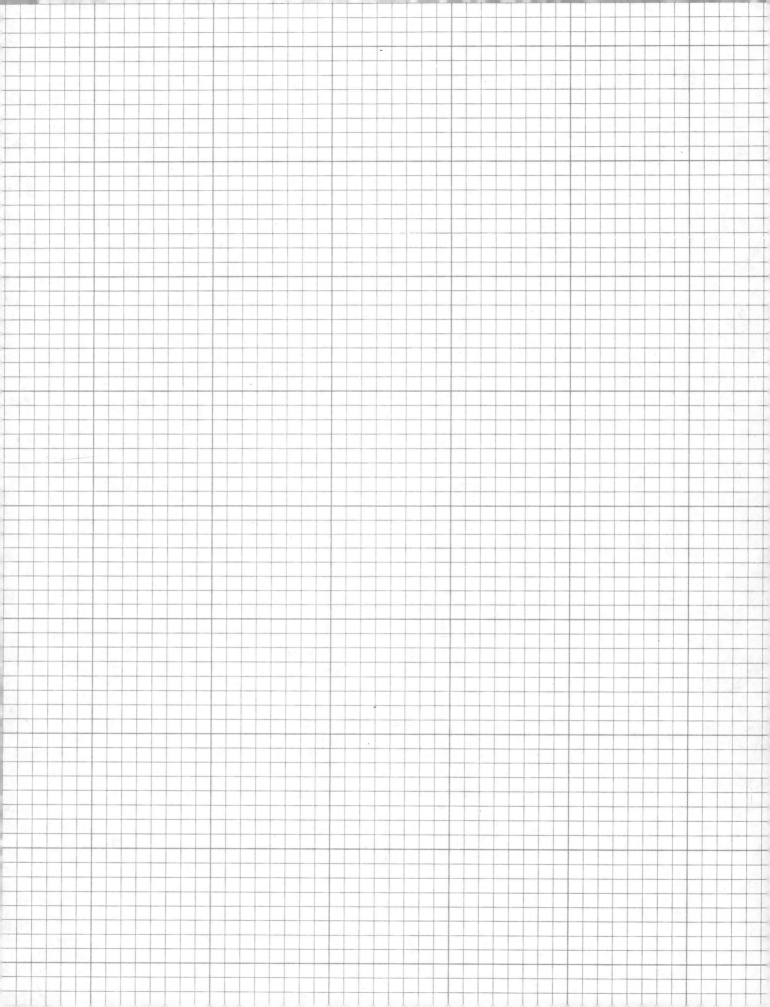

In Vivo, continued

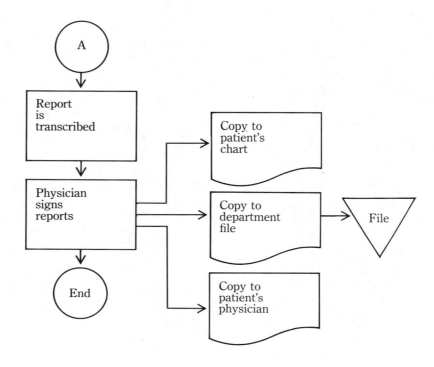

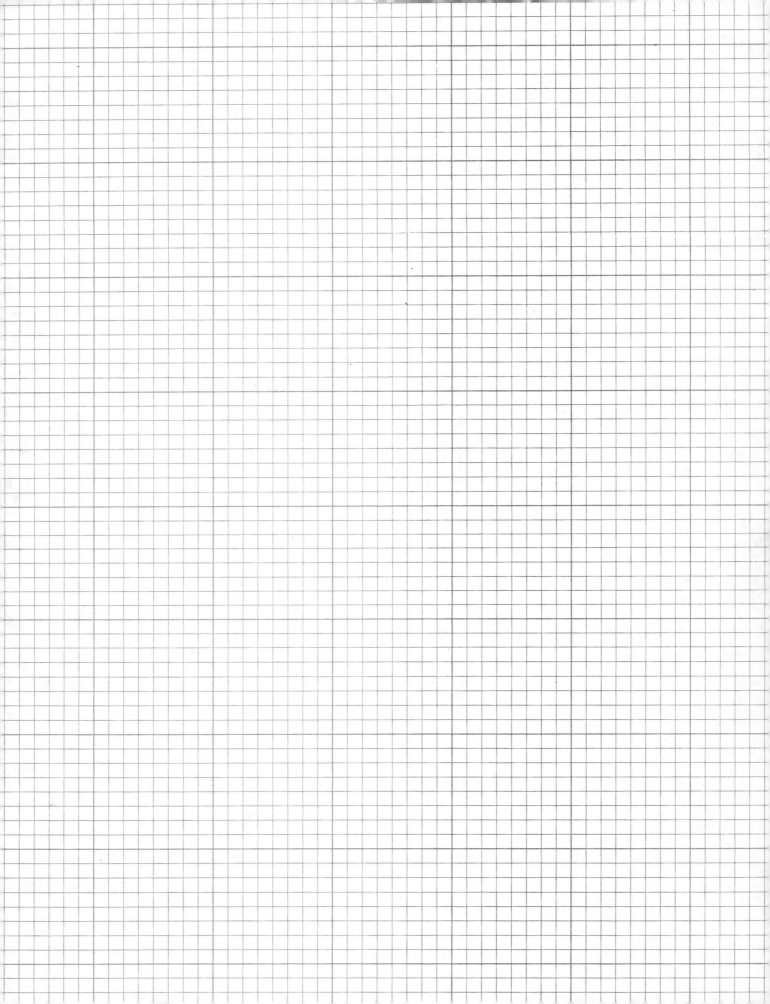

Input Inventory 3.1.4

A. Nuclear Medicine Supervisor

your document title
↓

		A	B	C	
1.	Requisition (in vitro).	☐	☐	☐	_____
2.	Outside agency requisition.	☐	☐	☐	_____
3.	Clinical-information form.	☐	☐	☐	_____
4.	Scheduling form.	☐	☐	☐	_____
5.	Requisition (in vivo).	☐	☐	☐	_____

USE INPUT DOCUMENT ANALYSIS FORM

A = same document title   B = minor variations   C = significant differences

Master File Inventory 3.1.4

A. Nuclear Medicine Supervisor

Notes
↓

		A	B	C	
1.	Patient file.	☐	☐	☐	_____
2.	Tape log.	☐	☐	☐	_____
3.	Patient log.	☐	☐	☐	_____
4.	Outside agency log.	☐	☐	☐	_____
5.	Suspense file for dictation.	☐	☐	☐	_____
6.	Assay sheet.	☐	☐	☐	_____

USE MASTER FILE ANALYSIS FORM

A = essentially similar   B = minor variations   C = significant differences

Report Inventory 3.1.4

A. Nuclear Medicine Supervisor

your document title
↓

		A	B	C	
1.	Monthly activity report.	☐	☐	☐	_____
2.	In vitro report.	☐	☐	☐	_____
3.	In vivo report.	☐	☐	☐	_____
4.	Schedule.	☐	☐	☐	_____

5. Reports to federal agencies regarding the use of radioactive material.

A B C

☐ ☐ ☐

your document title ↓

_____

6. Assay sheet file.

☐ ☐ ☐

_____

USE REPORT ANALYSIS FORM

A = essentially similar   B = minor variations   C = significant differences

System Performance Standards 3.1.4

	Units	A	B
1. Once a procedure is ordered, how much time elapses before a report is in the patient's record?	hours_____	☐	☐
2. Once a procedure is ordered, how much time elapses before the procedure is complete?	hours_____	☐	☐
3. When a patient is brought to the department, how long is the waiting time until the procedure is done?	mean time in minutes_____	☐	☐
4. What is the utilization of the cameras?	mean number of minutes cameras are in use daily divided by the product of 1,440 minutes and the total number of cameras in the department _____	☐	☐
5. How long does it take to find a report of a past patient?	minutes_____	☐	☐
6. How many times are procedures ordered but not carried out?	number of times per week____	☐	☐
7. How much work is done by outside agencies?	number of tests per month performed by outside agencies divided by total number of in vitro procedures _____	☐	☐
8. Are the requisition and the results form the same document?	yes or no _____	☐	☐
9. Once a requisition reaches the department, how much time elapses before the Business Office receives a copy?	hours_____	☐	☐
10. Are charge tickets for outside-agency procedures sent to the Business Office at the time the samples are sent out?	yes or no _____	☐	☐

USE PERFORMANCE STANDARDS ANALYSIS FORM

A = we have a standard   B = we do not have a standard

System Cost Factors 3.1.4

1. How much time do technicians spend calculating results? $ _____

2. How many clerical staffers does the department have? $ _____

3. Are all government-mandated inspection and inventory forms up-to-date? $ _____

USE SYSTEM COST ANALYSIS FORM *(also see Instructions, p. 15)*

System 3.1.5:
Respiratory Services
Description 3.1.5

The department engages in a variety of activities which, clinically, can be divided into three areas — overseeing the use of breathing-assist equipment, such as ventilators and oxygen tents; administering therapeutic treatments that involve inhaling medicated or pressurized gases; and performing diagnostic tests on respiratory systems.

A B C
☐ ☐ ☐ _____

Equipment Distribution

The request for a ventilator or other piece of equipment begins with a physician's order. The Nursing Station completes a requisition and sends it to the department.

☐ ☐ ☐ _____

Respiratory Therapy maintains a usage card for each piece of breathing-assist equipment it is responsible for setting up. The card typically contains the name of the item, its serial number, and its date of purchase. In addition, it has columns for recording the date the equipment was dispatched, the name of the patient using the equipment, the patient's room and bed number, and the date the equipment was returned to the department. These cards are kept in alphabetical order in an equipment-ready file.

☐ ☐ ☐ _____

When the requisition arrives, a departmental clerk removes a card for the type of equipment requested from the ready file and records the patient's name and the other necessary information. A technician is then dispatched to set up the equipment. A nurse normally records on the patient's chart the time the equipment was set up.

☐ ☐ ☐ _____

The Respiratory Therapy Clerk attaches the requisition to the equipment card and places the card in the equipment-in-use file, which is arranged by Nursing Station.

☐ ☐ ☐ _____

In most hospitals, patients are charged a per-day fee for the use of this equipment. A clerk reviews the equipment-in-use file daily and prepares a charge form for each piece of equipment in use. The charge form is sent to the Business Office.

☐ ☐ ☐ _____

A = essentially similar   B = minor variations   C = significant differences

On a periodic basis, a technician goes to the patient's room to make sure that the equipment is working properly.

A B C
□ □ □ _____

When the equipment is no longer needed, the patient's physician orders its removal. The Nursing Station notifies the department of the order by telephone, and a technician is dispatched to disconnect the equipment. Nursing charts the removal, and the technician returns the equipment to the department. The technician writes the date on the equipment card, then returns the card to the equipment-ready file.

□ □ □ _____

Treatment Administration

The patient's physician orders a treatment regimen, telling what procedures to perform, how often they should be performed each day, and if possible, when they should be stopped. Typically, the regimen is arranged after consultation with physicians and senior technicians in the department.

□ □ □ _____

The Nursing Station sends a requisition to the department. A clerk prepares a treatment record for the patient. This is normally a single card, containing the patient's name, patient number, and room and bed number; the type of treatment to be administered; its frequency; and, if known, the date treatment is to be stopped. The rest of the card is used to log the administration of treatments.

□ □ □ _____

The card is sent to a supervisor, who places it in a treatment file, which is arranged according to Nursing Station. The cards are removed or relocated as discharge and transfer information is received.

□ □ □ _____

The supervisor prepares a daily work schedule for the department's technicians. Working from the treatment record file, the supervisor assigns each technician to a Nursing Station or group of stations. The technicians each have responsibility for administering all treatments of a particular type to assigned patients in their areas.

□ □ □ _____

There are two common approaches for recording the actual administration. The technician may take the treatment records and record the treatment directly on the card. The technician then replaces the cards in the file on return to the department.

□ □ □ _____

With the other approach, the supervisor gives each technician a worklist. After performing each treatment, the technician initials the work-

---

A = essentially similar   B = minor variations   C = significant differences

list on the appropriate line and enters the time. This document is then returned to a clerk, who transfers the information onto the treatment records.

A B C

☐ ☐ ☐   _____

Regardless of the approach, the technician will record each treatment in the patient's medical record.

☐ ☐ ☐   _____

A clerk reviews the treatment records daily and prepares a charge ticket for each patient in the file. These are sent to the Business Office.

☐ ☐ ☐   _____

When the regimen is complete, a final charge ticket is sent to the Business Office. A clerk removes the patient's treatment record from the file and places it in alphabetical order in a past-treatment file.

☐ ☐ ☐   _____

Diagnostic Procedures

The diagnostic procedures performed by the department are often referred to as Pulmonary Function Testing.

☐ ☐ ☐   _____

The patient's physician orders a particular test. The Nursing Station completes a requisition and sends it to the department, along with a form containing clinical information (admitting diagnosis, reason for the test, etc.)

☐ ☐ ☐   _____

A clerk logs the requisition and schedules the procedure. The Nursing Station and Transportation are notified of the date and time.

☐ ☐ ☐   _____

As tests are scheduled, a clerk logs each patient's scheduled procedure. From this, the clerk prepares a Master Schedule.

☐ ☐ ☐   _____

On the scheduled day, the patient is brought to the department and logged in. The patient is then taken to the procedure room, along with the requisition and the clinical form. The procedure is performed, and the patient, after being logged out, is returned to his or her room.

☐ ☐ ☐   _____

A technician reviews the requisition and sends one copy to a clerk, who enters the appropriate charges and sends it to the Business Office. The remaining copy of the requisition, along with the clinical-information form and any quantitative results produced by the test, is given to the Respiratory Therapy physician, who reviews the material and dictates a report. The material goes to a suspense file, while the tape containing the dictation goes to a transcriber.

☐ ☐ ☐   _____

A = essentially similar   B = minor variations   C = significant differences

When the typed report is returned, it is matched with the material in the suspense file and given to the physician, who reviews the package and signs the report. One copy is sent to the patient's medical record; another copy, along with the remaining documents, is placed in alphabetical order in a results file. The remaining copies are sent to the patient's physicians.

A B C
☐ ☐ ☐ _____

Technicians for ED patients and Outpatient Respiratory Therapy provide treatments to patients in the ED. In arrest situations, for instance, they clear the patient's airway and take other appropriate steps to maintain the respiratory cycle.

☐ ☐ ☐ _____

Treatments are also rendered to outpatients. This is normally done on a recurring basis. In addition, diagnostic tests are administered to outpatients. (Charging follows the flow detailed in the outpatient system.)

☐ ☐ ☐ _____

Blood Gas

This test involves drawing a blood sample and measuring the quantity of oxygen and other gases it contains. In some hospitals, Respiratory Therapy performs this test. In others, the responsibility belongs to the Laboratory. In still others, the Laboratory draws the blood and delivers it to Respiratory Therapy for analysis.

☐ ☐ ☐ _____

Regardless of how responsibility is distributed, the flow remains about the same. The patient's physician orders the tests. The Nursing Station telephones the department responsible for drawing the blood and notifies the department of the requisition. The nurse then prepares a requisition and holds it until a phlebotomist arrives.

☐ ☐ ☐ _____

The phlebotomist draws the sample and, typically, enters the patient's name, patient number, and room and bed number, and the date and time on a label, which is attached to the sample vial. The phlebotomist then picks up the requisition and takes it with the sample to the department where the test is to be performed. The test is run, and results are entered onto the requisition.

☐ ☐ ☐ _____

The technician notifies the Nursing Station of the results and sorts the copies of the requisition. One copy goes to the patient's medical record; another goes to a clerk, who enters the charges and sends the form on to the Business Office; and the third copy is filed in alphabetical order in a blood-gas results file.

☐ ☐ ☐ _____

A = essentially similar   B = minor variations   C = significant differences

Flow Chart 3.1.5a

Equipment

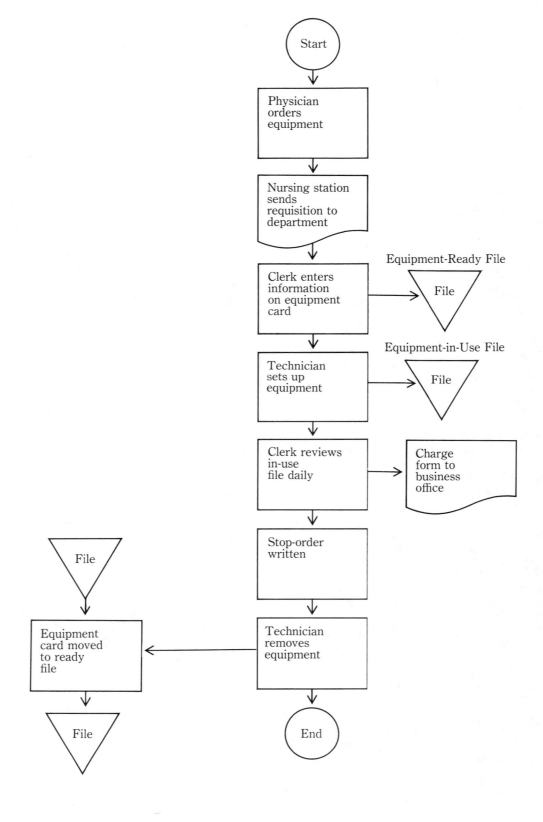

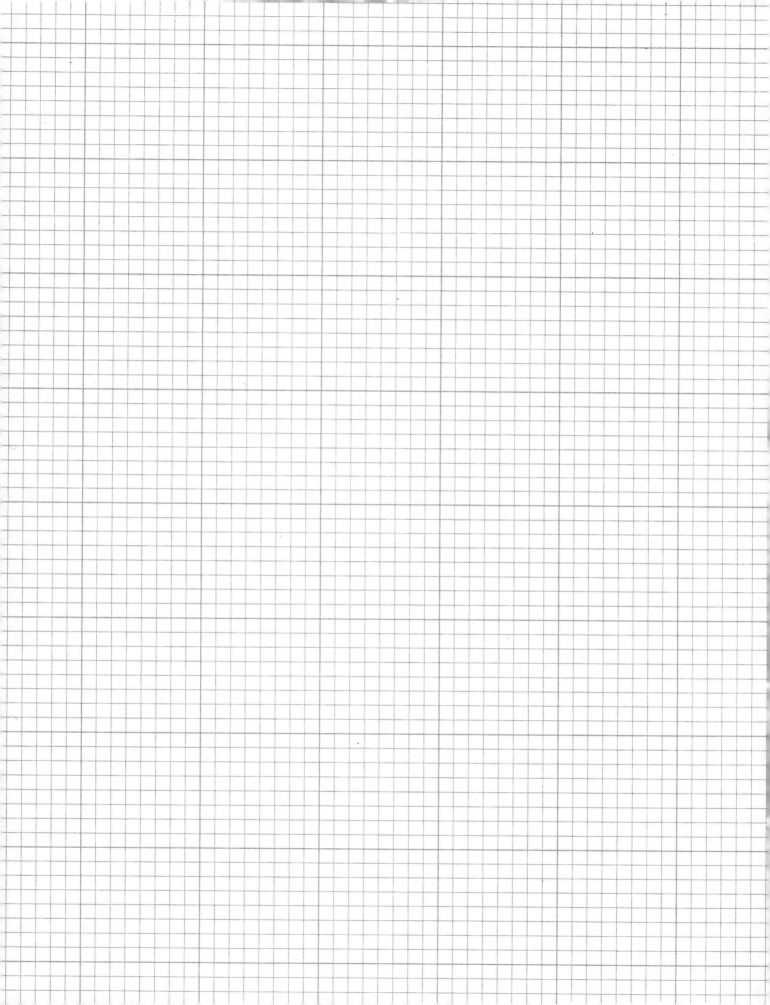

Flow Chart 3.1.5b

Treatment

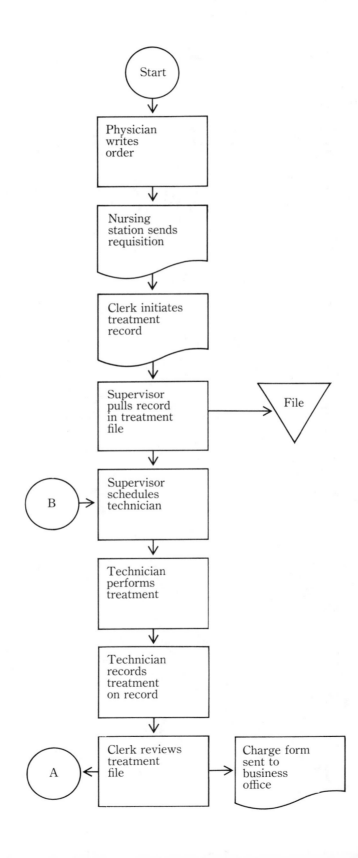

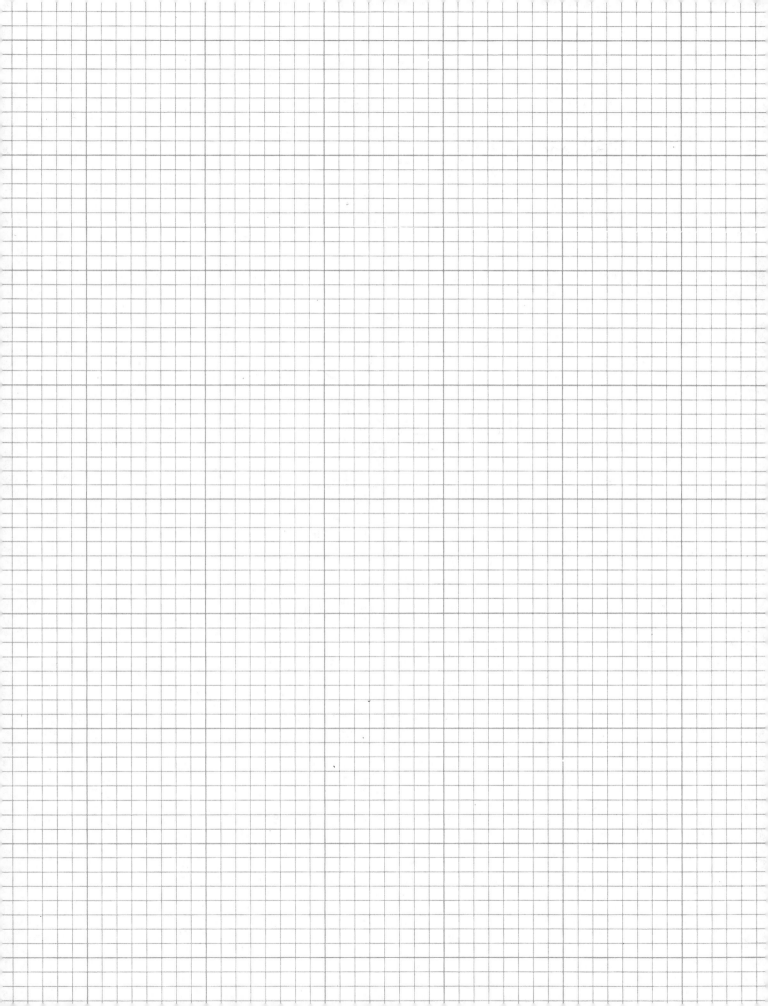

Treatment, continued

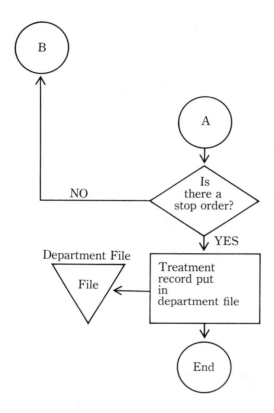

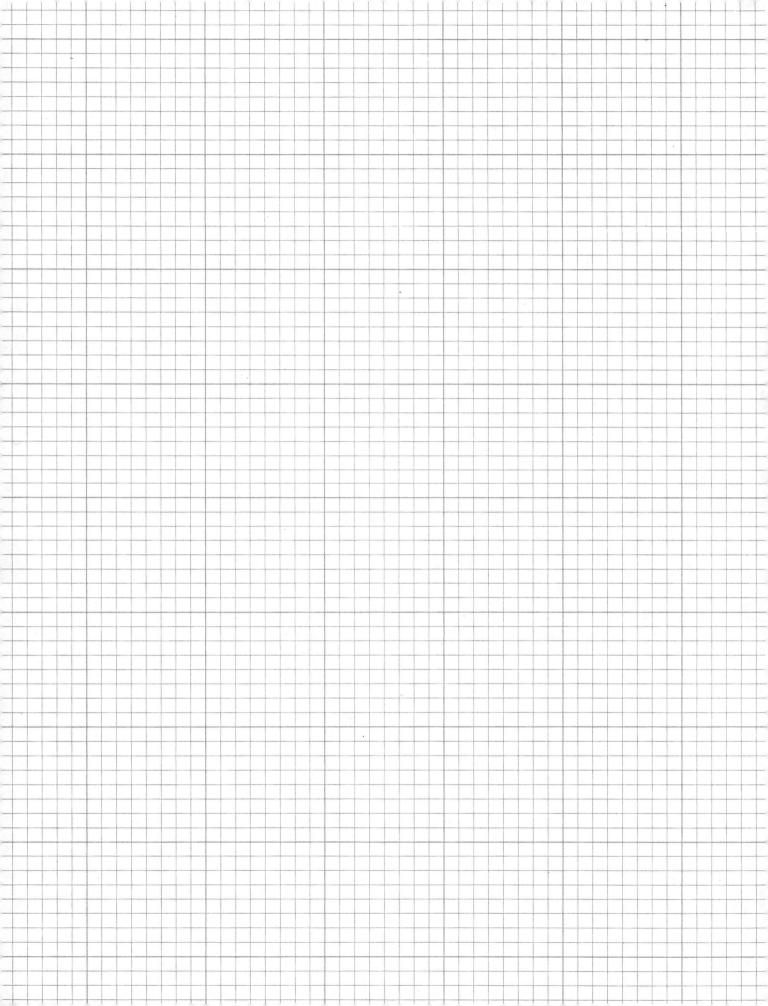

Flow Chart 3.1.5c

Diagnostic Procedures

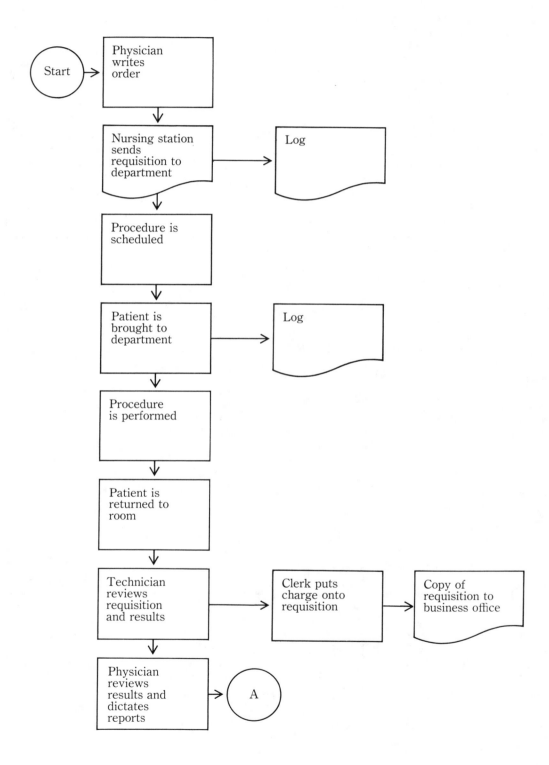

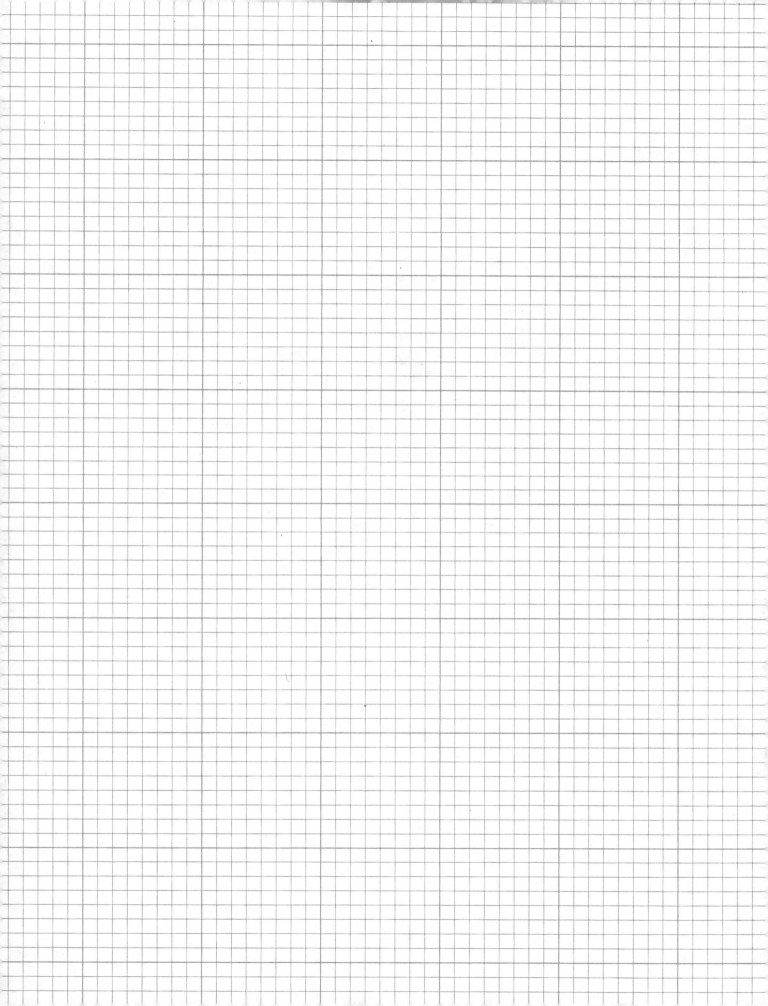

Diagnostic Procedures, continued

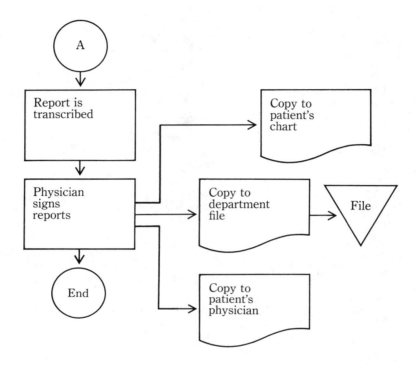

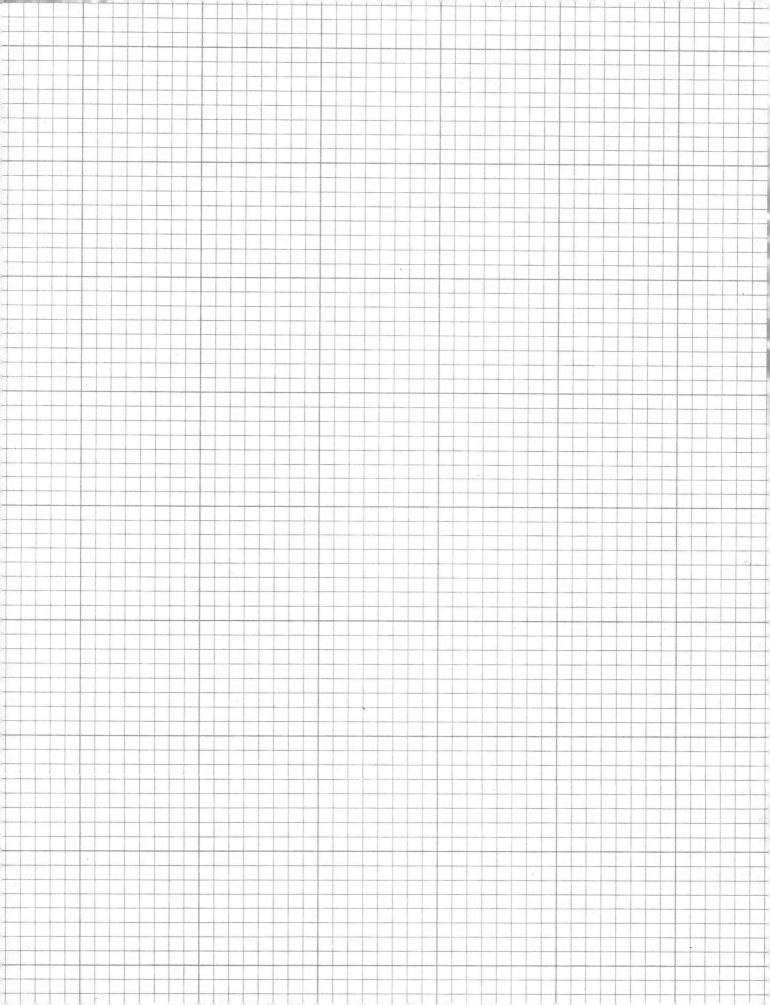

Flow Chart 3.1.5d

Blood Gas

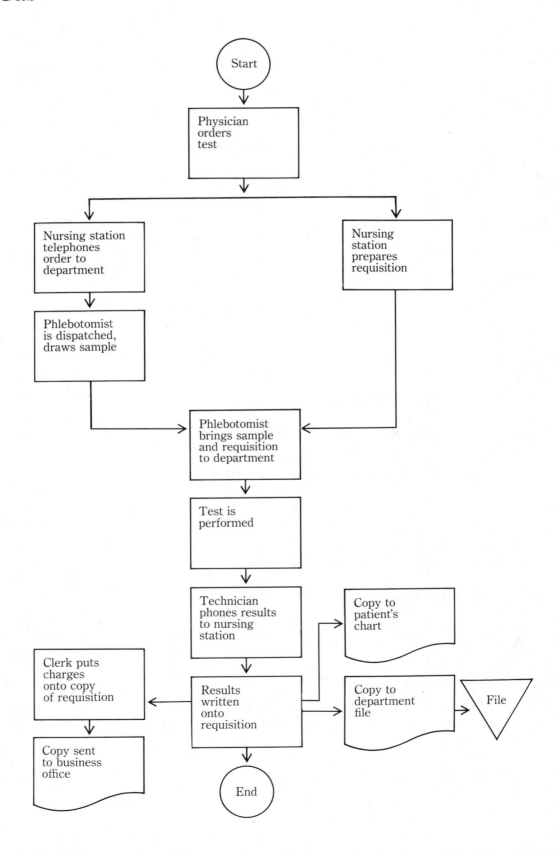

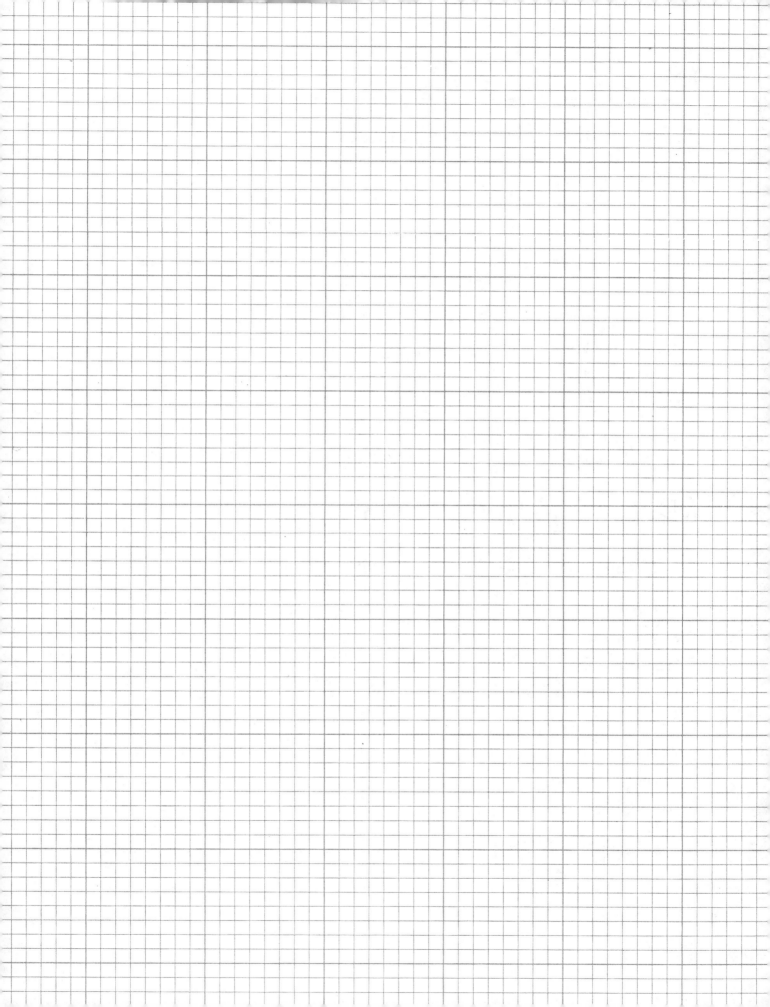

Input Inventory 3.1.5

A. Respiratory Therapy Supervisor

your document title
↓

		A	B	C	
1.	Equipment requisition.	☐	☐	☐	_____
2.	Equipment usage card.	☐	☐	☐	_____
3.	Equipment charge form.	☐	☐	☐	_____
4.	Treatment requisition.	☐	☐	☐	_____
5.	Treatment record card.	☐	☐	☐	_____
6.	Treatment charge form.	☐	☐	☐	_____
7.	Requisition for diagnostic procedure.	☐	☐	☐	_____
8.	Clinical-information form.	☐	☐	☐	_____
9.	Blood-gas requisition.	☐	☐	☐	_____

USE INPUT DOCUMENT ANALYSIS FORM

A = same document title   B = minor variations   C = significant differences

Master File Inventory 3.1.5

A. Respiratory Therapy Supervisor

Notes
↓

		A	B	C	
1.	Equipment-ready file.	☐	☐	☐	_____
2.	Equipment-in-use file.	☐	☐	☐	_____
3.	Treatment-record file (current).	☐	☐	☐	_____
4.	Treatment-record file (past).	☐	☐	☐	_____
5.	Census.	☐	☐	☐	_____
6.	Diagnostic reports.	☐	☐	☐	_____
7.	Blood-gas requisitions.	☐	☐	☐	_____
8.	Patient log.	☐	☐	☐	_____

USE MASTER FILE ANALYSIS FORM

A = essentially similar   B = minor variations   C = significant differences

Report Inventory 3.1.5

A. Respiratory Therapy Supervisor

your document title ↓

		A	B	C	
1.	Monthly activity report.	☐	☐	☐	_____
2.	Results of diagnostic work.	☐	☐	☐	_____

USE REPORT ANALYSIS FORM

A = essentially similar   B = minor variations   C = significant differences

System Performance Standards 3.1.5

Units

			A	B
1.	From the time the Nursing Station requisitions equipment, how long does it take to have the equipment set up?	minutes_____	☐	☐
2.	What is the accuracy of the equipment-in-use file?	number of errors (missing, inaccurate or misplaced cards) divided by total number of cards in the file _____	☐	☐
3.	How often is equipment brought to a room after a patient has been transferred?	number of times per month _____	☐	☐
4.	How many ordered treatments are not performed?	mean number per week _____	☐	☐
5.	What is the ratio of technicians to treatments given daily?	daily number of treatments per technician _____	☐	☐
6.	From the time the Nursing Station prepares a requisition, how long does it take for a diagnostic procedure to be performed?	hours_____	☐	☐
7.	How long do patients wait in the department for diagnostic procedures?	minutes_____	☐	☐
8.	From the time a blood-gas order is telephoned to the department, how long does it take to get a result to the Nursing Station?	minutes_____	☐	☐
9.	How many results files does the department maintain?	number_____	☐	☐

USE PERFORMANCE STANDARDS ANALYSIS FORM

A = we have a standard   B = we do not have a standard

System Cost Factors 3.1.5

1. How does the department charge for medications used in treating patients? $ _____

2. Can the supervisor pinpoint the location of each technician at any given time (via sign-in sheets or other reporting mechanisms)? $ _____

3. How many clerical staffers work in the department? $ _____

USE SYSTEM COST ANALYSIS FORM *(also see Instructions, p. 15)*

System 3.1.6:
EKG/EEG Services

Description 3.1.6

Hospitals administer EKGs in two ways – the patient is brought to the department for the procedure or arrives as an outpatient; or an EKG technician is dispatched to the patient. In either case, the information flow is the same.

A B C
□ □ □

The Flow

A requisition for an EKG is sent to the department following a physician's order. This requisition contains the patient's name, room and bed number, the name of the test, and the physician's name. The requisition also details clinical information needed to evaluate the EKG trace. In some situations, a separate form is used to supply this information. Typically this form consists of a short clinical history of the patient, admitting diagnosis, and a listing of current medications.

□ □ □

An EKG clerk logs the requisition into the department, recording the patient's name, the test requested, the date, the room and bed number, and the time the requisition was received.

□ □ □

The clerk then records the charge for the procedure on the requisition and sends one copy to the Business Office.

□ □ □

If the patient is expected to come to the department, the clerk calls the Nursing Station and schedules the procedure.

□ □ □

If the procedure is to be performed in the patient's room, the clerk prepares a dispatch ticket and gives it to an EKG technician.

□ □ □

The technician goes to the patient with an EKG machine, connects the machine to the patient, and records an EKG strip. The technician immediately writes the patient's name, the date and time, and his or her initials on the strip.

□ □ □

The technician then brings the strip back to the department, where it is cut into segments and mounted on a specially designed form. The strip then goes to an EKG clerk, who attaches the

---

A = essentially similar   B = minor variations   C = significant differences

221

remaining copy of the requisition to the mounting form and sends the material to a cardiologist.

A B C
☐ ☐ ☐ _____

The cardiologist interprets the strip and dictates a report.

☐ ☐ ☐ _____

The requisition and strip are returned to an EKG clerk, while the dictation is sent to a transcriber. When the transcribed report is returned, the cardiologist signs it and gives it to the clerk.

☐ ☐ ☐ _____

One copy of the report is attached to the strip and requisition and filed in one of three ways — alphabetically, by the patient's EKG number, or by the patient's hospital record number.

☐ ☐ ☐ _____

Another copy of the report, along with a copy of the EKG strip, is taken to the Nursing Station and placed on the patient's chart. The remaining copies are mailed to the patient's physicians.

☐ ☐ ☐ _____

EEG

The flow of information and paperwork for an EEG is identical to that used for an EKG.

☐ ☐ ☐ _____

In most hospitals, the same department handles both EKGs and EEGs. Normally, a specially trained technician's sole responsibility is to operate the EEG equipment.

☐ ☐ ☐ _____

Flow Chart 3.1.6

EKG

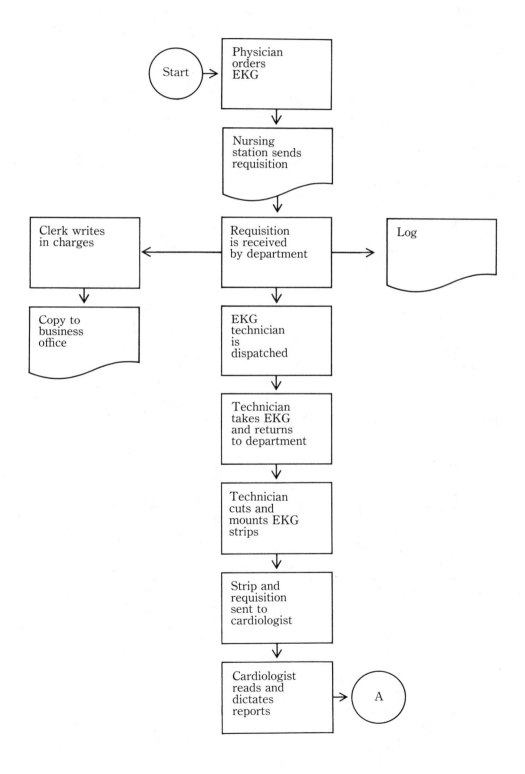

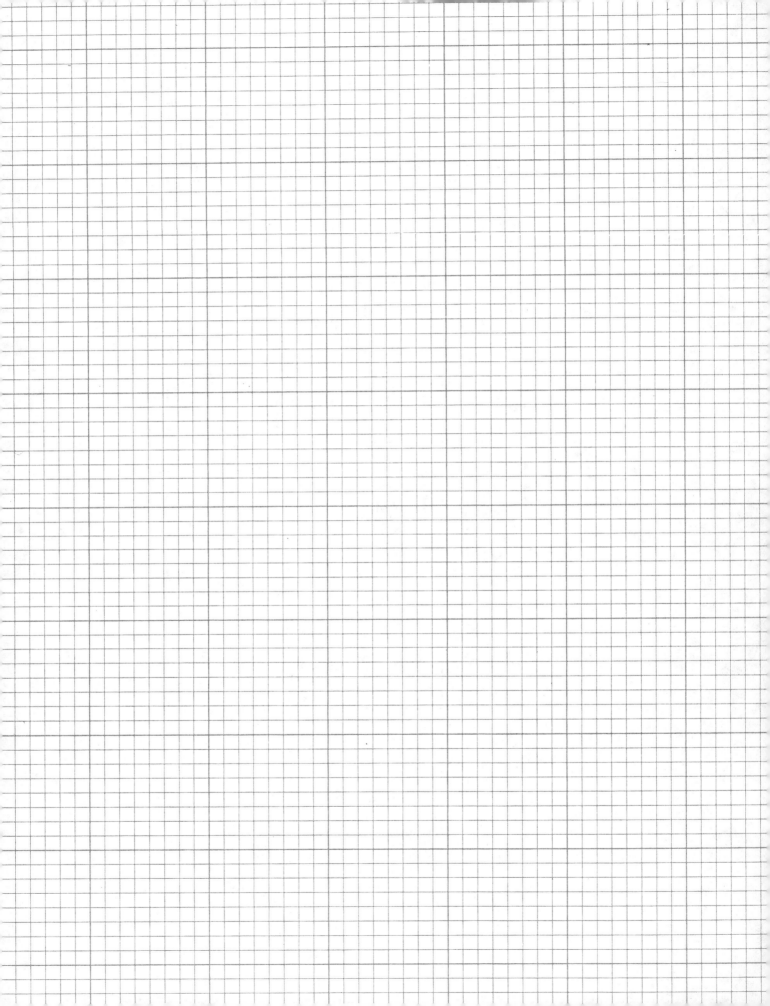

EKG, continued

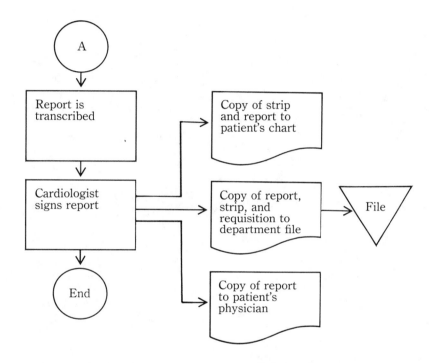

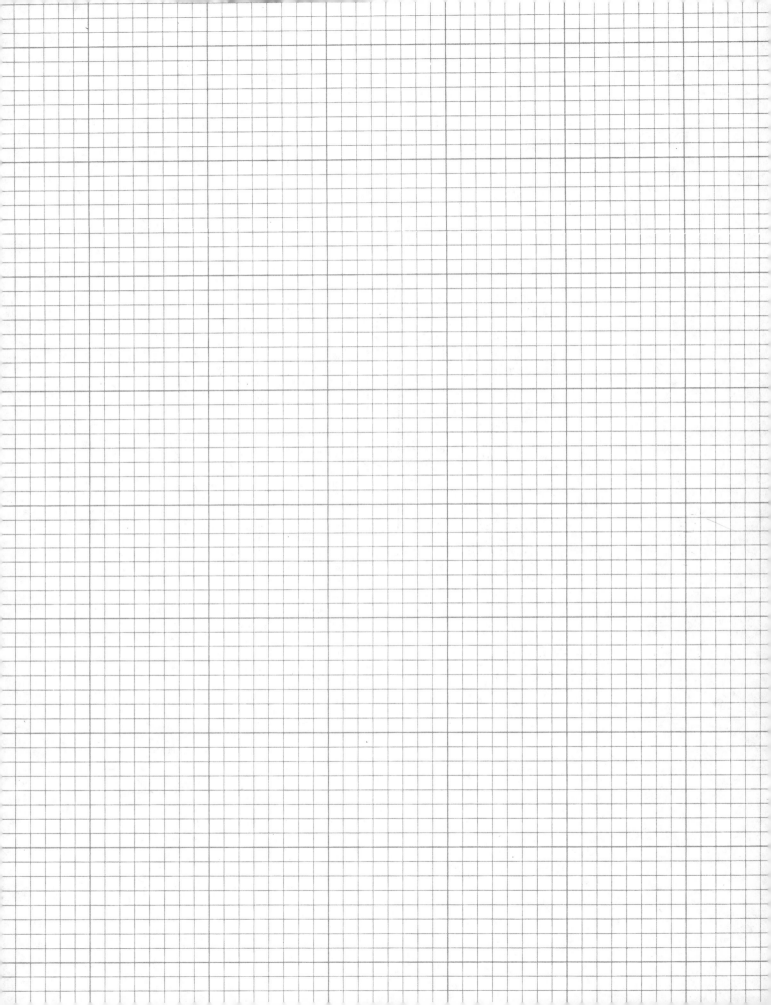

Input Inventory 3.1.6

A. EKG Supervisor

your document title
↓

    A B C

1. Requisition.   ☐ ☐ ☐   _____

2. Clinical information form.   ☐ ☐ ☐   _____

3. Mounting form.   ☐ ☐ ☐   _____

4. Dispatch ticket.   ☐ ☐ ☐   _____

USE INPUT DOCUMENT ANALYSIS FORM

A = same document title	B = minor variations	C = significant differences

Master File Inventory 3.1.6

A. EKG Supervisor

Notes
↓

    A B C

1. EGK Log.   ☐ ☐ ☐   _____

2. Patient file.   ☐ ☐ ☐   _____

3. Department schedule.   ☐ ☐ ☐   _____

USE MASTER FILE ANALYSIS FORM

A = essentially similar	B = minor variations	C = significant differences

Report Inventory 3.1.6

A. EKG Supervisor

your document title
↓

    A B C

1. EKG Report.   ☐ ☐ ☐   _____

2. Productivity report.   ☐ ☐ ☐   _____

USE REPORT ANALYSIS FORM

A = essentially similar	B = minor variations	C = significant differences

System Performance Standards 3.1.6

		Units	A	B
1.	From the time a requisition is received, how long does it take for a technician to reach the patient?	minutes_____	☐	☐
2.	How many times must a technician be sent back to the patient because the EKG is unreadable?	number of times per week____	☐	☐
3.	From the time a strip is brought to the department, how long does it take to get a report onto the patient's chart?	hours_____	☐	☐
4.	How long do patients wait in the department before procedures are run?	minutes_____	☐	☐

USE PERFORMANCE STANDARDS ANALYSIS FORM

A = we have a standard   B = we do not have a standard

System Cost Factors 3.1.6

1. What is the cost of duplicating EKGs for the department's file? $ _____

2. How many clerical staffers does the department employ? $ _____

3. How much of the technician's time is spent in clerical duties? $ _____

USE SYSTEM COST ANALYSIS FORM *(also see Instructions, p. 15)*

System 3.2:
Rehabilitation Services
Description 3.2

The department has two major activities. It renders therapy as part of a physical rehabilitation program, and it performs electromyographs (EMGs), a diagnostic procedure in which electrical signals from muscles are measured and analyzed.

A B C
☐ ☐ ☐ _____

Therapy

The flow begins when the patient's physician writes an order for physical therapy. The Nursing Station prepares a requisition and sends it to the department.

☐ ☐ ☐ _____

Normally, the physician either consults with the department before writing the order or is contacted by the department once the order is received. The purpose of this interaction is to establish a treatment program for the patient.

☐ ☐ ☐ _____

After this program has been developed, it is written onto a treatment record, which is placed in the patient's departmental file along with the requisition. A supervisor also establishes a time file to ensure that prescribed treatments are carried out on the proper days. The card file contains one card for each patient undergoing treatment. Each card contains a patient's name, patient number, room and bed number, and a brief description of the therapy program. The cards are filed chronologically by the next service date.

☐ ☐ ☐ _____

In the evening, a supervisor removes all cards for the following day. The supervisor prepares a schedule and notifies the Nursing Stations and Transportation. A clerk, working from the schedule, pulls the files of all patients who are listed.

☐ ☐ ☐ _____

On the scheduled day, the patient is brought to the department. A therapist renders the appropriate service, records it both on the patient's treatment records and in the progress notes, returns the record to the patient's file, and gives the file to a clerk.

☐ ☐ ☐ _____

A = essentially similar   B = minor variations   C = significant differences

The patient is then returned to the Nursing Station, where a nurse records in the patient's record the fact that physical therapy was received.

A B C
□ □ □ _____

The clerk who receives the file prepares a charge ticket and sends it to the Business Office. The clerk then replaces the file and refiles the treatment card in a slot corresponding to the next therapy due date.

□ □ □ _____

There is no standard reporting mechanism. The department maintains close but informal contact with the patient's physician. The Department Head may establish a policy requiring that written reports be sent to the physicians of patients being treated. If this is the case, copies of those reports go into the departmental files.

□ □ □ _____

When a stop order is received from a patient's physician, the order is placed in the patient's file, and the patient's card is removed from its file and destroyed.

□ □ □ _____

Referred Outpatients

Normally, physical therapy begins when a patient is in the hospital and continues after discharge. The same treatment record, patient card and charging system are maintained, with the Business Office required to render an out-patient bill as opposed to entering the charge onto an inpatient account.

□ □ □ _____

EMGs

The patient's physician orders an EMG. The Nursing Station sends a requisition along with a clinical-information form to the department. A clerk logs in the requisition, schedules the service, and notifies the Nursing Station and Transportation.

□ □ □ _____

On the day before the service is to be rendered, the patient's name is placed on the schedule for the following day.

□ □ □ _____

On the day of treatment, the patient is brought to the department. The patient and the requisition are taken to the treatment area where a Physical Medicine physician administers the test. The Physical Medicine physician records the quantitative results as they are generated.

□ □ □ _____

After the test has been completed, the patient is taken back to the Nursing Station. A copy of the requisition is sent to a clerk, who enters the appropriate charges and forwards the form to the Business Office.

A B C
☐ ☐ ☐

The physician dictates a report. This tape, along with the remaining copies of the requisition, the clinical-information form, and the quantitative results, is sent to a transcriber. When the written report, including the quantitative results, is returned to the department, the physician reviews and signs it. One copy is placed in the patient's medical record. Another, along with the requisition and the clinical-information form, is placed in the patient's departmental file. The remaining copies are sent to the patient's attending and consulting physicians.

☐ ☐ ☐

Other Programs

In many hospitals the rehabilitation aspect of physical medicine programs is being expanded. Some institutions have programs for training people to cope with activities of daily living. Others include such specialized programs as speech, occupational, and recreation therapy in their overall rehabilitation program. The ordering, recording, and patient charging actions are the same as those undertaken for physical therapy treatments.

☐ ☐ ☐

It is also becoming common for the department to be involved in treating patients in their homes after discharge.

☐ ☐ ☐

A = essentially similar   B = minor variations   C = significant differences

Flow Chart 3.2a

Therapy

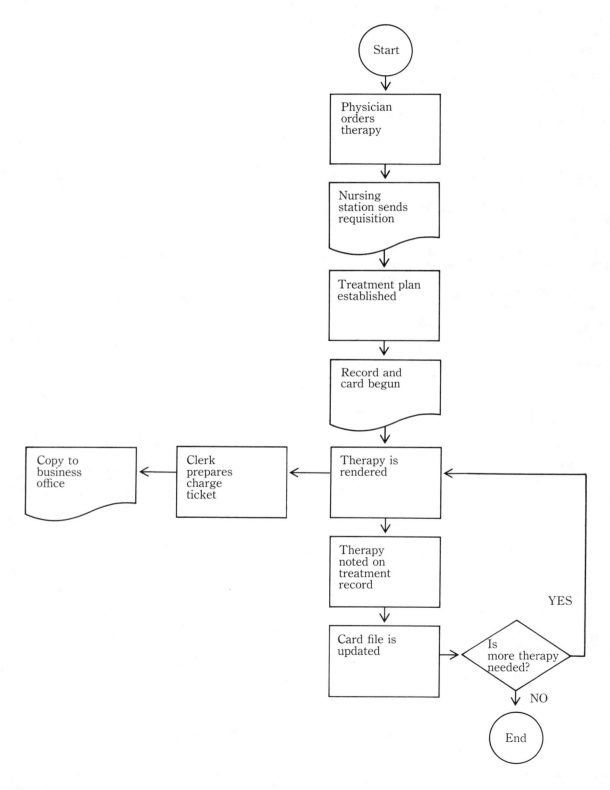

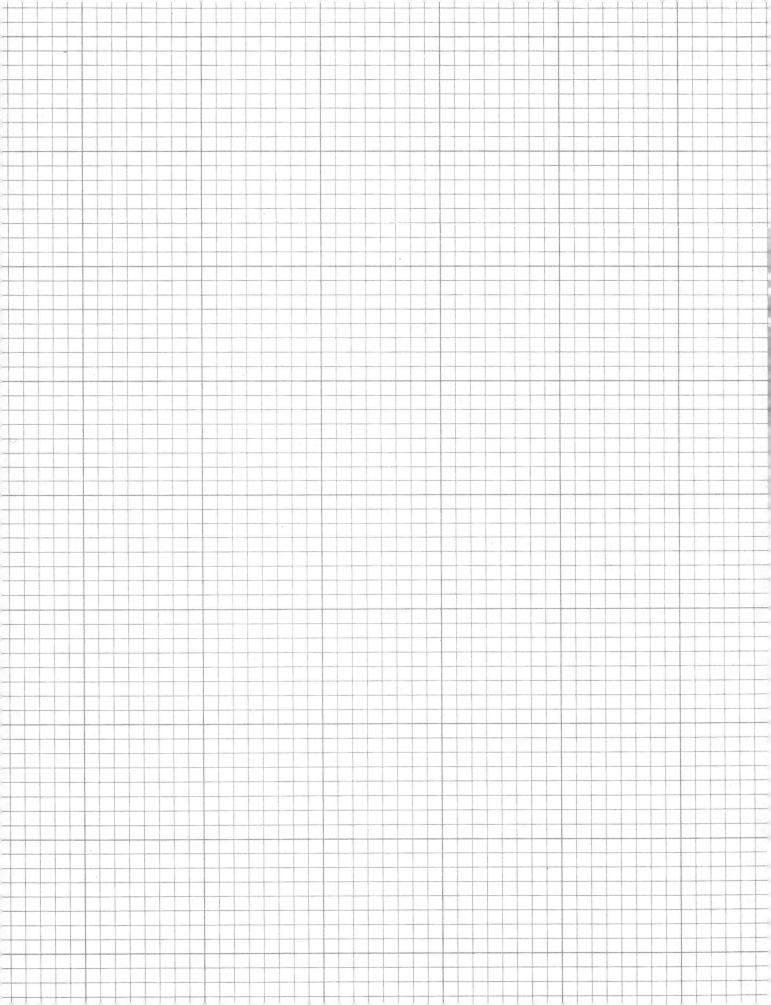

Flow Chart 3.2b

EMG

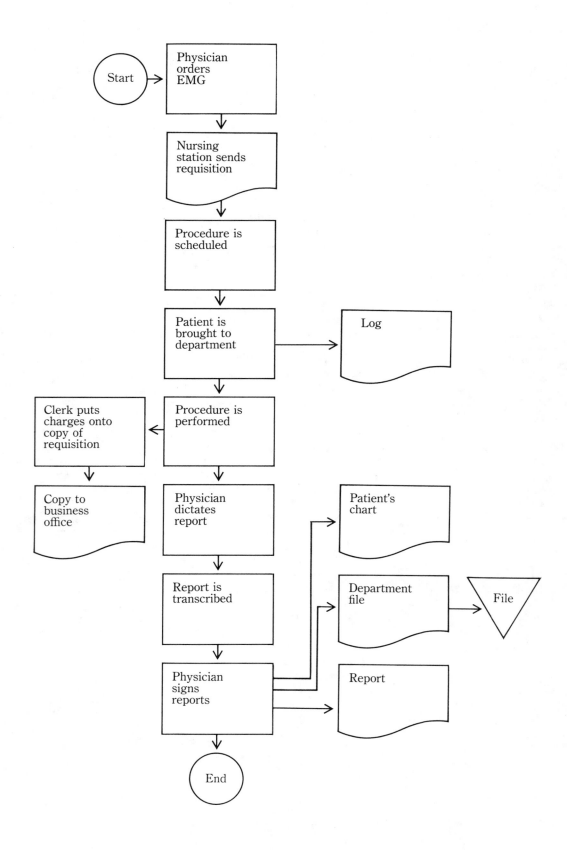

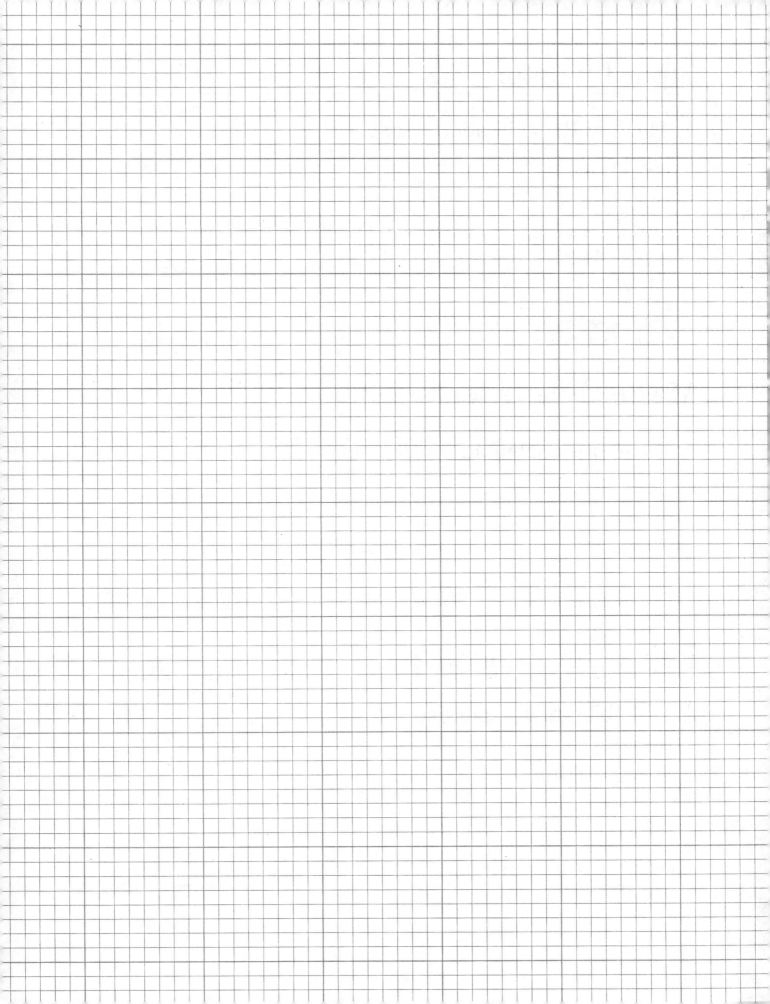

Input Inventory 3.2

A. Head of Rehabilitation Services

your document title ↓

	A B C	
1. Treatment record.	☐ ☐ ☐	_____
2. Patient card.	☐ ☐ ☐	_____
3. Charge ticket.	☐ ☐ ☐	_____
4. Therapy requisition.	☐ ☐ ☐	_____
5. EMG requisition.	☐ ☐ ☐	_____

USE INPUT DOCUMENT ANALYSIS FORM

A = same document title   B = minor variations   C = significant differences

Master File Inventory 3.2

A. Head of Rehabilitation Services

Notes ↓

	A B C	
1. Card file.	☐ ☐ ☐	_____
2. Patient file.	☐ ☐ ☐	_____
3. Patient log.	☐ ☐ ☐	_____

USE MASTER FILE ANALYSIS FORM

A = essentially similar   B = minor variations   C = significant differences

Report Inventory 3.2

A. Rehabilitation Supervisor

your document title ↓

	A B C	
1. Monthly activity report.	☐ ☐ ☐	_____
2. Progress report to physician.	☐ ☐ ☐	_____
3. EMG results.	☐ ☐ ☐	_____
4. Schedule.	☐ ☐ ☐	_____

USE REPORT ANALYSIS FORM

A = essentially similar   B = minor variations   C = significant differences

System Performance Standards 3.2

Units

1. What percentage of patients are seen after they are dismissed?

annual number of patients
seen after dismissal divided
by total number of inpatients   A B
treated _____ ☐ ☐

2. How many patients have a treatment plan?

percentage of total patients
per month who have a
treatment plan _____ ☐ ☐

3. Are visits to Physical Medicine recorded on patient's medical record?

yes or no _____ ☐ ☐

4. How long does it take for a charge ticket to reach the Business Office once an EMG is completed or therapy is rendered?

hours_____ ☐ ☐

5. What is the average waiting time for patients?

minutes_____ ☐ ☐

6. How many patients miss treatments scheduled as a part of their treatment plan?

percent of scheduled
treatments not
performed _____ ☐ ☐

USE PERFORMANCE STANDARDS ANALYSIS FORM

A = we have a standard   B = we do not have a standard

System Cost Factors 3.2

1. Do physical therapists transport patients? $ _____

2. How many clerical staffers does the department have? $ _____

USE SYSTEM COST ANALYSIS FORM *(also see Instructions, p. 15)*

System 3.3:
Surgical Services
Description 3.3

Notes
↓

The flow begins when the physician schedules the patient for surgery. This can take place either before the patient is admitted or after. In the former situation, the patient is admitted specifically for an operation; in the latter, the patient is usually admitted for diagnostic work that is intended to indicate whether surgery is needed.

A B C
☐ ☐ ☐ _____

Locations for performing surgery may be centralized or decentralized. With decentralization, it is common to find separate locations for urology, oral surgery, and caesarian deliveries as well as a general surgical suite. In such cases, the following communication flows are duplicated in their entirety.

☐ ☐ ☐ _____

There are a variety of techniques used for scheduling. Some hospitals use a first-come, first-served approach. Others use block scheduling, with each surgeon allocated a fixed amount of time at specific times and days. Still others have different methods.

☐ ☐ ☐ _____

When the case is scheduled, the Scheduling Clerk in Surgery writes the appropriate information into the scheduling book. Typically, this information includes the patient's name; the surgeon; the patient's physician; the patient's age, sex, room and bed number if known; and the procedure to be performed.

☐ ☐ ☐ _____

Each afternoon, the Scheduling Clerk uses the sheets for the next day to prepare the schedule for that day. A typical schedule shows in chronological order what procedures will be performed on which patient in each operating room. The schedule also shows the surgeon's name and the anesthesiologist's name.

☐ ☐ ☐ _____

After making several copies of the schedule, the clerk distributes them.

☐ ☐ ☐ _____

Aside from its obvious function, the schedule has a variety of other uses. It allows the Surgical Supervisor to assign technicians who will perform surgical preps. It alerts the Nursing Stations, so that nursing personnel can make sure that preoperative orders have been written and are being carried out.

☐ ☐ ☐ _____

A = essentially similar   B = minor variations   C = significant differences

238

It also alerts transporters of the need to pick up certain patients for surgery. And it serves as a guide to the surgical staff in the preparation of the operating suites for the various types of surgery.

A B C
□ □ □ _____

The patient is the focal point of much activity on the day before surgery. A variety of preoperative tests are performed. The anesthesiologist evaluates the patient. And it is the last opportunity for the surgeon to meet with the patient, explain what will be done, and obtain the patient's signature on a consent form.

□ □ □ _____

The Nursing Station also begins a surgical checklist, which will be part of the chart. The list includes all activities that must be accomplished before the surgery can begin. The list varies from hospital to hospital but usually contains such items as:

□ □ □ _____

1. Has the consent form been signed?

□ □ □ _____

2. Is the completed history and physical on the chart?

□ □ □ _____

3. Has the patient had a chest x-ray within the last (established number of) days?

□ □ □ _____

4. Are the results of all preoperative tests posted in the patient's record?

□ □ □ _____

5. Has an EKG been performed?

□ □ □ _____

6. Has the site of the incision been prepared?

□ □ □ _____

On the day of surgery, transporters pick up the patient and the medical record and deliver the patient to Surgery. Some set procedure is followed at the Nursing Station to assure that the right patient is taken. One approach is to require that a nurse accompany the transporters to the patient's room in order to identify the patient.

□ □ □ _____

At Surgery, a clerk logs the patient into the department. Surgical forms, including the Operating Room Record, the Anesthesia Record and the IV/Medication Sheet, are added to the patient's record. In addition, the checklist is reviewed to make sure it is complete.

□ □ □ _____

When the surgeon and the operating suite are ready, the patient is taken in, and the procedure is performed. During the operation, the anesthesiologist makes the appropriate notations on the Anesthesia Record.

□ □ □ _____

A = essentially similar   B = minor variations   C = significant differences

After the procedure is completed, the surgical team performs a sponge count and an instrument count. The results are entered onto the Operating Room Record. The Circulating Nurse makes any other required notations onto this record, gives one copy to a Surgery Clerk for filing, and places the other copy back into the patient's record.

A B C
☐ ☐ ☐ _____

The patient and his record are then taken to the Recovery Room, where a Recovery Room Record is begun.

☐ ☐ ☐ _____

In the meantime, the surgeon dictates a postoperative report. After it is transcribed, it is placed in the patient's record.

☐ ☐ ☐ _____

When the patient's condition has stabilized, a physician, usually the operating surgeon or the anesthesiologist, discharges the patient from the Recovery Room. Transporters are called to return the patient to his or her room.

☐ ☐ ☐ _____

Outpatient Surgery

Performing surgery on an outpatient basis is becoming increasingly popular. It results in less cost to the patient and releases a hospital bed.

☐ ☐ ☐ _____

There are two approaches taken in establishing an outpatient-surgery program. The hospital may establish a separate facility and hire a separate staff for this activity, or outpatient surgery may be integrated into the main Surgery Department.

☐ ☐ ☐ _____

The major difference in flow in the two approaches is that a separate facility handles its own scheduling, while an integrated facility maintains one scheduling book.

☐ ☐ ☐ _____

The overall flow for an outpatient going to surgery is very similar to that used for an inpatient. The patient's physician schedules the case. For outpatients, however, the physician must also make arrangements for preoperative testing to be handled on an outpatient basis.

☐ ☐ ☐ _____

If preoperative tests are scheduled prior to the day of surgery, the patient registers for them and receives them in the same manner as any other referred outpatient. However, in scheduling the tests, the physician's office notifies the departments involved that these are preoperative procedures. The departments then forward results to Surgery, where they are placed in a patient folder, sorted and filed alphabetically.

☐ ☐ ☐ _____

A = essentially similar   B = minor variations   C = significant differences

On the day of surgery, the patient arrives at a
registration point and completes an Outpatient
Surgery Registration Form. This can be the
hospital's standard Outpatient Registration
Form or an abbreviated version of its Admission
Form. There are at least two copies of this form
—one for the patient's record, the other for the
Business Office.

The patient, along with the Registration Form,
is taken to Surgery, where the patient is placed
in a preoperative area.

A surgical clerk initiates a medical record, which
includes the Registration Form, results forms
from the clinical department, and a checklist.

Working from the form, a nurse prepares the
patient for surgery. This preparation includes
confirming that all required preoperative testing
has been completed and that the consent form
has been signed, administering preoperative
medication, and making sure that all other items
on the checklist have been completed.

The patient is then taken into an operating suite.
From this point until the patient is ready to
leave the Recovery Room, the flow is identical
to that used for an inpatient.

Notes

A B C
☐ ☐ ☐ _____

☐ ☐ ☐ _____

☐ ☐ ☐ _____

☐ ☐ ☐ _____

☐ ☐ ☐ _____

A = essentially similar   B = minor variations   C = significant differences

Flow Chart 3.3

Surgery

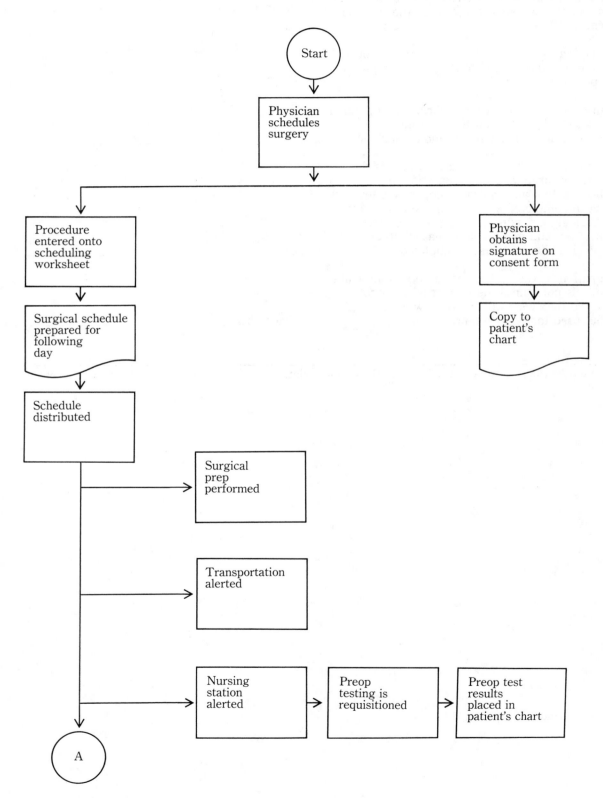

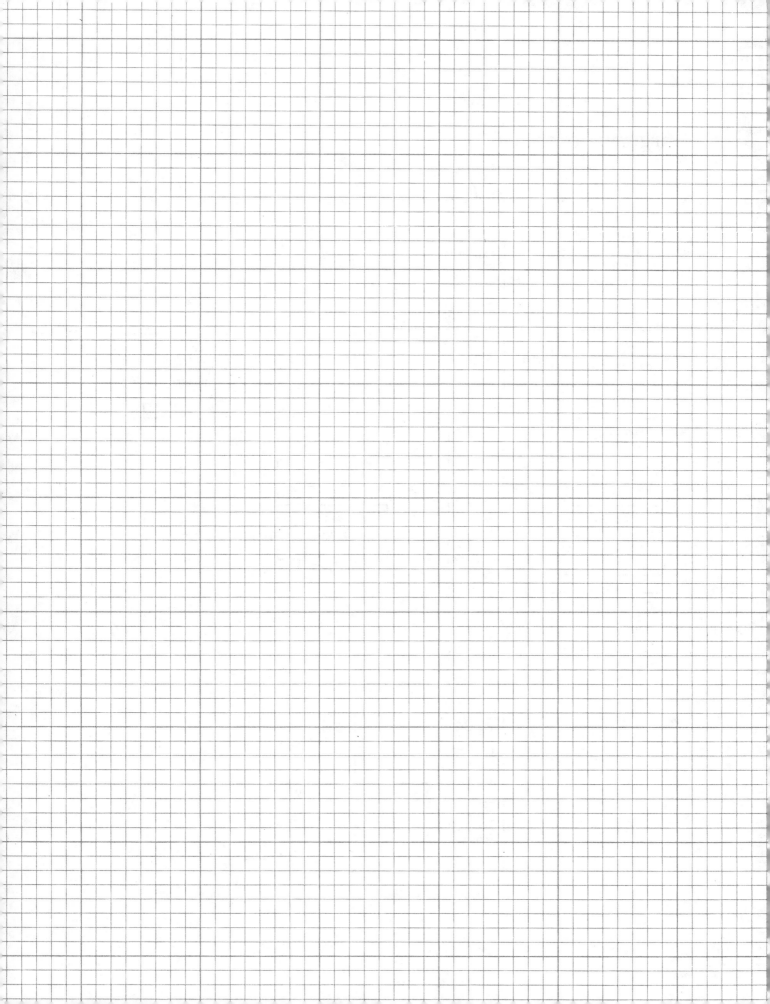

Surgery, continued

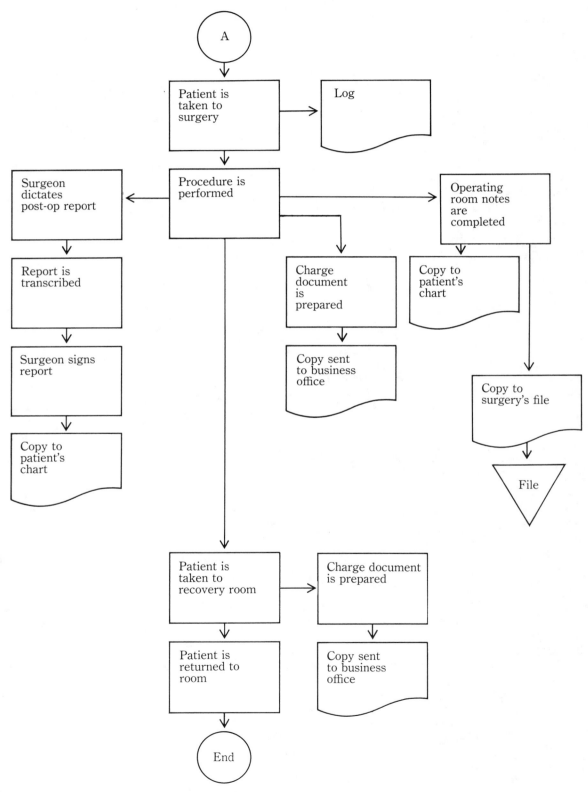

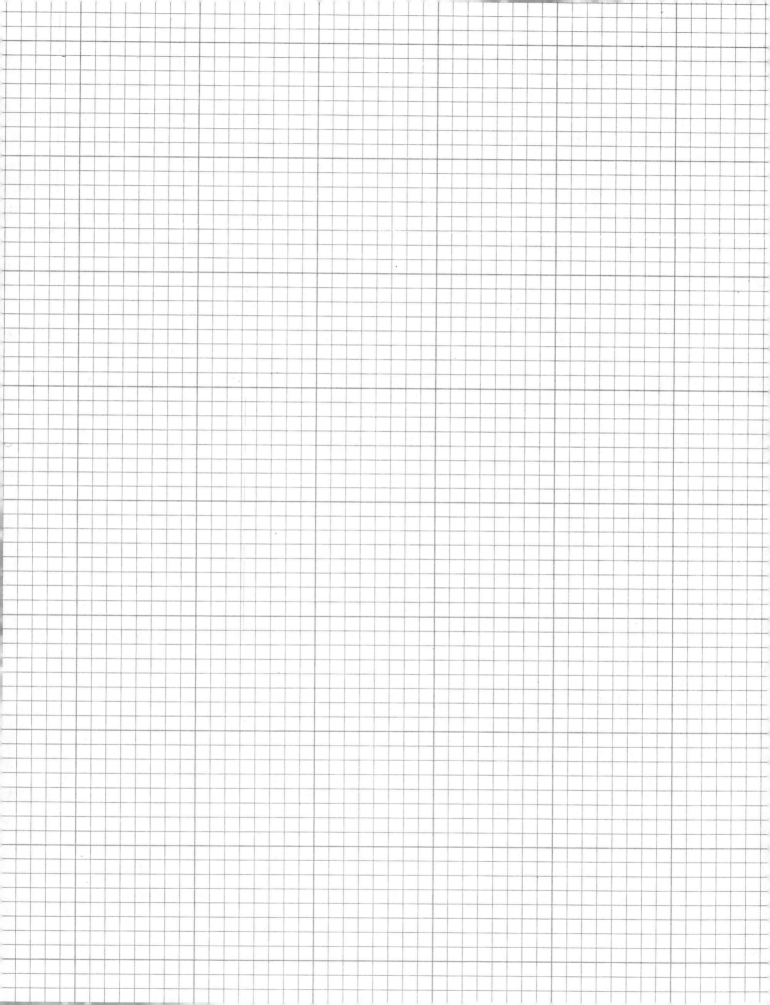

Input Inventory 3.3

A. Surgical Supervisor

your document title ↓

	A	B	C	
1. Checklist.	☐	☐	☐	_____
2. Operating Room Record.	☐	☐	☐	_____
3. Anesthesia Record.	☐	☐	☐	_____
4. Consent Form.	☐	☐	☐	_____
5. IV/Medication Sheet.	☐	☐	☐	_____
6. Recovery Room Record.	☐	☐	☐	_____
7. Outpatient Registration Form.	☐	☐	☐	_____

USE INPUT DOCUMENT ANALYSIS FORM

A = same document title   B = minor variations   C = significant differences

Master File Inventory 3.3

A. Surgical Supervisor

Notes ↓

	A	B	C	
1. Schedule sheets.	☐	☐	☐	_____
2. Surgical Log.	☐	☐	☐	_____
3. Operating Room forms.	☐	☐	☐	_____

USE MASTER FILE ANALYSIS FORM

A = essentially similar   B = minor variations   C = significant differences

Report Inventory 3.3

A. Surgical Supervisor

your document title ↓

	A	B	C	
1. Schedule.	☐	☐	☐	_____
2. Prep Technician Assignment Sheet.	☐	☐	☐	_____
3. Postop Report.	☐	☐	☐	_____

USE REPORT ANALYSIS FORM

A = essentially similar   B = minor variations   C = significant differences

System Performance Standards 3.3

Units

		A	B
1. What is the waiting time for scheduling elective surgery?	days _____	☐	☐
2. Can a physician schedule an admission and a surgery with one telephone call?	yes or no _____	☐	☐
3. How long does it take to clean an operating suite and prepare it for the next case?	minutes_____	☐	☐
4. When is the surgery schedule available for distribution?	time of day in military time __	☐	☐
5. During Surgery's eight busiest hours, what percentage of the time are the suites unoccupied?	percentage _____	☐	☐
6. How many operations are postponed because a consent is not signed or preop test results or the history and physical are not in the medical record?	number per month _____	☐	☐
7. How many operations are delayed because the patient is taken to Surgery late?	number per month _____	☐	☐

USE PERFORMANCE STANDARDS ANALYSIS FORM

A = we have a standard   B = we do not have a standard

System Cost Factors 3.3

1. How many clerical staffers are employed by Surgery? $ _____

2. What is the cost of copying the Surgical Schedule? $ _____

3. How many patients are on the waiting list? $ _____

4. Of the patients on the waiting list, how many cases are cancelled and not rescheduled? $ _____

USE SYSTEM COST ANALYSIS FORM *(also see Instructions, p. 15)*

Patient Records Management Systems

System 4.1: Transcription

Description 4.1

Transcription is the conversion of dictated material into printed reports. The items most commonly transcribed are reports of diagnostic procedures, such as radiology tests; clinical histories and physical examinations; surgical reports; and discharge reports.

A B C
□ □ □

Two organizational approaches are used to set up a transcription capability. In some hospitals, one department handles all transcribing. Typically, this department is part of Medical Records.

□ □ □

In other hospitals, all departments with transcription needs have their own transcribers. Normally, these departments are Medical Records, Radiology, Clinical Laboratory, Nuclear Medicine, EKG/EEG, Physical Medicine, and Respiratory Therapy. With this approach, Medical Records remains responsible for transcribing histories and physicals, surgical reports, and discharge summaries.

□ □ □

Flow

Regardless of the organizational approach, the flow remains basically the same. The reporting physician dictates a report into a recording machine. This may be a hand-held cassette recorder, a dictating machine, the microphone of a centralized dictation system or a telephone tied into a central dictating system. A single hospital may use more than one approach.

□ □ □

If the report is dictated into a smaller recorder or dictating machine, a clerk removes the tape or belt from the unit, completes a label stating what type of report the tape or belt contains, attaches the label to the tape or belt, and sends it to Transcription.

□ □ □

The Transcription Supervisor logs the tape or belt into the department and assigns it to a transcriber.

□ □ □

From the label, the transcriber knows what type of form should be placed into the typewriter (history and physical form, radiology report

---

A = essentially similar   B = minor variations   C = significant differences

251

form, etc.). The transcriber then transcribes the material and returns both the tape or belt and the transcribed reports to the supervisor.

A B C
☐ ☐ ☐ _____

With a centralized system, the recording devices are in one location, usually Medical Records. As tapes are generated by the system, the supervisor logs them into the department and assigns them to individual transcribers. Since an individual tape may contain more than one type of report, the transcriber must listen to the physician's introductory remarks before putting the proper form into the typewriter.

☐ ☐ ☐ _____

Once the transcriber has transcribed all material on the tape, he or she returns the tape and the reports to the supervisor.

☐ ☐ ☐ _____

When the supervisor receives completed reports, whether they are the output of a centralized or a noncentralized system, he or she reviews the reports for accuracy, reviews the tape or belt to ensure that all reports have been transcribed, logs the tape or belt out of the department, and oversees the distribution of the reports.

☐ ☐ ☐ _____

The standard distribution is as follows:

1. Histories, physicals, and surgical reports are placed in the patient's medical record, which is filed at the Nursing Station.

☐ ☐ ☐ _____

2. Discharge summaries are placed in the patient's medical record, which, for discharged patients, is filed in Medical Records.

☐ ☐ ☐ _____

3. Reports of diagnostic tests are returned to the clinical department, which is responsible for further distribution. This normally involves placing one copy in the patient's record, one copy in the patient's departmental file, and one copy in an envelope for mailing to the patient's attending physician.

☐ ☐ ☐ _____

Prioritizing

In hospitals with centralized systems, there usually are at least two sets of lines connected to the recording equipment. Physicians are then able to dictate over any of the lines from any of the input microphones.

☐ ☐ ☐ _____

Having more than one line serves two purposes. It decreases the possibility that recording equipment will be tied up at any particular time. Even more important is the fact that it allows the hospital to designate one line as a priority, or

---

A = essentially similar   B = minor variations   C = significant differences

STAT, line. This line is used only for reports where speed of transcribing is essential. Transcription gives top priority to reports coming in on this line.

A B C
□ □ □

An example of the type of report given this treatment would be the history and physical of a newly admitted patient scheduled for surgery the next day. Many hospitals require that the history and physical of such a patient be attached to the chart before surgery is performed. Any transcription delay, therefore, could result in a postponement of the operation.

□ □ □

Standards

The key standards for judging the performance of transcribers are their speed and their accuracy. Most hospitals have playback systems with monitors and timers that allow the supervisor to measure how much time a transcriber spent on a given tape. By counting the number of report lines transcribed from that tape, the supervisor can measure a line-per-minute speed for the transcriber. Accuracy is determined simply by reviewing the reports.

□ □ □

Word Processing

Word processing means computerized control of text entry. In the place of typewriters are cathode ray tube terminals (CRTs) along with one or more printers. Word processing systems can greatly speed the transcribing process. They can, for example, store standard reports, check for spelling, and simplify error correction.

□ □ □

Use of word processing need not be limited to Medical Records. Some hospitals have found roles for such systems in Personnel, Administration, Maintenance, and the Nursing Office.

□ □ □

Other Dictation

The Transcription Department may also have other responsibilities. Some hospitals allow the chairmen of medical staff committees to dictate minutes into the centralized dictation system. Other hospitals may extend similar services to the medical staff.

□ □ □

A = essentially similar   B = minor variations   C = significant differences

Flow Chart 4.1

Transcription

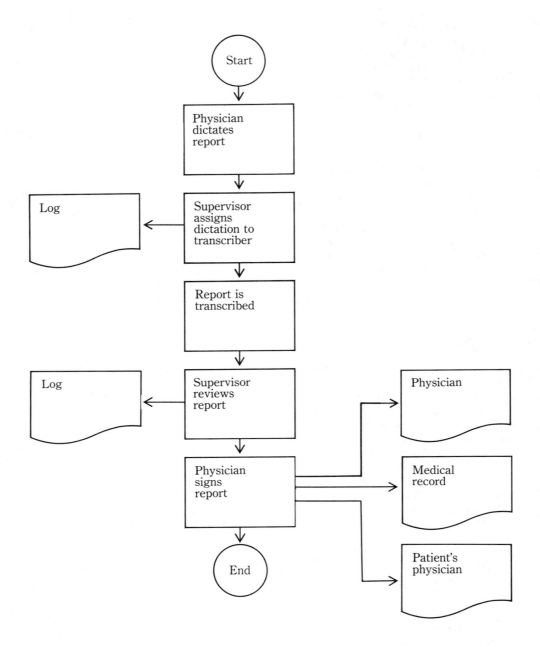

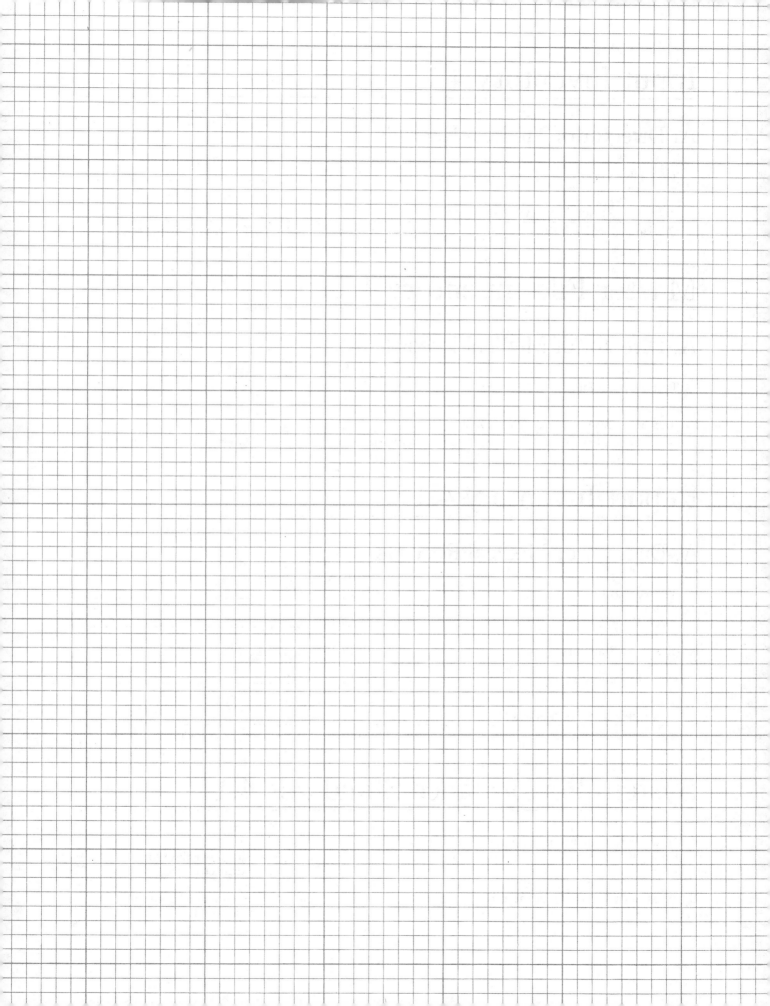

Input Inventory 4.1

A. Director of Medical Records

your document title
↓

                    A B C

Tape labels.   ☐ ☐ ☐ _____

USE INPUT DOCUMENT ANALYSIS FORM

A = same document title   B = minor variations   C = significant differences

Master File Inventory 4.1

A. Director of Medical Records

Notes
↓

                    A B C

Transcription log.   ☐ ☐ ☐ _____

USE MASTER FILE ANALYSIS FORM

A = essentially similar   B = minor variations   C = significant differences

Report Inventory 4.1

A. Director of Medical Records

your document title
↓

                    A B C

1. History and Physical. ☐ ☐ ☐ _____

2. Surgical report.   ☐ ☐ ☐ _____

3. Discharge Summary. ☐ ☐ ☐ _____

4. Monthly activity report. ☐ ☐ ☐ _____

USE REPORT ANALYSIS FORM

A = essentially similar   B = minor variations   C = significant differences

System Performance Standards 4.1

Units

1. How many lines per minute does the average transcriber produce?

                             mean rate (lines per day) for A B
                             all medical transcribers_____ ☐ ☐

2. What is the accuracy of the transcribers?

                             number of errors per hundred
                             lines of transcription _____ ☐ ☐

3. Once a nonstat report is dictated, how much time elapses before the report is transcribed?

minutes_____   ☐ ☐

4. Once a stat report is dictated, how much time elapses before the report is transcribed?

minutes_____   ☐ ☐

5. How often is surgery delayed or postponed because a history and physical are not part of the patient's medical record?

number of times per month _____   ☐ ☐

6. Once a patient is discharged, how much time elapses before a discharge summary is made part of the patient's record?

hours_____   ☐ ☐

7. How often are physicians prevented from dictating because all dictation lines are busy?

number of times per week____   ☐ ☐

8. How many medical transcribers are employed?

number_____   ☐ ☐

9. How many clinical reports are prerecorded and stored in a memory typewriter?

number_____   ☐ ☐

USE PERFORMANCE STANDARDS ANALYSIS FORM

A = we have a standard   B = we do not have a standard

System Cost Factors 4.1

1. How many departments have medical transcribers? $ _____

2. What is the value of all hospital transcription equipment? $ _____

3. Do medical transcribers transcribe nonmedical reports, such as minutes and letters? $ _____

USE SYSTEM COST ANALYSIS FORM *(also see Instructions, p. 15)*

System 4.2:
Indexing, Storage, and Retrieval
Description 4.2

Notes
↓

The Medical Records Department has three major activities: compiling and filing complete and accurate medical records, generating statistical reports based on medical record and census information, and retrieving stored records rapidly.

A B C
□ □ □ _____

Record Content

The typical medical record contains the following documents:

1. A history and physical form.

□ □ □ _____

2. Consent forms signed by the patient.

□ □ □ _____

3. The Admission Form.

□ □ □ _____

4. A graphics form, containing all vital signs recorded during the patient's stay.

□ □ □ _____

5. A medication record.

□ □ □ _____

6. Physician order forms.

□ □ □ _____

7. Physician progress notes.

□ □ □ _____

8. Results of diagnostic tests.

□ □ □ _____

9. Nursing notes.

□ □ □ _____

10. Specialized forms used for certain Nursing Stations, such as Intensive Care Unit (ICU) and Obstetrics, and for patients with certain diagnoses (e.g., a chemotherapy record for a cancer patient).

□ □ □ _____

11. Surgical reports.

□ □ □ _____

12. Medicare certifications and other forms related to utilization review and quality assurance.

□ □ □ _____

13. Clinical progress notes, such as a Physical-Medicine form.

□ □ □ _____

Some hospitals have adopted a different approach to recording the problems and treatments related to a specific patient. This type of

---

A = essentially similar   B = minor variations   C = significant differences

record, called the Problem-Oriented Medical Record, is based on identifying each problem a patient has and then associating each problem with the treatments the patient receives, the progress the patient makes, and the recommended treatment regimen. All hospital personnel taking care of the patient use the same record for entering notations of care and observations concerning the patient. The traditional approach relies more on a straight chronological listing of orders, results, and progress notes.

A B C
□ □ □ _____

Notification upon Admission

At the time of admission, a Medical Records Clerk reviews the files to determine if the patient has been admitted previously. If this is the case, the patient's old records are sent to the Nursing Station.

□ □ □ _____

Nursing Station to File

The flow of the Medical Record begins when the attending physician writes a discharge order. Once the patient leaves the Nursing Station, a nurse removes the patient's record from its chart holder, inspects the record for accuracy, enters the date and time of discharge on the record's copy of the Admitting Form, and then either sends the record to Medical Records or places it in a discharged-patient suspense file. The purpose of this file is to allow the Nursing Station to match late-arriving results and reports with the proper patient record. Otherwise, these late documents must be sent on to Medical Records for sorting and mounting.

□ □ □ _____

If the Station does keep a suspense file, records in the file are sent to Medical Records after a fixed period of time, which is usually about three days.

□ □ □ _____

At Medical Records, a control clerk logs each record for a newly discharged patient. Normally, the clerk will get a copy of the daily discharge list and line out each patient's name as his or her record is received. Logging the record into the department involves recording the patient's name and number, the date of discharge, and the date that the record was received.

□ □ □ _____

The clerk then puts the record into a permanent folder, reviews the record for accuracy, attaches a checklist to the front of the folder, and makes appropriate entries onto the checklist. The purpose of the checklist is to ensure that all

A = essentially similar   B = minor variations   C = significant differences

indexing, abstracting, and processing is
complete before the record is placed in
the permanent file.

A B C
☐ ☐ ☐

The control clerk then sends the record to
another clerk who places it in a physician-
suspense file, arranged alphabetically by
attending physician. The record stays there until
all physicians involved with the patient have
entered appropriate information, including the
discharge diagnosis, dictated and signed clinical
reports and the discharge summary. The clerk
handling this file is responsible for giving the file
to physicians when they come to the department
to work on records and for refiling the record
after a physician has made any entries.

☐ ☐ ☐

Periodically, the clerk reviews the file, counts
the number of reports being held for each
physician, and sends a delinquent-records report
to an appropriate official (e.g., the Director of
Medical Affairs, the Chief of Staff).

☐ ☐ ☐

In most hospitals, having delinquent records
results in the physician's losing admitting
privileges. Admitting receives a copy of the
delinquency report.

☐ ☐ ☐

The admissions ban can be lifted only when an
administrative officer approves an emergency
admission or Medical Records notifies Admitting
that the physician is no longer delinquent.

☐ ☐ ☐

Once the record has all the needed physician
input, it is sent back to the Control Clerk. At
this point a variety of tasks involving coding,
abstracting, indexing, and reviewing must be
done. The number of clerks involved in this
process varies from hospital to hospital. In some
institutions, only one or two clerks are used to
perform all these tasks. In others, practically
each task is performed by a different, specialized
clerk.

☐ ☐ ☐

The first step is reviewing the chart and coding
onto the Admitting Form, or face sheet, the discharge diagnoses and all surgical procedures
performed.

☐ ☐ ☐

Then, a variety of index cards are prepared.
Typically, a hospital maintains four index files:

☐ ☐ ☐

1. Patient File—one card for each patient.
   Each card contains demographic information — name, address, telephone number,
   etc. — plus one line of information for each
   hospital stay. This information typically
   includes the admission date, the discharge
   date, and the major discharge diagnosis.

☐ ☐ ☐

A = essentially similar   B = minor variations   C = significant differences

2. Disease File—one card for each disease code. The cards are filed numerically by disease code. The patient's number is written onto the card corresponding to the patient's major discharge diagnosis.

A B C
☐ ☐ ☐

3. Surgical File—one card for each surgical code, according to the surgical procedure performed. The cards are filed numerically by surgical code. The patient's number is written onto each card, with the cards corresponding to a surgical procedure performed on the patient in the hospital.

☐ ☐ ☐

4. Physician File—one card for each physician on the medical staff. The patient's name and number are written onto each card, with the cards corresponding to a physician who was a prime attending physician during the patient's stay.

☐ ☐ ☐

The patient file is kept in one place indefinitely. The other three files are kept for a year. At the end of each year, the past year's files are stored, and new ones are begun.

☐ ☐ ☐

After indexing is completed, statistical information is extracted from the record. Facts such as the length of stay, the presence of a hospital-acquired infection, and the performance of an autopsy are gathered and collated.

☐ ☐ ☐

Finally, the abstracting is done. Most hospitals gather information that is used in generating quality-control reports. The most common of these reports are those sent out by the Professional Activities Service (PAS). A clerk completes an abstracting form for each discharged patient. The form is sent to PAS, where it is processed. The resulting reports list the volume of various clinical activities and present statistical indicators that allow the hospital to compare its level of service with the service levels of other hospitals of similar size and service range in the same geographical area.

☐ ☐ ☐

Some hospitals use other abstracting services, but the type of reports received are similar.

☐ ☐ ☐

A second type of abstracting involves gathering data for Professional Standards Review Organizations (PSROs). In the future these organizations, established by the U.S. Congress, will generate more data needs.

☐ ☐ ☐

A = essentially similar   B = minor variations   C = significant differences

After abstracting is completed, the record is returned to the Control Clerk, who logs the fact that the record is ready for permanent filing. The clerk then gives the record to a filing clerk.

A B C
□ □ □

The permanent patient-record file is kept in either alphabetical or numerical order.

□ □ □

Numbering Systems

Hospitals use two numbering systems. The most common approach is to assign a patient a number for each admission.

□ □ □

The other approach is called the unit record system. Each patient has only one number, which is used each time the particular patient returns.

□ □ □

The advantage of the unit system is that it allows all records to be filed together, under one number. The disadvantage is that it is more expensive to operate.

□ □ □

Some hospitals use a combination of these two techniques. Admitting assigns a new account number at each admission. Medical Records assigns a record number for intradepartmental use.

□ □ □

Retrieval

Many different individuals have the right to obtain a patient's record. The attending physician needs to review it in order to record. Medical Staff Committees must have access in order to ensure that proper care is being rendered. Records are needed for educational purposes. Research also uses historical medical records information (normally on a depersonalized basis without identification of a patient by name). Finally records may be subpoenaed.

□ □ □

When any request for a record is made, the file clerk first determines if the person making the request has a right to see the record. This normally involves following written procedures, which are primarily designed to protect patient privacy. When questions arise, the Medical Records Supervisor is consulted.

□ □ □

The clerk then retrieves the record and logs it out of the file. The sign-out sheet contains the patient's name and number, the date the record is being taken from the file, and the signature of the person receiving the record.

□ □ □

A = essentially similar   B = minor variations   C = significant differences

The clerk also places a sign-out card in the files, marking where the record should be. This card also shows who has the record and when it was taken.

A B C
□ □ □ _____

When the record is returned, the return date is entered into the sign-out log, and the record is refiled.

□ □ □ _____

Microfilm

After a patient record has been held in the permanent file for a fixed period of time, it may be microfilmed. The original record is then destroyed.

□ □ □ _____

Census Reports

Medical Records often is responsible for maintaining census and occupancy statistics. The department compiles the needed data by examining admission, discharge, and transfer reports.

□ □ □ _____

A = essentially similar   B = minor variations   C = significant differences

Flow Chart 4.2

The Medical Record

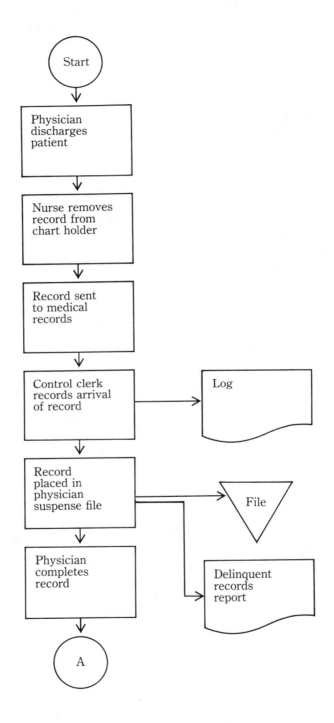

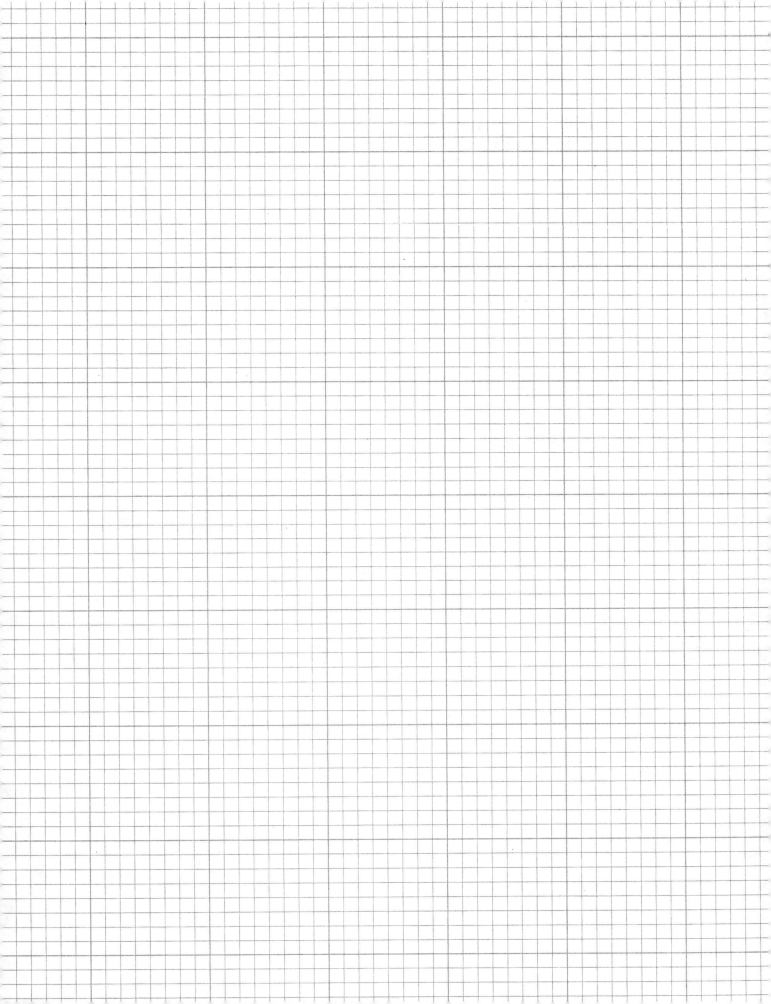

The Medical Record, continued

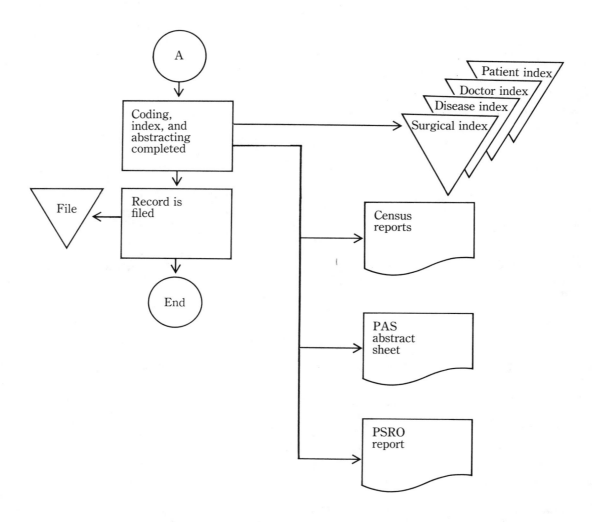

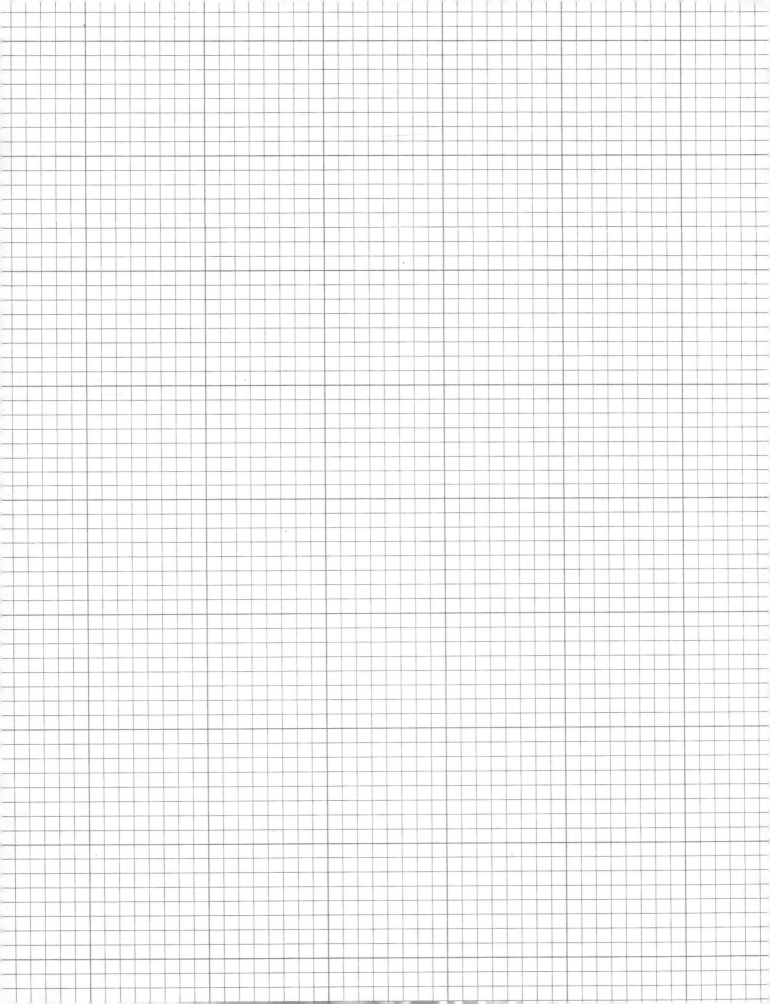

Input Inventory 4.2

A. Director of Medical Records

your document title
↓

	A	B	C	
1. Checklist.	☐	☐	☐	_____
2. Patient index card.	☐	☐	☐	_____
3. Disease index card.	☐	☐	☐	_____
4. Physician index card.	☐	☐	☐	_____
5. Surgical procedure index card.	☐	☐	☐	_____
6. Record-out card.	☐	☐	☐	_____
7. Abstracting sheet.	☐	☐	☐	_____

USE INPUT DOCUMENT ANALYSIS FORM

A = same document title   B = minor variations   C = significant differences

Master File Inventory 4.2

A. Medical Record Supervisor

Notes
↓

	A	B	C	
1. Log book (discharges).	☐	☐	☐	_____
2. Physician-suspense file.	☐	☐	☐	_____
3. Patient index.	☐	☐	☐	_____
4. Disease index.	☐	☐	☐	_____
5. Surgical procedure index.	☐	☐	☐	_____
6. Physician index.	☐	☐	☐	_____
7. Abstract sheets.	☐	☐	☐	_____
8. Reports from abstracting service.	☐	☐	☐	_____
9. Patient records (permanent).	☐	☐	☐	_____
10. Log of patient-number assignments.	☐	☐	☐	_____

B. Head Nurse

Discharge-patient suspense file.	☐	☐	☐	_____

USE MASTER FILE ANALYSIS FORM

A = essentially similar   B = minor variations   C = significant differences

Report Inventory 4.2

A. Director of Medical Records

your document title ↓

	A B C	
1. Delinquent-records report.	☐ ☐ ☐	_____
2. Statistical reports.*	☐ ☐ ☐	_____
3. Census reports.*	☐ ☐ ☐	_____

USE REPORT ANALYSIS FORM

A = essentially similar	B = minor variations	C = significant differences

*Obtain list of reports plus samples.

System Performance Standards 4.2

Units

			A	B
1. How many results and report forms must be attached to Medical Records by Medical Records personnel?	number per week _____		☐	☐
2. From the time a record reaches the department, how long does it take for all physician input to be completed?	mean number of days_____		☐	☐
3. From the time all physician input is complete, how long does it take for a record to reach the permanent file?	days _____		☐	☐
4. Does the department have a way of knowing if a Nursing Station fails to send on the record of a discharged patient?	yes or no _____		☐	☐
5. How long does it take to retrieve a filed record?	minutes_____		☐	☐
6. Are there written procedures stating who may have access to patient records?	yes or no _____		☐	☐
7. How often are records misfiled?	times per month _____		☐	☐
8. How many records must be renumbered after an initial number is found to be incorrect?	number per month _____		☐	☐

USE PERFORMANCE STANDARDS ANALYSIS FORM

A = we have a standard	B = we do not have a standard

System Cost Factors 4.2

1. How many staffers are employed in Medical Records? $ _____

2. How many square feet are needed for storing medical records? $ _____

3. How much time is spent copying medical records? $ _____

USE SYSTEM COST ANALYSIS FORM *(also see Instructions, p. 15)*

System 4.3:
Quality Assurance
Description 4.3

The generation of reports on the quality of care rendered by the hospital takes place both inside and outside of the institution.

A B C
□ □ □

Externally, reports are produced by firms such as the Professional Activity Services (PAS), and Professional Standards Review Organizations (PSROs). These groups generate statistical summaries of the processes and outcome of care rendered by a hospital.

□ □ □

The internal generation comes from the activities of medical staff committees charged with monitoring the quality of care.

□ □ □

External

Medical Records completes and submits the forms required by external agencies. In turn, these agencies prepare reports and return them to the hospital.

□ □ □

Typically, these reports go to the Chief Executive Officer, the Director of Medical Affairs, and the Chief of Staff.

□ □ □

Internal

Each hospital has a variety of committees whose activities are primarily involved in reviewing medical records to determine if complete and proper care was rendered. These committees represent the hospital's major efforts in the area of quality assurance.

□ □ □

Typically, the major committees are:

1. The Medical Records Committee, which has overall responsibility for ensuring that staff physicians complete records properly.

□ □ □

2. The Tissue Committee, which reviews the records of surgical patients who had organs or other tissues removed to determine the appropriateness of the surgical procedure.

□ □ □

A = essentially similar   B = minor variations   C = significant differences

3. The Mortality Review Committee, which considers the records of patients who died in the hospital.

A B C
☐ ☐ ☐

4. The Utilization Review Committee, which reviews hospital records, paying particular attention to the medical necessity of a hospital admission and the actual length of stay as compared with the length of stay normally associated with the discharge diagnosis.

☐ ☐ ☐

In addition, each medical staff department may conduct a review of the quality of care delivered by the physician members of that department.

☐ ☐ ☐

If a committee identifies questionable medical care, it invites the physician involved to respond to the committee's questions.

☐ ☐ ☐

The review process continues through the Staff Executive Committee, the Joint Conference Committee, and the Board of Trustees until the questions are resolved or appropriate disciplinary action has been taken.

☐ ☐ ☐

Certification/Recertification

Depending on the type of third-party coverage and the admitting diagnosis, an admission may be subject to a certification/recertification process. The purpose of this process is to verify the necessity for both admission and continued hospitalization.

☐ ☐ ☐

The specific procedures, as well as the actual number of certification/recertification flows, vary from area to area. In general, however, they follow the same pattern.

☐ ☐ ☐

For a nonemergency admission, the admitting diagnosis and other pertinent information are reviewed by a physician or a Utilization Technician. If the reviewer questions the admission, he or she may ask the admitting physician to complete a certification document justifying the admission. To resolve disagreements between the reviewer and physician, an appeals process exists.

☐ ☐ ☐

Once the patient is admitted, a recertification process comes into play. For Medicare patients, review is required at fixed time intervals. To meet PSRO regulations, reviews may be required at intervals associated with the admitting diagnosis.

☐ ☐ ☐

Notes
↓

A = essentially similar   B = minor variations   C = significant differences

The recertification process normally involves a review of the patient's record by a Utilization Technician. In cases where standards are not being met, the technician brings the case to the attention of a physician-staffed committee.

A B C
□ □ □ _____

The admitting physician has the opportunity to justify continued hospitalization and the level of care being rendered. If, however, the committee feels that further hospitalization is not justified, it will decertify the patient and notify both the patient and physician of this decision. Decertification normally means notifying the involved third parties that the committee feels continued hospitalization is no longer justified. This, in turn, results in the withdrawal of coverage by the third party.

□ □ □ _____

Delineation of Privileges

When a physician is appointed to a medical staff, he or she is given permission to perform certain procedures. In return, the physician is forbidden from exceeding certain limits. For example, surgeons may only perform operations they are certified to perform.

□ □ □ _____

At present, most hospitals rely on informal procedures to determine if physicians are staying within the bounds of their privileges.

□ □ □ _____

A = essentially similar   B = minor variations   C = significant differences

Flow Chart 4.3

Review of Quality

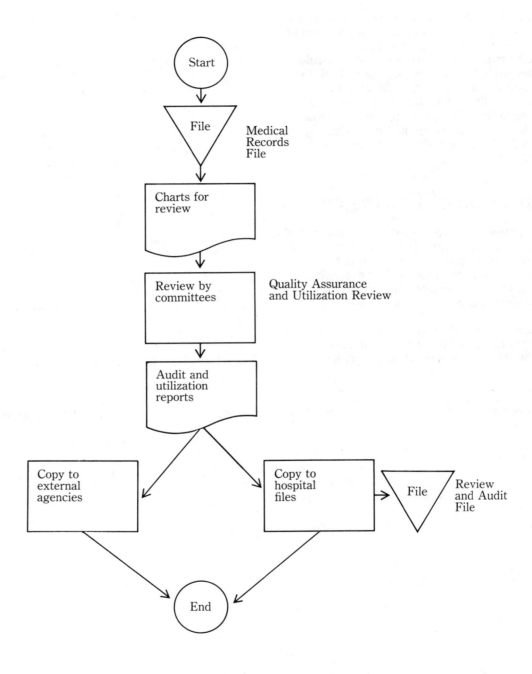

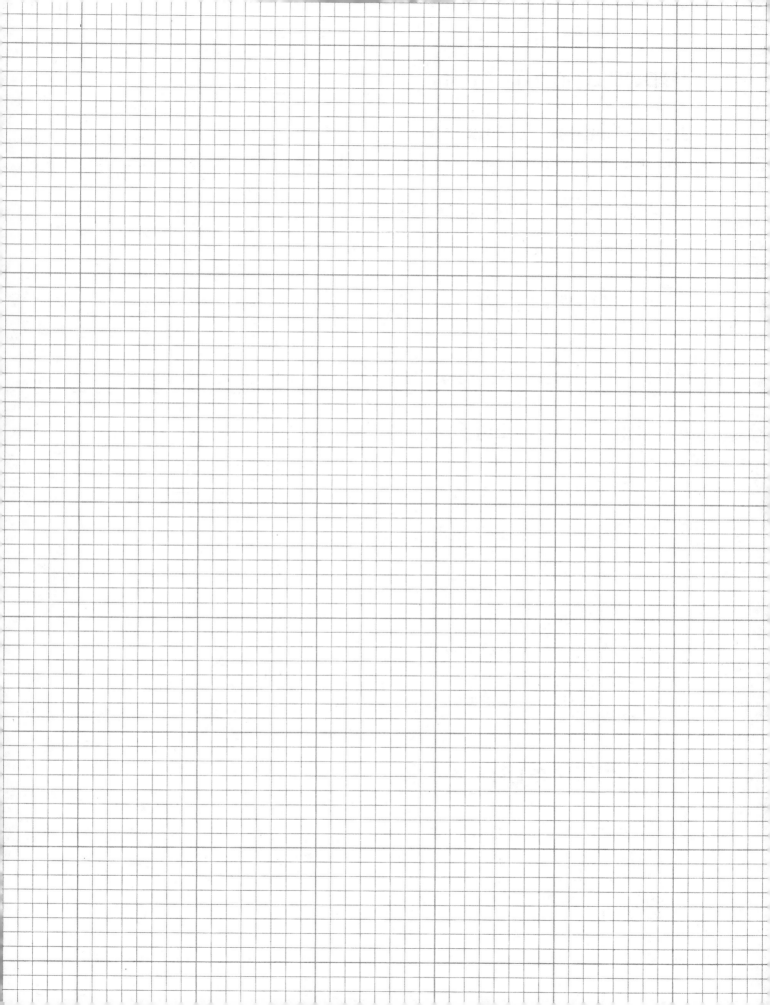

Input Inventory 4.3

A. Utilization Technician

your document title
↓

A B C

Certification/recertification form. □ □ □ _____

B. Medical Records Supervisor

Input documents for agencies generating
statistical reports. □ □ □ _____

USE INPUT DOCUMENT ANALYSIS FORM

A = same document title   B = minor variations   C = significant differences

Master File Inventory 4.3

Notes
↓

A. Utilization Technician

A B C

1. Certification and recertification criteria. □ □ □ _____

2. Minutes of review committee. □ □ □ _____

B. Medical Records Supervisor

Reports from external agencies. □ □ □ _____

C. Medical Staff Office

Listing of privileges for each medical staff
member. □ □ □ _____

USE MASTER FILE ANALYSIS FORM

A = essentially similar   B = minor variations   C = significant differences

Report Inventory 4.3

your document title
↓

A. Utilization Technician

A B C

Notification of decertification. □ □ □ _____

USE REPORT ANALYSIS FORM

A = essentially similar   B = minor variations   C = significant differences

System Performance Standards 4.3

Units

1. What proportion of admissions undergo the recertification process?

     percentage of admissions   A B
     per month_____   ☐ ☐

2. What proportion of admissions have third party payments discontinued as a result of utilization review activities?

     percentage of admissions per month _____   ☐ ☐

3. In how many cases, when the hospital's Utilization Review activity does not terminate coverage, does a third party refuse to pay or retrospectively deny financial coverage because the admission or length of stay is deemed to be excessive?

     percentage of admissions denied _____   ☐ ☐

4. How many retrospective denials are appealed with the result that 50 percent or more of the disallowed coverage is reinstated?

     cases reinstated per year ____   ☐ ☐

5. How many physicians are admonished in writing or have admitting privileges altered or rescinded as a result of medical audit activity?

     number per year _____   ☐ ☐

USE PERFORMANCE STANDARDS ANALYSIS FORM

A = we have a standard   B = we do not have a standard

System Cost Factors 4.3

1. What is the direct budget for utilization review? $ _____

2. What is the direct budget for medical quality control activities? $ _____

3. What is the dollar write-off resulting from retrospective denials of third party coverage as a result of utilizations deemed to be excessive or inappropriate? $ _____

4. How many paid physician workhours are spent in the medical quality control activity? $ _____

5. How many unpaid physician workhours are spent in the medical quality control activity? $ _____

USE SYSTEM COST ANALYSIS FORM *(also see Instructions, p. 15)*

Financial Management Systems

System 5.1.1:
Charging

Description 5.1.1

Census Interface

When the patient is admitted, an account for that patient is established. Admitting notifies the Business Office of the new patient's arrival. The Business Office then prepares an account card on which charges will be tabulated.

A B C
□ □ □   _____

When the patient is transferred or discharged, the Nursing Station notifies both the Business Office and Admitting, as well as other affected departments (e.g., Dietary, Information Desk).

□ □ □   _____

The Business Office must know about transfers in order to adjust room rates. Discharge notification signals this office to begin preparing the patient's bill.

□ □ □   _____

Types of Charges

Once the patient is admitted, the Business Office begins to accumulate notices of chargeable services rendered and supplies used in caring for the patient. Such charges can be categorized as follows:

□ □ □   _____

1. Room charge.

□ □ □   _____

2. Room accessories, such as telephone and television.

□ □ □   _____

3. Patient Services/Nursing Originated. A document filled out at the Nursing Station goes to the Business Office as a charge notification. Common examples of Nursing Originated charges are those for Radiology, Laboratory, Nuclear Medicine, EKG, EEG, and Blood Bank.

□ □ □   _____

4. Patient Services/Department Originated. A document generated by the ancillary department notifies the Business Office.

□ □ □   _____

5. Surgery Related.

□ □ □   _____

A = essentially similar   B = minor variations   C = significant differences

A B C

6. Drugs.
☐ ☐ ☐
_____

7. Central Service Supplies.
☐ ☐ ☐
_____

8. Storeroom supplies.
☐ ☐ ☐
_____

9. Physician charges (in cases where the hospital issues bills for physician services).
☐ ☐ ☐
_____

Room Payments

A fixed rate is established for each hospital bed, and the patient is charged that rate for each day the bed is occupied. When the discharge notice is received, the Business Office computes the number of days the patient was in the hospital.
☐ ☐ ☐
_____

Room Accessories

These are computed in much the same manner as the room rate. At admission, the patient selects accessories. Daily service charges for these are posted to the patient's account by the Business Office. Admitting tells the Business Office what accessories the patient is using. At discharge, accessory charges are computed and posted.
☐ ☐ ☐
_____

Patient Services/Nursing Originated

Upon receipt of a physician's order, the Nursing Station completes a requisition, which goes to the department that will render the service.
☐ ☐ ☐
_____

The department involved sends one copy of this requisition to the Business Office for posting. Before forwarding it, the department ascertains that all services rendered are written on the form checked off, with prices written on the form.
☐ ☐ ☐
_____

Patient Services/Department Originated

Upon receipt of a physician's order, the Nursing Station completes a requisition, which goes to the department involved. But without notification from these departments, the Nursing Station cannot determine either the exact nature of the service or the frequency of the treatment.
☐ ☐ ☐
_____

Respiratory Therapy and Physical Medicine are examples of such departments.
☐ ☐ ☐
_____

A = essentially similar   B = minor variations   C = significant differences

Such departments must either record the service rendered and its price on a copy of the requisition or initiate a separate charge document. The procedure used depends on the department and the hospital.

A B C
□ □ □ _____

The copy of the requisition or new charge document is then sent to the Business Office for posting.

□ □ □ _____

Surgery

A master sheet containing all services and supplies used in Surgery is prepared by Surgery and sent to the Business Office for posting.

□ □ □ _____

Drugs

The Nursing Station, working from a physician's order, sends a requisition to the Pharmacy. Pharmacy prices the requisition and sends a copy to the Business Office for posting.

□ □ □ _____

In some hospitals, the physician's order itself is the requisition. A copy of the order sheet is pulled from the chart by the Nursing Station and then sent to Pharmacy. Pharmacy completes a charge document and sends it to the Business Office for posting.

□ □ □ _____

Central Service Supplies

The Nursing Station completes a requisition and sends it to Central Service, where it is priced, with a copy then sent to the Business Office for posting.

□ □ □ _____

Delivery of the item requested occurs in one of two ways – Central Service delivers it after receiving the requisition or the item is taken from the Nursing Station floor stock. In the latter case, the requisition is not only a charge document, but also a restocking notification.

□ □ □ _____

Storeroom Supplies

Some patient-care items are dispensed through the Storeroom rather than through Central Service.

□ □ □ _____

The Nursing Station obtains them via a Storeroom requisition, stocks them, and dispenses them to patients as needed. The Nursing Station then completes a charge document and sends it to the Business Office.

□ □ □ _____

A = essentially similar   B = minor variations   C = significant differences

Flow Chart 5.1.1a

Room Charge/Room Accessories

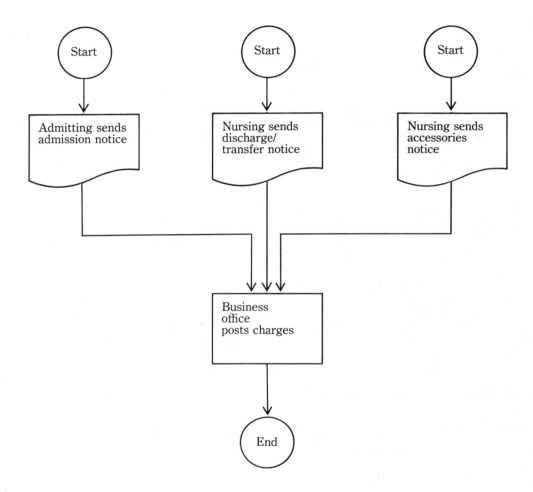

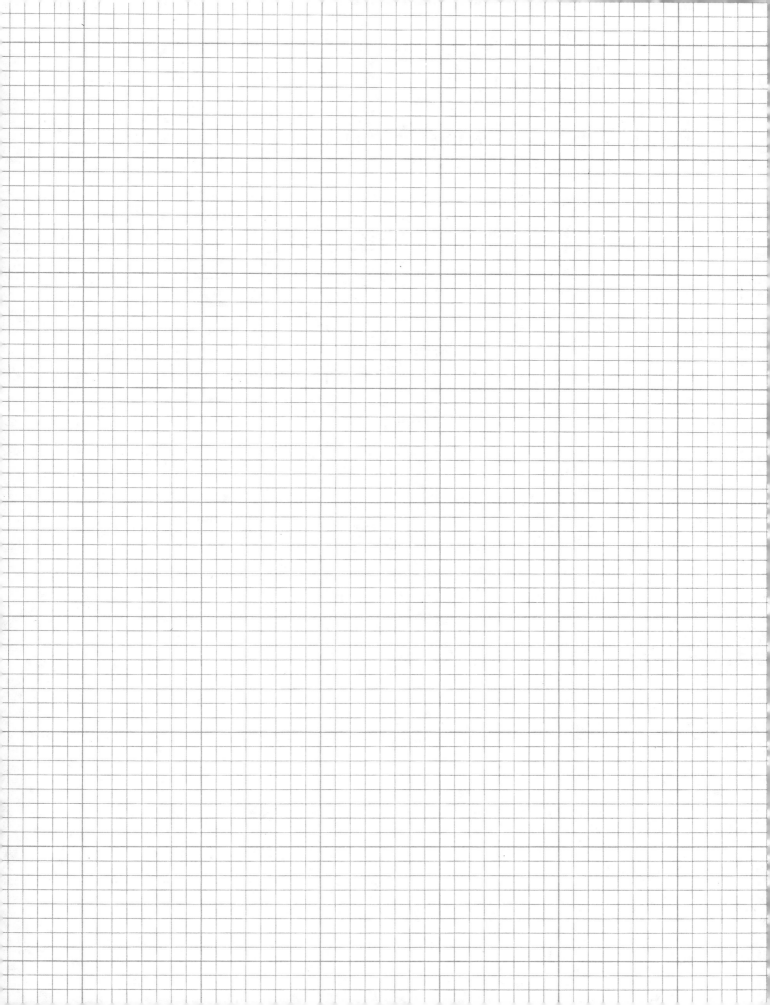

Flow Chart 5.1.1b

Patient Services/Nursing Originated

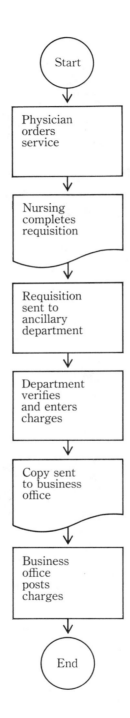

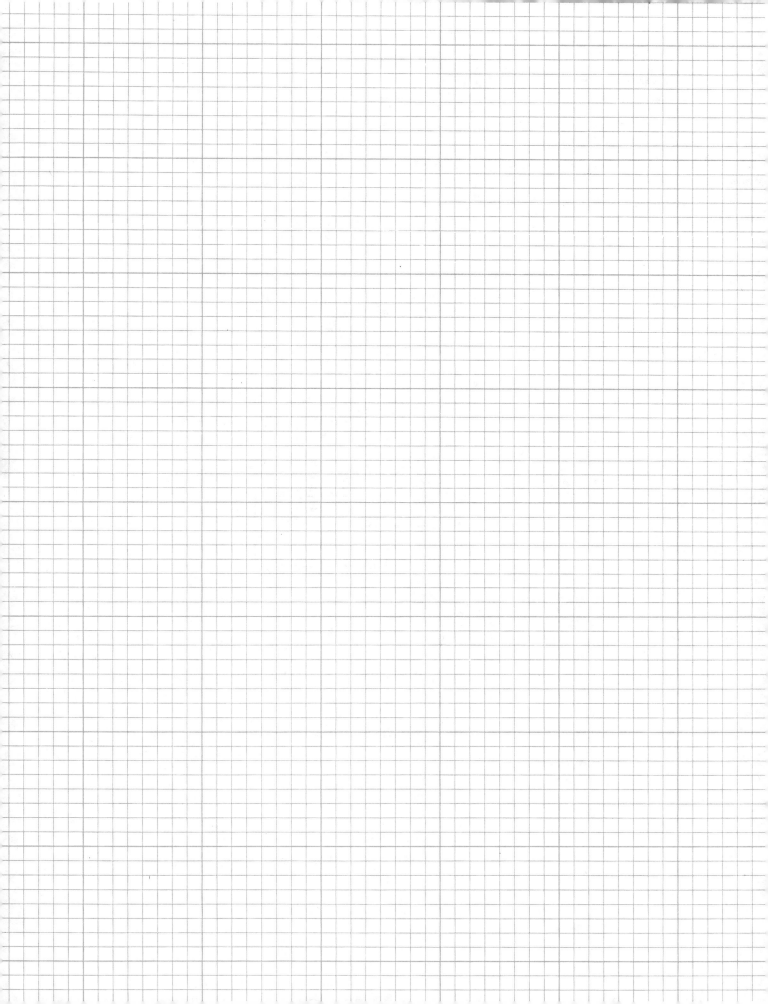

Flow Chart 5.1.1c

Census Interface

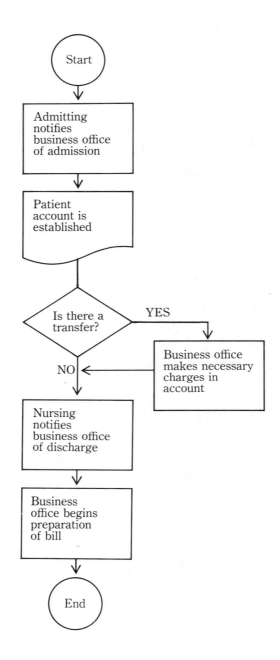

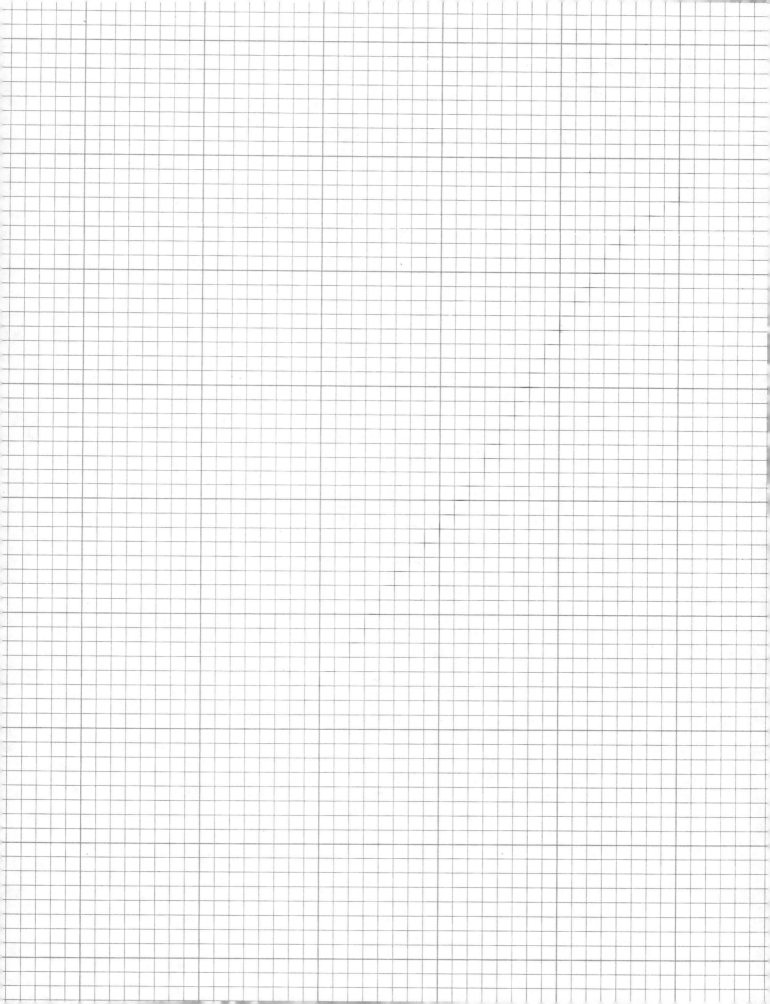

Flow Chart 5.1.1d

Patient Services/Department Originated

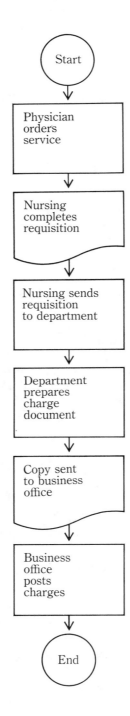

Start

Physician
orders
service

Nursing
completes
requisition

Nursing sends
requisition
to department

Department
prepares
charge
document

Copy sent
to business
office

Business
office
posts
charges

End

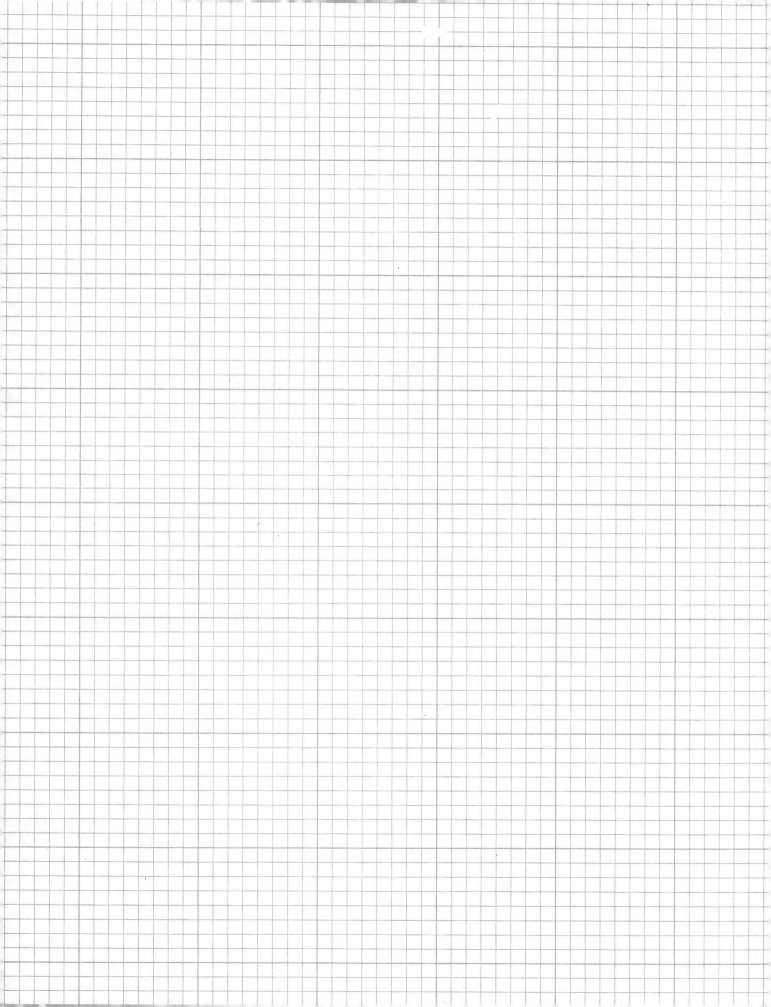

Flow Chart 5.1.1e

Surgery

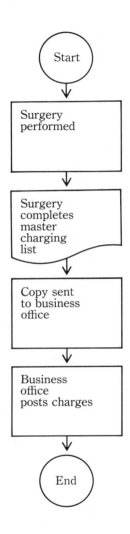

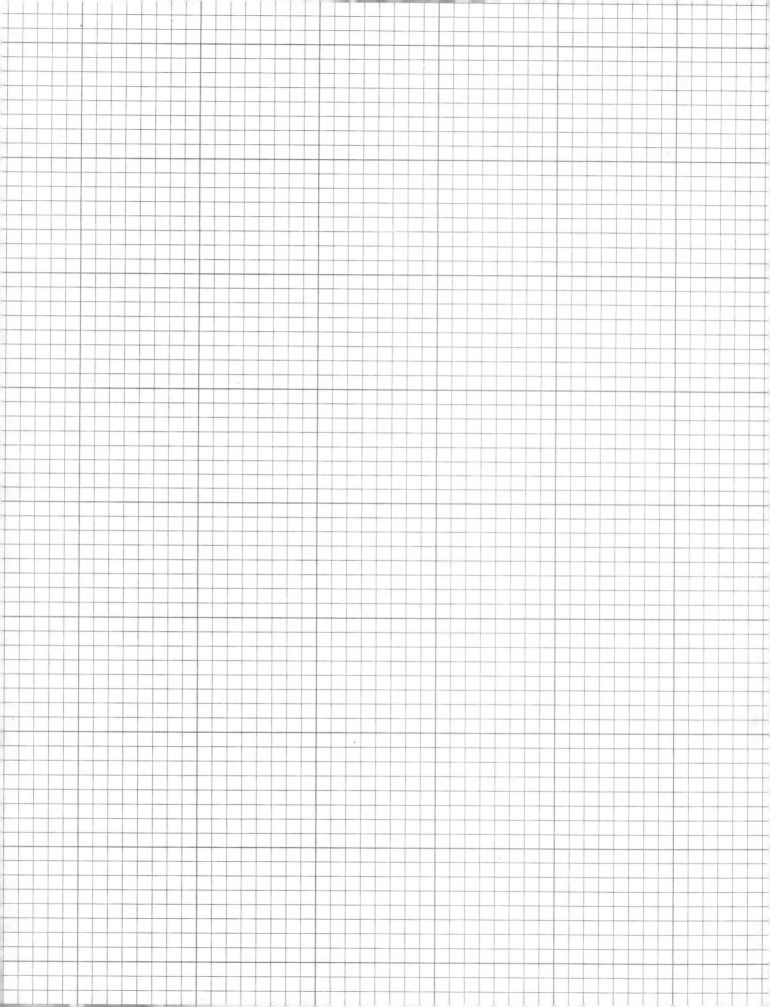

Flow Chart 5.1.1f

Central Service Supplies

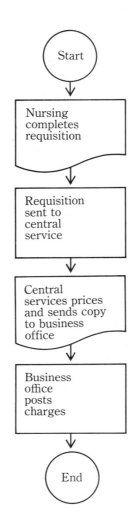

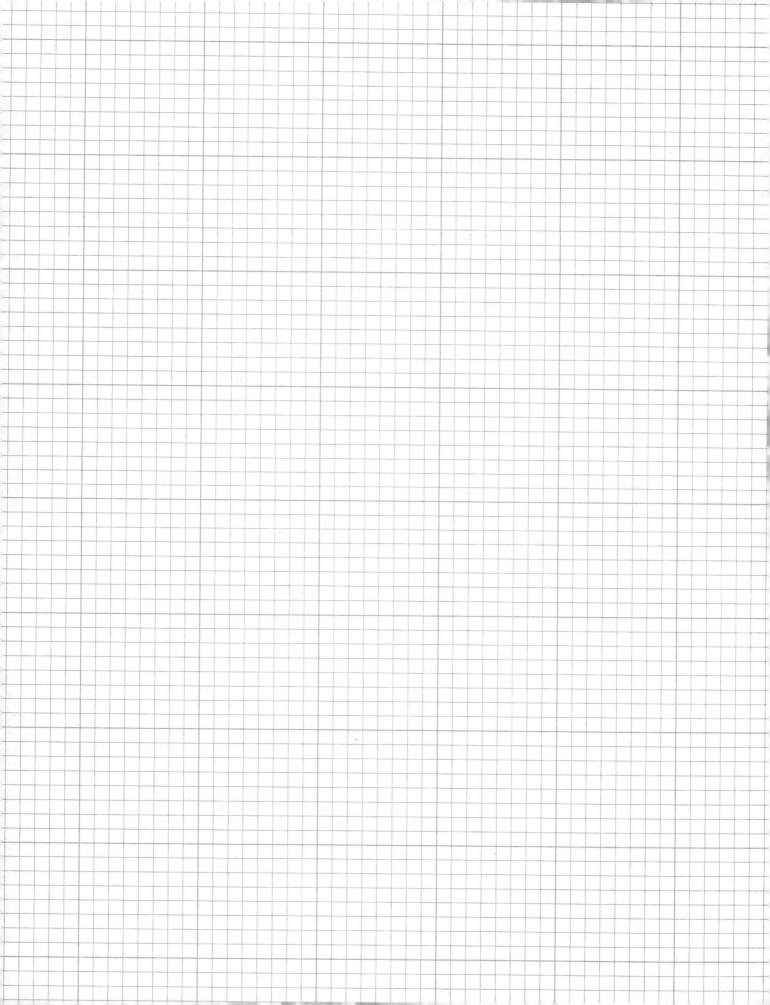

Flow Chart 5.1.1g

Storeroom Supplies

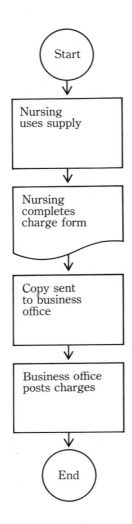

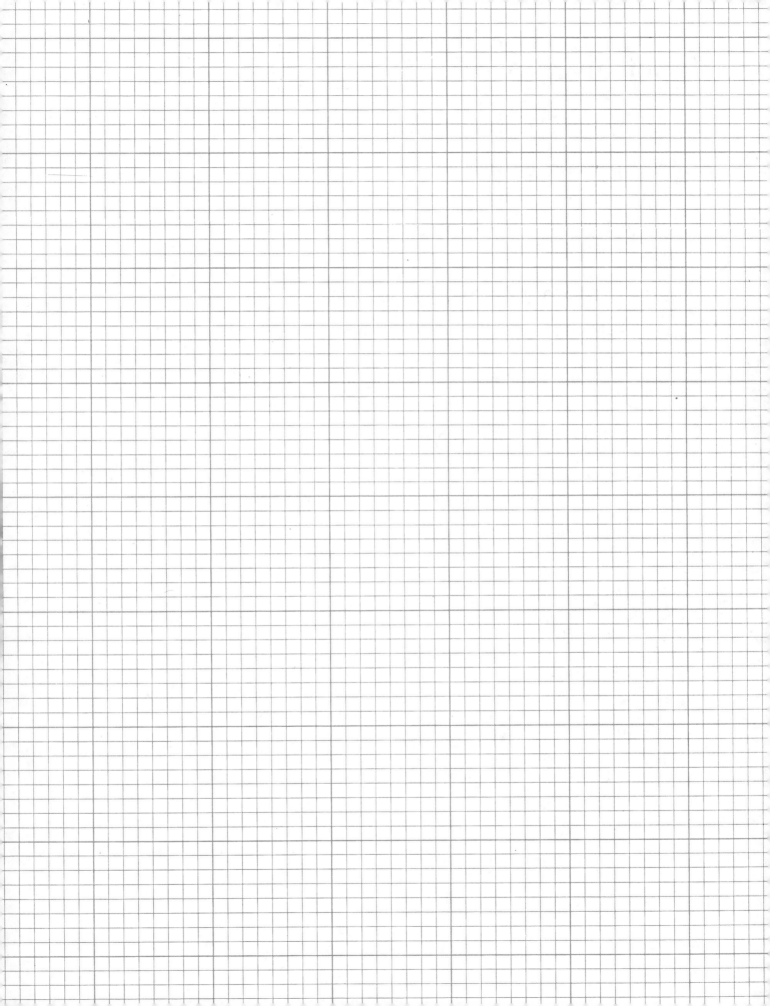

Input Inventory 5.1.1

your document title ↓

A. Admitting Department Head

1. Form used to notify the Business Office which room accesories the patient has selected.

A B C
□ □ □ _____

2. Form used to notify the Business Office that a patient has been admitted. (Normally, this is a copy of the admitting form.)

□ □ □ _____

B. Supervisor of the Posting Section

1. Account Card.

□ □ □ _____

2. Tally sheets used to keep track of daily charges, such as an ICU surcharge or an isolette charge.

□ □ □ _____

C. Clinical Department Heads

Form sent to the Business Office to record charges.

□ □ □ _____

D. Head Nurse

1. Requisition forms for all Clinical Departments

□ □ □ _____

- Radiology
- Laboratory
- Blood Bank
- Respiratory Therapy
- EKG
- EEG
- Physical Medicine
- Central Service
- Pharmacy
- Nuclear Medicine
- Storeroom

□ □ □ _____

2. Requisition from all Nursing Stations (Medical-Surgical, Pediatrics, ICU, Labor and Delivery, etc.). Request a sample of requisitions specifically designed for each unit.

□ □ □ _____

3. Physician Order Sheet.

□ □ □ _____

E. Surgery Department Head

A B C

1. Master Charge Sheet. ☐ ☐ ☐ _____

2. Any other document submitted to the
Business Office for charge purposes. ☐ ☐ ☐ _____

USE INPUT DOCUMENT ANALYSIS FORM

A = same document title	B = minor variations	C = significant differences

Master File Inventory 5.1.1

Notes
↓

A. Supervisor of the Posting Section

A B C

1. Account cards and charge tickets for current
patients. ☐ ☐ ☐ _____

2. Account cards and charge tickets for
discharged patients. ☐ ☐ ☐ _____

3. Incoming charge tickets. ☐ ☐ ☐ _____

B. Head Nurse

Copies of requisition forms. ☐ ☐ ☐ _____

C. Clinical Department Heads

Copies of requisitions from the Nursing
Stations, and copies of department-originated
charge tickets. ☐ ☐ ☐ _____

USE MASTER FILE ANALYSIS FORM

A = essentially similar	B = minor variations	C = significant differences

Report Inventory 5.1.1

A. Director of Finance

A B C

1. Daily and monthly revenue by revenue
center. ☐ ☐ ☐ _____

2. Price book. A listing of all chargeable
services and supplies, along with their prices.
Determine the mechanisms for: ☐ ☐ ☐ _____

- Entering new items and changing the prices for old items.

A B C
☐ ☐ ☐

your document title ↓
_____

- Establishing a charging mechanism for new items.

☐ ☐ ☐   _____

B. Director of Purchasing

Listing of all chargeable supplies sent directly to a Nursing Station.

☐ ☐ ☐   _____

USE REPORT ANALYSIS FORM

A = essentially similar	B = minor variations	C = significant differences

System Performance Standards 5.1.1

	Units	A	B
1. How long does it take for charge tickets to reach the Business Office?	days _____	☐	☐
2. How long does it take to post charges?	number of days from the time the charge arrives _____	☐	☐
3. Does the hospital have an accurate and up-to-date price book?	number of months since price book was completely repriced and reissued _____	☐	☐

USE PERFORMANCE STANDARDS ANALYSIS FORM

A = we have a standard	B = we do not have a standard

System Cost Factors 5.1.1

1. Lost Charges

   A. How much revenue is lost because services are rendered but no charge ticket is submitted? $ _____

   B. How much revenue is lost because an order is placed but the service is never performed? $ _____

   C. How much revenue is lost because an order is placed but cannot be carried out because the patient is discharged before the service department responds? $ _____

   D. How much revenue is lost because price changes aren't recognized? $ _____

   E. How much revenue is lost because new services and supplies are instituted without a charging mechanism being established? $ _____

2. What is the dollar volume lost because Central Service items are used but not billed? $ _____

3. How many charges are not posted because the patient's name and number are illegible on the requisition? $ _____

4. How many times are charges posted to the wrong account? $ _____

5. What is the cost of embossers used at the Nursing Station? $ _____

6. How much nursing time is used in completing requisitions? $ _____

7. How much time is spent in each clinical department preparing charge tickets for submittal to the posting area? $ _____

USE SYSTEM COST ANALYSIS FORM *(also see Instructions, p. 15)*

System 5.1.2: Credits

Description 5.1.2

Notes
↓

If a patient is erroneously charged for a service or supplies, a credit must be made on his or her account card. Normally errors occur when it is decided that a service or supply is not needed after a charge document has been sent to the Business Office for posting.

A B C
□ □ □ _____

A single form, called a Credit Slip, is used by all departments and by Nursing Stations.

□ □ □ _____

The Flow

For Radiology, Laboratory, Nuclear Medicine, EKG, EEG, Respiratory Therapy, Blood Bank, and Physical Medicine, the department initiates the Credit Slip. It is filled out with such essential items as patient's name and number, name of service, and charge; and sent to the Department Head or another supervisor for approval. It then goes to the Business Office for posting.

□ □ □ _____

For Central Service items, the Nursing Station fills out the Credit Slip and sends it to Central Service for pricing and review by the Department Head.

□ □ □ _____

With storeroom items, the Nursing Station fills out the Credit Slip completely and sends it directly to the Business Office.

□ □ □ _____

For drugs, the Nursing Station sends the unused medications back to Pharmacy, along with a card giving the patient's name and account number. Pharmacy fills out a Credit Slip, which is reviewed by the Department Head. If approved, it then goes to the Business Office for posting.

□ □ □ _____

Review

A supervisor in the Business Office, usually the Business Office Manager, reviews Credit Slips before passing them on to the posting section.

□ □ □ _____

A = essentially similar   B = minor variations   C = significant differences

Flow Chart 5.1.2

Credits

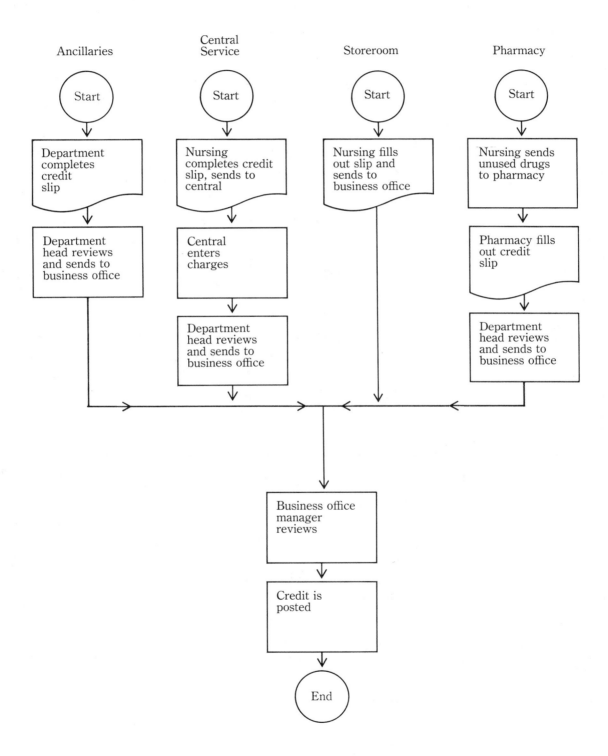

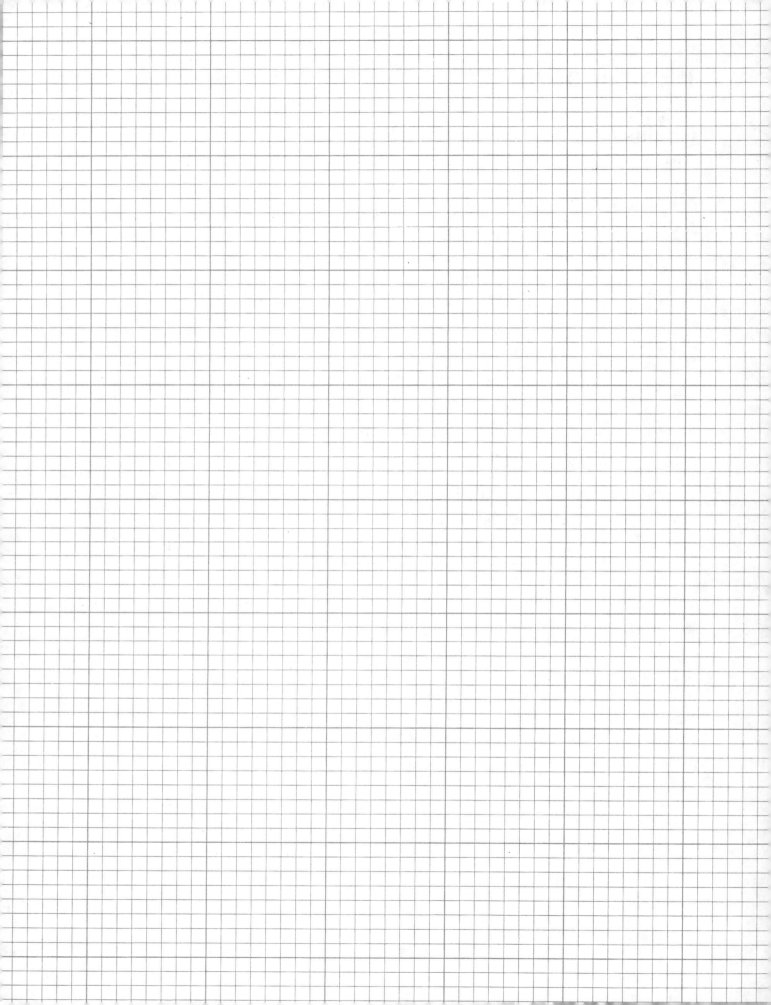

Input Inventory 5.1.2

A. Business Office Manager

your document title
↓

Credit Slip.

A B C
☐ ☐ ☐ _____

B. Head Nurse

Form used to identify patient when unused
drugs are returned to Pharmacy.

☐ ☐ ☐ _____

USE INPUT DOCUMENT ANALYSIS FORM

A = same document title   B = minor variations   C = significant differences

Master File Inventory 5.1.2

(none)

Report Inventory 5.1.2

A. Business Office Manager

your document title
↓

Daily listing of credits issued by each
department.

A B C
☐ ☐ ☐ _____

USE REPORT ANALYSIS FORM

A = essentially similar   B = minor variations   C = significant differences

System Performance Standards 5.1.2

	Units	A	B
1. How many people must give written approval before a credit is issued?	number of persons _____	☐	☐
2. What is the ratio of credits to total revenue?	percentage _____	☐	☐
3. What is the amount of credits issued?	monthly average in thousands of dollars _____	☐	☐
4. What is the amount of credits issued by Pharmacy?	monthly average in thousands of dollars _____	☐	☐

USE PERFORMANCE STANDARDS ANALYSIS FORM

A = we have a standard   B = we do not have a standard

System Cost Factors 5.1.2

1. How much revenue is lost because unjustified credits are submitted without validation by a supervisor? $ _____

2. How much delay is there in receiving payments because of questions from patients and insurance companies concerning missing charges? $ _____

USE SYSTEM COST ANALYSIS FORM *(also see Instructions, p. 15)*

System 5.1.3:
Billing

Description 5.1.3

Notice of Discharge

When the patient is discharged, the Nursing
Station notifies the Business Office. This notification triggers preparation of the patient's bill.

A B C
☐ ☐ ☐ _____

Late Charges

A requisition or other charge document that
arrives at the Business Office for posting after
the patient has been discharged is called a late
charge. Billing must be delayed until all charges
are collected and posted.

☐ ☐ ☐ _____

Therefore the time it takes for all charges to
reach the posting area establishes the minimum
time needed to produce a patient's bill.

☐ ☐ ☐ _____

Bill Preparation

Once late charges are in, the Business Office,
working from the account card, prepares a
detailed bill, which shows all services used by
the patient, along with a tabulation of the
charges for those services and supplies.

☐ ☐ ☐ _____

In most instances, the account card itself
contains this itemized tabulation, and it is
necessary only to add the late charges and check
the bill for accuracy.

☐ ☐ ☐ _____

Proration

Part of preparing the bill is determining how
much each insurance company involved with the
patient will pay, and how much will be left for
the patient to pay. This computation is called
proration.

☐ ☐ ☐ _____

The hospital may choose to start by billing the
entire amount to the major insurance carrier,
then bill what the first insurance company does
not pay to the second, and so on until an unpaid
balance remains for patient to pay.

☐ ☐ ☐ _____

A = essentially similar   B = minor variations   C = significant differences

Verification

Verification involves contacting insurance companies, usually by telephone, to determine if a patient actually has the coverage he or she claims.

A B C
□ □ □ _____

Medical Records

In order to bill many insurance companies, such as Blue Cross and the Medicare intermediary, it is necessary to have a discharge diagnosis on the bill.

□ □ □ _____

Obtaining this involves interaction between the Business Office and Medical Records.

□ □ □ _____

The most common approach is to have Medical Records enter the diagnosis on the bill. Another approach is to have Medical Records produce a daily listing of patients discharged and their discharge diagnoses.

□ □ □ _____

The time needed to get a discharge diagnosis depends on how long it takes physicians to enter the diagnosis on the face sheet of the patient's medical record.

□ □ □ _____

In-House Bills

An important collection tool is the bill produced on demand while the patient is still in the hospital. This allows the hospital to monitor the noninsured portion of each patient's bill and take action when that portion becomes excessive.

□ □ □ _____

Medicare

For Medicare patients in the hospital on December 31, the hospital must produce a year-end bill and start another bill for the period beginning January 1. Such a bill is called a straddle bill.

□ □ □ _____

Producing the Bill

Once all services are itemized, the actual bill, or bills, is produced.

□ □ □ _____

The itemized listing of services, supplies, and charges is usually done on a general-purpose billing form. A copy of this goes into the patient's file. If the patient has commercial insurance coverage (i.e., insurance other than

---

A = essentially similar   B = minor variations   C = significant differences

Blue Cross or a government-sponsored plan), a copy of the general-purpose bill goes to the insurance company.

A B C
☐ ☐ ☐ _____

Blue Cross, Medicare, Medicaid, and Workmen's Compensation require bills prepared on special forms.

☐ ☐ ☐ _____

Sending the Bill

Once all forms associated with the account of a discharged patient are completed, the bills are mailed. Account records are then transferred to the Business Office's collection section.

☐ ☐ ☐ _____

Notices or Statements

The itemized listing of services, supplies, and charges prepared at discharge is called a bill. Subsequent mailings to patients and to insurance companies concerning overdue accounts are called notes or statements.

☐ ☐ ☐ _____

A = essentially similar B = minor variations C = significant differences

Flow Chart 5.1.3

Billing

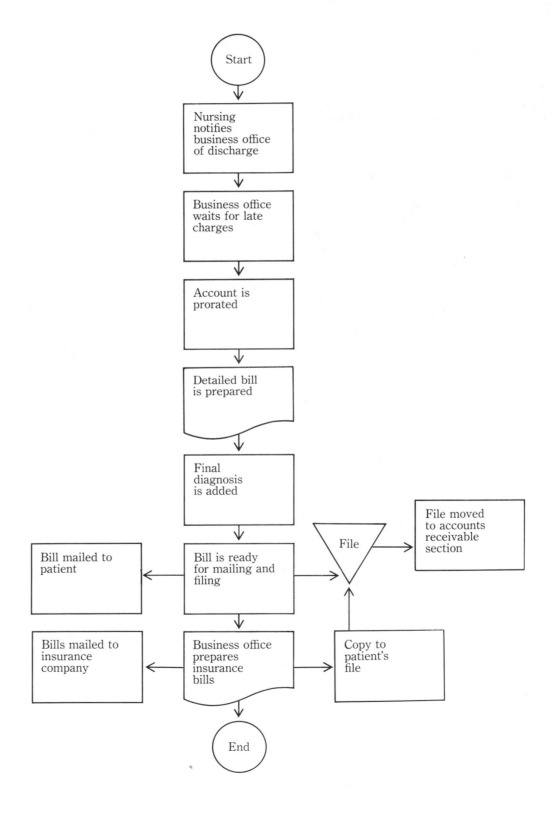

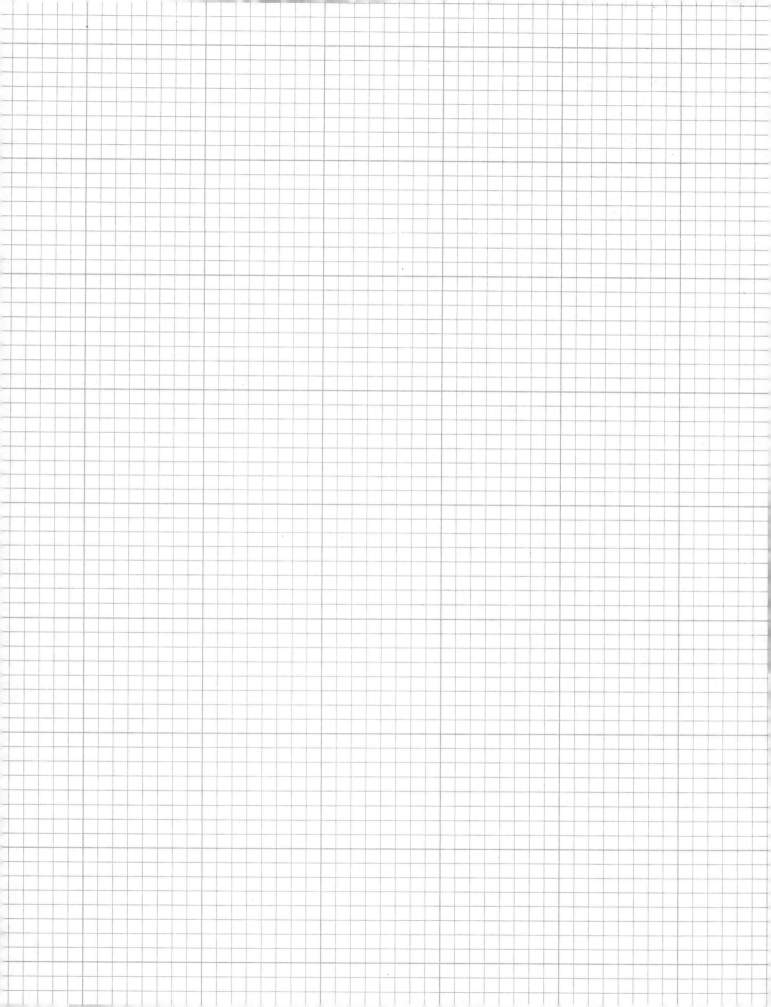

Input Inventory 5.1.3

A. Business Office Manager

your document title ↓

A B C

1. All billing forms, including:

☐ ☐ ☐ _____

- General-purpose bill
- Blue Cross bill
- Medicare bill
- Medicaid bill
- Welfare bill
- Workmen's Compensation bill
- Special bills for certain commercial insurance companies

☐ ☐ ☐ _____

2. Form used for estimating amount of bill each insurance company will pay.

☐ ☐ ☐ _____

3. Form used to record verification of insurance.

☐ ☐ ☐ _____

4. Form used to record discharge diagnosis. This form is prepared in Medical Records and sent to the Business Office.

☐ ☐ ☐ _____

USE INPUT DOCUMENT ANALYSIS FORM

A = same document title	B = minor variations	C = significant differences

Master File Inventory 5.1.3

A. Business Office Manager

Notes ↓

1. Description of each type of insurance policy encountered by the hospital. For each policy, the hospital should know the name and mailing address of the carrier, the amount and limits of coverage, the method of computing and the deductible or coinsurance figure.

A B C

☐ ☐ ☐ _____

2. Discharged patients not yet billed. These are the accounts being held for late charges.

☐ ☐ ☐ _____

USE MASTER FILE ANALYSIS FORM

A = essentially similar	B = minor variations	C = significant differences

Report Inventory 5.1.3

A. Business Office Manager

your document title
↓

1. Daily listing of bills produced. This should show patient name, amount billed to each carrier, amount billed to the patient, total amount billed, and the insurance category or subcategory.

A B C
☐ ☐ ☐ _____

2. Medical Records Control. Listing of accounts forwarded to Medical Records for insertion of discharge diagnosis.

☐ ☐ ☐ _____

USE REPORT ANALYSIS FORM

A = essentially similar	B = minor variations	C = significant differences

System Performance Standards 5.1.3

Units

		A	B
1. How long are accounts held pending the arrival of late charges?	days _____	☐	☐
2. How long does it take from the time a patient is discharged to produce a bill?	days _____	☐	☐
3. How many bills are returned unpaid by insurance companies and other third parties?	monthly average number ____	☐	☐
4. What percentage of bills being sent to third parties have been verified as to coverage?	percentage of total third-party bills _____	☐	☐
5. How many bills are being held pending determination of a final diagnosis?	number of bills _____	☐	☐

USE PERFORMANCE STANDARDS ANALYSIS FORM

A = we have a standard	B = we do not have a standard

System Cost Factors 5.1.3

1. How much time and money is spent in copying bills and associated documents? $ _____

2. What special equipment is used in preparing bills (bursters, stamping machines, etc.)? $ _____

3. How much time is lost in filing and retrieving bills? $ _____

4. What effect does the inability to prorate have on the hospital's days in receivables and collection rate? $ _____

5. How many patients, particularly outpatients and ED patients, would pay their bills at the time of dismissal if a complete bill could be prepared instantaneously? $ _____

USE SYSTEM COST ANALYSIS FORM *(also see Instructions, p. 15)*

System 5.1.4:
Accounts Receivable
Description 5.1.4

Reports

A major portion of accounts receivable activity involves preparing and distributing reports on transactions involving individual accounts. Accounts receivable reports also summarize the overall collection effort of the hospital.

A B C
☐ ☐ ☐ _____

Reports on individual accounts highlight the amount owed by the involved insurance companies, the amount owed by the patient, the age of the account as computed from the date of discharge, and the dates of the most recent payments from the insurance companies and the patient.

☐ ☐ ☐ _____

The most common accounts receivable reports are the Aged Trial Balances, which first sort the accounts by primary payment source – Blue Cross, Medicaid, patient, etc. – then sort within those categories by age of the account.

☐ ☐ ☐ _____

Statements

If the patient does not pay within some pre-determined time after receiving the bill, a series of statements is sent to him or her. Each statement contains a harsher dunning message than the preceding one.

☐ ☐ ☐ _____

Payments

The Account Receivable activity also includes posting and reporting payments.

☐ ☐ ☐ _____

Payments come to the hospital in two ways – checks mailed in and cash turned in at a Cashier Station. Checks from insurance companies may cover more than one patient's account. When they do, they are accompanied by a pay listing that tells how much to apply to each account.

☐ ☐ ☐ _____

A = essentially similar   B = minor variations   C = significant differences

Transfers

Receivables fall into three major categories —
insurance-pay, patient-pay, and bad debt. Within
the insurance-pay section, there are several
subcategories — usually Medicare, Blue Cross,
Medicaid, Workmen's Compensation, and local
welfare.

A B C

☐ ☐ ☐ _____

Accounts may move from category to category.
The category or subcategory at any given time
is determined by who is responsible for the
largest percentage of the account. For example,
an account may start out in the Blue Cross
subcategory, but if Blue Cross pays its portion,
the account then is transferred to another
category or subcategory.

☐ ☐ ☐ _____

Eventually, after all insurance companies have
paid their share, the balance is transferred to the
patient-pay category.

☐ ☐ ☐ _____

If the patient does not pay within the time
period specified by the hospital, the account is
transferred to bad debt and turned over to a
collection agency. The hospital must maintain
follow-up records of accounts turned over to the
collection agency.

☐ ☐ ☐ _____

A = essentially similar   B = minor variations   C = significant differences

316

Flow Chart 5.1.4

Accounts Receivable

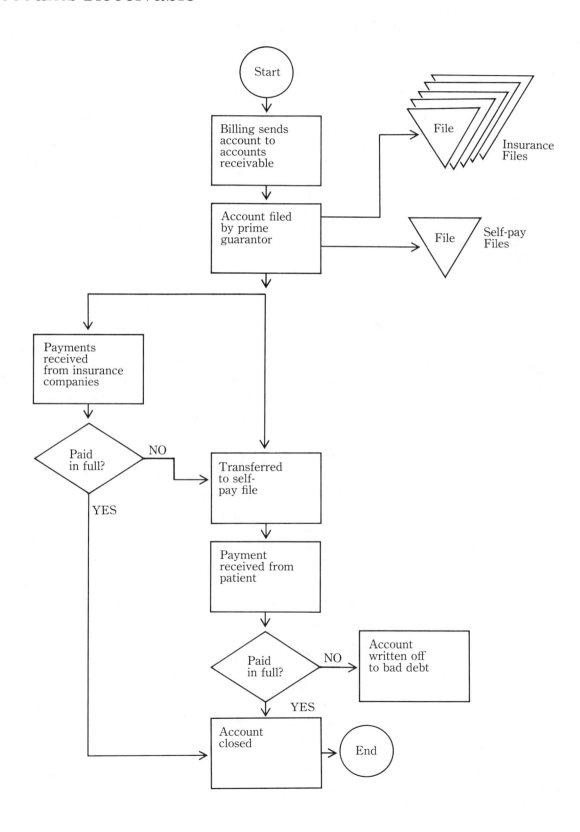

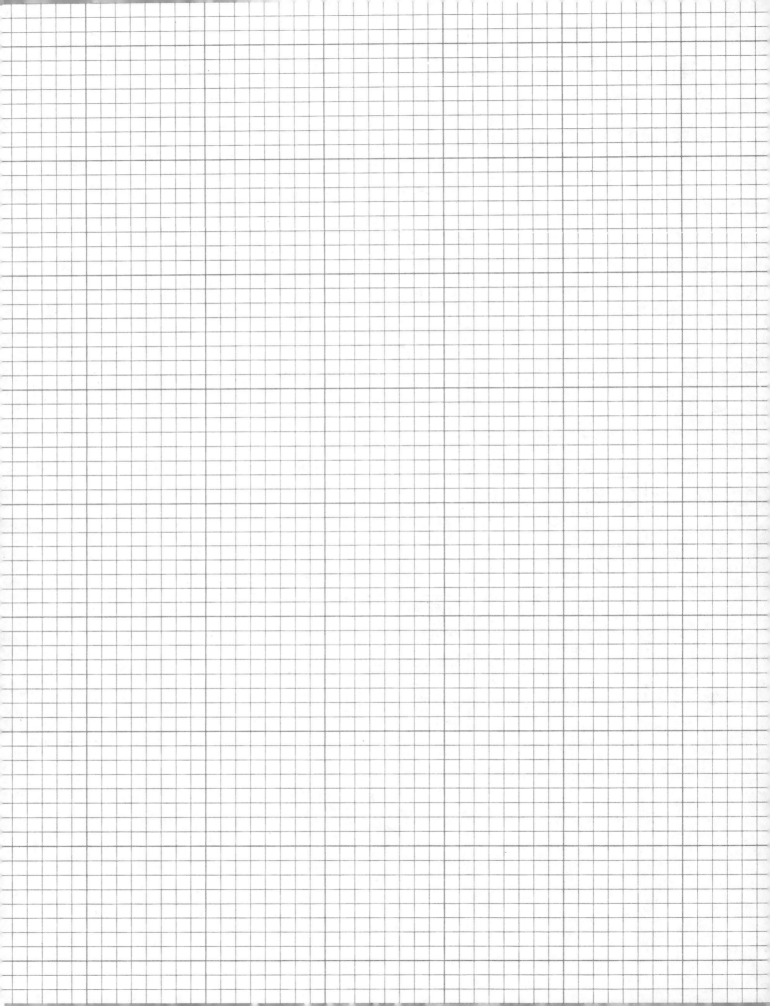

Input Inventory 5.1.4

A. Business Office Manager

your document title
↓

1. Log for recording receipt of account payments

    A   B   C
    ☐   ☐   ☐   _____

2. Account history. This is a form on which a Billing or Credit Clerk records the results of conversations with the account guarantor and with involved insurance companies.

    ☐   ☐   ☐   _____

USE INPUT DOCUMENT ANALYSIS FORM

A = same document title	B = minor variations	C = significant differences

Master File Inventory 5.1.4

A. Business Office Manager

Notes
↓

1. Patient Accounts. There are two common methods of filing accounts while they are in the Accounts Receivable section:

    A   B   C
    ☐   ☐   ☐   _____

- All accounts are filed together in alphabetical order.

    ☐   ☐   ☐   _____

- Accounts are sorted according to their insurance classification, then filed alphabetically within that classification.

    ☐   ☐   ☐   _____

2. Patient Accounts/Bad Debt. This file contains accounts that are delinquent and have been turned over to a Collection Agency or to an attorney.

    ☐   ☐   ☐   _____

USE MASTER FILE ANALYSIS FORM

A = essentially similar	B = minor variations	C = significant differences

Report Inventory 5.1.4

A. Business Office Manager

your document title
↓

1. Trial Balances. These come in a variety of formats. Ask for trial balances and any other listings of accounts used in posting payments and pursuing collection efforts.

    A   B   C
    ☐   ☐   ☐   _____

2. Daily report of cash (currency and checks) received and posted.

    ☐   ☐   ☐   _____

3. Listing of accounts transferred from one insurance category to another, or from an insurance category to the patient-pay category.

A B C
☐ ☐ ☐ _____

4. Listing of accounts transferred to the bad debt category.

☐ ☐ ☐ _____

5. Listing of money owed the hospital from previous accounts. This report should be checked before any refunds are made.

☐ ☐ ☐ _____

6. Collection rate by insurance category.

☐ ☐ ☐ _____

USE REPORT ANALYSIS FORM

A = essentially similar	B = minor variations	C = significant differences

System Performance Standards 5.1.4

Units

1. How many statements are sent to a patient each month?

number of statements sent in a 30-day period to a self-pay patient _____

A B
☐ ☐

2. How many accounts are turned over to a collection agency?

monthly average number ____

☐ ☐

3. How much money is written off?

monthly average in thousands of dollars _____

☐ ☐

4. How many times is a trial balance prepared?

number of times each year __

☐ ☐

5. How many types of trial balances are prepared?

number_____

☐ ☐

6. What is the number of days in receivables for third-party accounts?

days _____

☐ ☐

7. What is the number of days in receivables for self-pay accounts?

days _____

☐ ☐

8. What is the collection rate?

percentage _____

☐ ☐

USE PERFORMANCE STANDARDS ANALYSIS FORM

A = we have a standard	B = we do not have a standard

System Cost Factors 5.1.4

1. How much time is spent in preparing trial balances?

$ _____

2. What is the amount of adjustment each time a trial balance is prepared?

$ _____

3. How much time is needed to process payments (i.e., find the account and post the payment) and deposit them? $ _____

4. How much money is refunded to patients without checking to see if they owe for previous visits or stays? $ _____

USE SYSTEM COST ANALYSIS FORM *(also see Instructions, p. 15)*

System 5.2: Budgeting

Description 5.2

Budgeting is a two-part process, with the first part involving actual preparation. Once each year, a master budget for the institution is established, with most of the preparation responsibility resting with the Office of Financial Affairs. The second part of the budgeting process is the ongoing preparation and distribution of reports that show how well each department is performing in relation to budgetary projections.

A B C
☐ ☐ ☐ _____

Preparation

Practically every hospital prepares one budget yearly, with the budgetary period coinciding with the hospital's fiscal year. At a fixed time before the beginning of the fiscal year, the Chief Financial Officer distributes budgetary worksheets to all departments. These forms are intended to gather each department's projections for the next year's activity, personnel requirements, supply needs, revenue to be generated, and equipment needs.

☐ ☐ ☐ _____

Normally, the Department Heads are required to explain their revenue projections, defend their equipment and supply cost requests, and justify any increases in personnel.

☐ ☐ ☐ _____

The worksheets arrive at the Office of Financial Affairs, where they are reviewed and consolidated into a proposed master budget. This document is then reviewed and modified by various individuals or groups of individuals – a Budget Committee, Department Heads, physicians, and Medical Staff representatives. Eventually the budget is sent to the Chief Executive. If the Chief Executive approves it, he or she then presents it to the hospital's governing body.

☐ ☐ ☐ _____

After the budget has been approved by all parties, the Office of Financial Affairs returns copies to the individual departments. At least one complete master copy is kept by the Director of Fiscal Affairs.

☐ ☐ ☐ _____

Cash Budget

After the Director of Finance completes the master budget, he or she prepares a cash budget. This document is used in determining cash outlays, short term borrowing needs, new equipment purchases, and expenditures for other capital items.

A B C
☐ ☐ ☐ _____

Analysis

Over the course of the fiscal year, the Director of Finance continually analyzes the performance of each department in relation to its budget.

☐ ☐ ☐ _____

The Director of Finance obtains the needed information from a large number of reports coming from all parts of the institution. For example, Purchasing usually generates a report on all items purchased by each department. This document helps the director evaluate a department's actual supply use as compared with its projected use.

☐ ☐ ☐ _____

In most hospitals, the Director of Finance produces budget analysis reports monthly. Typically, they show month-to-date and year-to-date performance.

☐ ☐ ☐ _____

These are distributed to Department Heads and to appropriate administrative officers.

☐ ☐ ☐ _____

Another important output of the budgetary process is a series of long-range (five years and longer) forecasts based on the analysis of demographic, technological, epidemiological, economic, and sociological data. These forecasts are used to develop a hospital master plan, plan capital investments, and prepare for Certificate-of-Need (see System 1).

☐ ☐ ☐ _____

A = essentially similar   B = minor variations   C = significant differences

Flow Chart 5.2a

Preparation

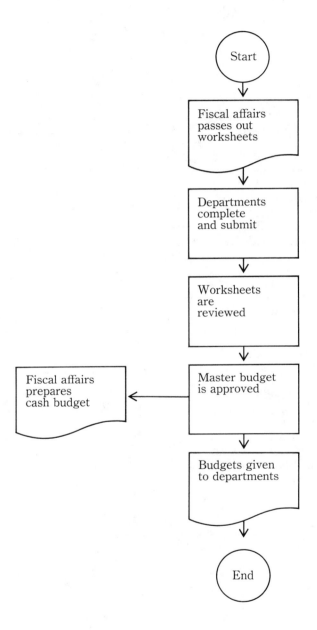

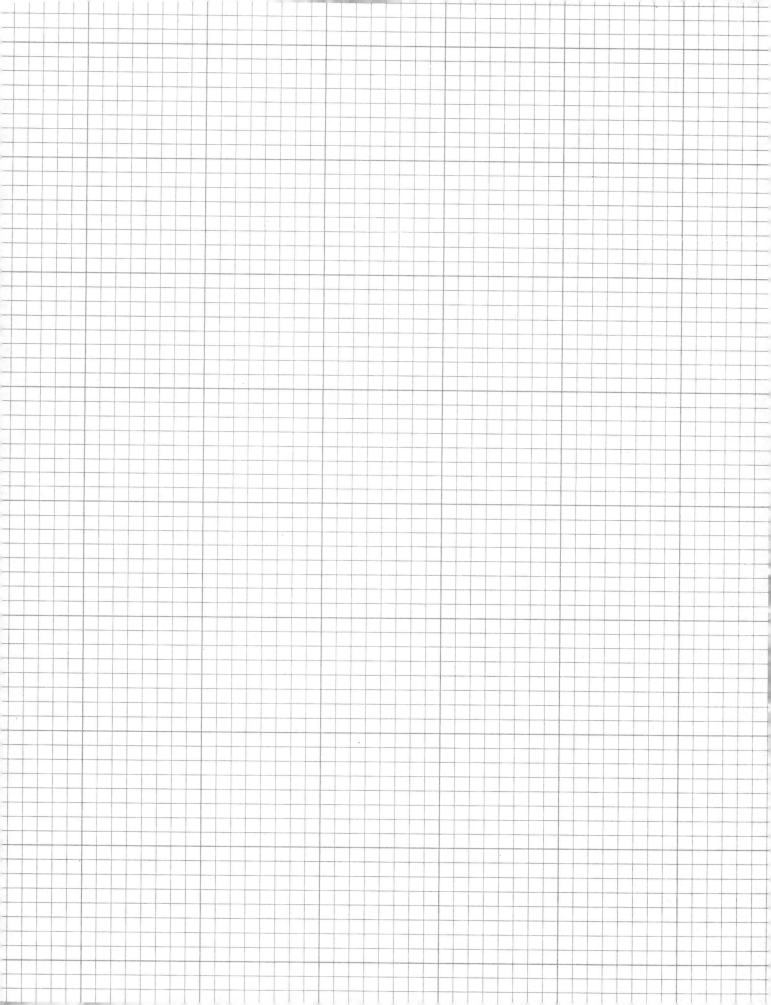

Flow Chart 5.2b

Budget Analysis

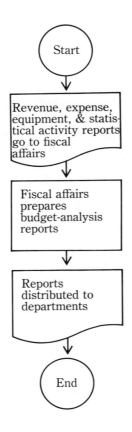

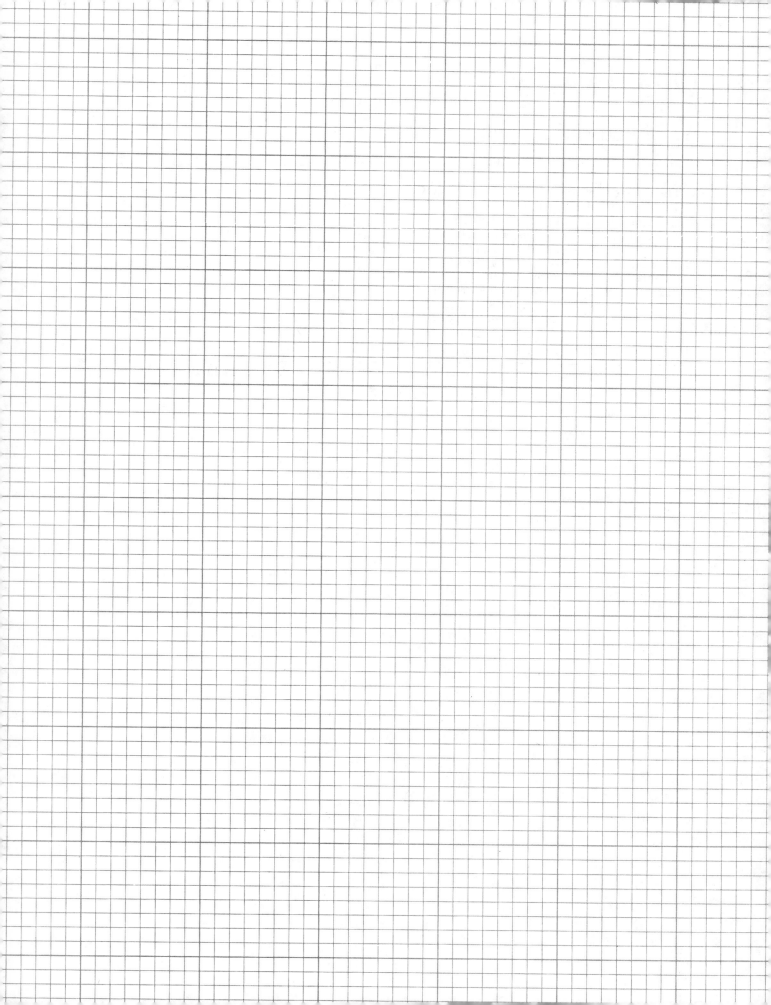

Input Inventory 5.2

A. Director of Finance

A B C

1. Budget Worksheets.

☐ ☐ ☐ _____

2. The number and variety of reports the flow into the Financial Affairs Office for use in preparing the budget analysis Reports vary widely from hospital to hospital. The form on the following page should be used to determine what information the Director of Financial Affairs receives and the source of this information. The code number refers to the code number of the report shown on its Input or Report inventory form.

☐ ☐ ☐ _____

USE INPUT DOCUMENT ANALYSIS FORM

A = same document title   B = minor variations   C = significant differences

BUDGET INVENTORY

Name of Report	Report Code	Key Information Report Contains	Who Submits it?	How Often

Master File Inventory 5.2

A. Director of Finance

Notes
↓

        A B C

1. Budgetary Worksheets.   ☐ ☐ ☐ _____

2. Master Budget.   ☐ ☐ ☐ _____

3. Budgetary Analysis Forms.   ☐ ☐ ☐ _____

4. Source documents for Analysis Forms.   ☐ ☐ ☐ _____

5. Historical Data:

   - workhours
   - revenue
   - output
   - expenses   ☐ ☐ ☐ _____

USE MASTER FILE ANALYSIS FORM

A = essentially similar   B = minor variations   C = significant differences

Report Inventory 5.2

A. Director of Finance

your document title
↓

        A B C

1. Master budget.   ☐ ☐ ☐ _____

2. Cash budget.   ☐ ☐ ☐ _____

3. Budget Analysis Forms.   ☐ ☐ ☐ _____

USE REPORT ANALYSIS FORM

A = essentially similar   B = minor variations   C = significant differences

System Performance Standards 5.2

                                Units   A B

1. Does the hospital have a budget?   yes or no _____ ☐ ☐

2. How often are budget analysis reports prepared?

   0 – never
   1 – monthly
   2 – quarterly
   3 – semiannually
   4 – yearly _____ ☐ ☐

3. How much in advance must Department Heads submit their budget worksheets?

   number of months before
   the start of the next
   fiscal year _____ ☐ ☐

4. How close did the hospital come last year to meeting its revenue projections? percentage _____ Units A ☐ B ☐

5. How close did the hospital come to meeting its expense projections last year? percentage _____ ☐ ☐

6. How many days after the close of an accounting period are budget analysis reports released to cost center managers? days _____ ☐ ☐

USE PERFORMANCE STANDARDS ANALYSIS FORM

A = we have a standard   B = we do not have a standard

System Cost Factors 5.2

1. How many workhours are spent in preparing the budget? $ _____

2. How many workhours are spent in preparing the analysis reports? $ _____

USE SYSTEM COST ANALYSIS FORM *(also see Instructions, p. 15)*

System 5.3: Accounts Payable

Description 5.3

When orders for material or services are placed, the Accounts Payable Section receives a copy of the Purchase Order (PO). This establishes an account payable.

The Accounts Payable Section must know the quantities, item description, unit price, vendor, and terms of purchase. In addition, Purchasing notifies this section when services have not been performed or ordered, or items do not meet specifications.

When the ordered item is received or when the service has been performed, Purchasing sends Accounts Payable a completed receiving copy of the PO. This authorizes Accounts Payable to initiate payment.

To minimize the number of checks written and to improve control, some hospitals only issue one check per month per vendor. Other hospitals take this one step further and only pay after a single monthly summary bill, or statement, has been received.

When this document is received, Accounts Payable prepares a payment voucher, which is sent to the Treasurer, who prepares a check and sends it to the vendor.

Each voucher is verified by an Accounts Payable Voucher Control Number and a Voucher Control Number log. Accounts Payable assigns the number and maintains the log.

The voucher itself must be supported by a copy of the PO, a copy of the receiving report, and the vendor's invoice. This material is filed in voucher-number sequence.

Once payment has been made, the Treasurer sends Accounts Payable a copy of the voucher. Accounts Payable then notifies the Accounting Section which posts the payment.

Notes

A B C

Reports

The reports prepared by Accounts Payable are primarily concerned with the management of

---

A = essentially similar   B = minor variations   C = significant differences

332

cash, the amounts paid to individual vendors over a certain time period, the amounts of purchase returns, the services not performed and the purchase discounts not taken.

A B C
☐ ☐ ☐ _____

Periodic forecasts of Accounts Payable to be paid assist the Treasurer in managing cash disbursements.

☐ ☐ ☐ _____

The Discounts Lost Report records the name of the vendor, the amount of the Purchase Discount Lost, and an explanation as to why the discount was lost.

☐ ☐ ☐ _____

Additional management information is secured by monthly reports, which analyze by vendor and by item how much was spent and the reason for all Purchase Returns and Contractual Services Not Properly Performed. This information provides management with indications as to when to negotiate changes in contractual terms, when to negotiate contracts with new vendors, when to consider changing particular material items, and when to consider performing services inhouse rather than using outside contractors.

☐ ☐ ☐ _____

These reports are primarily distributed outside the section for decision-making use by the Purchasing Department, the Treasurer, the Director of Finance, and the administrative staff.

☐ ☐ ☐ _____

A = essentially similar   B = minor variations   C = significant differences

Flow Chart 5.3

Accounts Payable

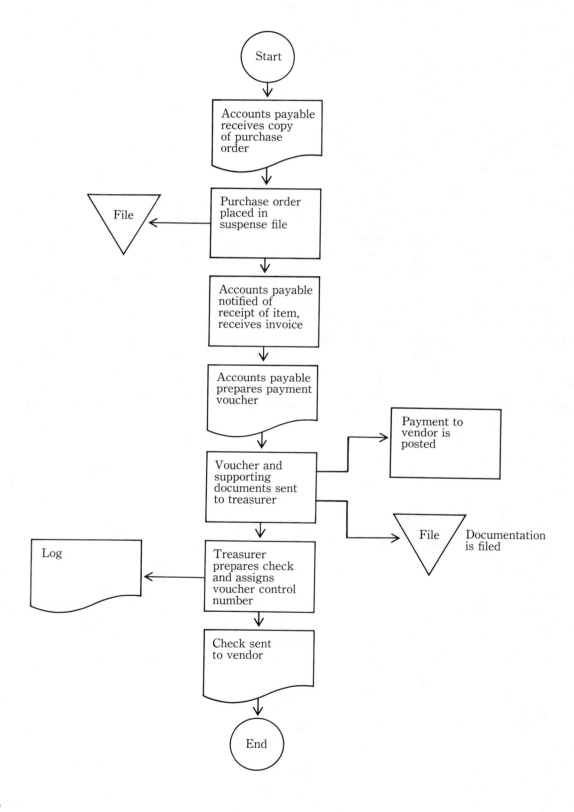

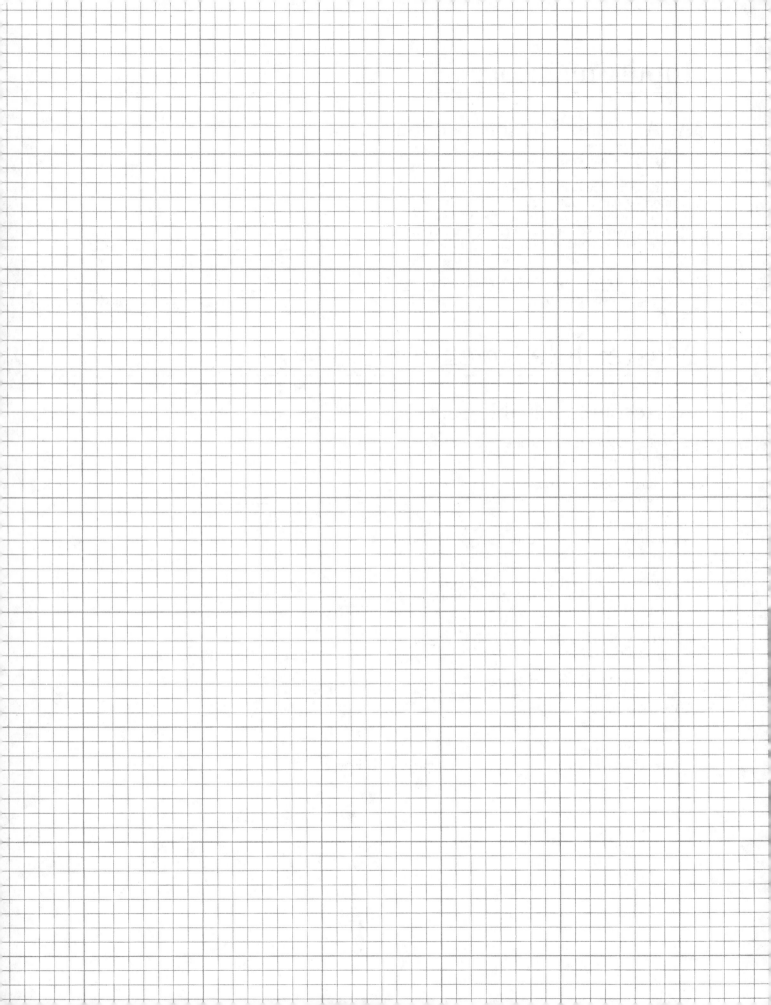

Input Inventory 5.3

A. Accounts Payable Section

your document title
↓

A B C

1. Payment vouchers. ☐ ☐ ☐ _____

2. Vendor history. This is the form on which all
information pertaining to the vendor is
maintained (e.g., normal and special vendor
terms, conversations with vendor regarding
payments on billings, prior annual business). ☐ ☐ ☐ _____

USE INPUT DOCUMENT ANALYSIS FORM

A = same document title	B = minor variations	C = significant differences

Master File Inventory 5.3

A. Accounts Payable Section

Notes
↓

A B C

1. Vendor Accounts. These are filed in alphabetical sequence. ☐ ☐ ☐ _____

2. Purchase Discounts Lost. These are filed in
alphabetical sequence by vendor. ☐ ☐ ☐ _____

3. Accounts Payable to be Paid. These are filed
in vendor alphabetical sequence by date when
payment is due. The only accounts shown
here are those accounts for which a payment
voucher has not yet been prepared even
though a vendor invoice or statement has
been received. ☐ ☐ ☐ _____

4. Purchase Returns. These are filed in vendor
alphabetical sequence. ☐ ☐ ☐ _____

5. Contractual Services Not Properly Performed. These are filed in vendor alphabetical sequence. ☐ ☐ ☐ _____

USE MASTER FILE ANALYSIS FORM

A = essentially similar	B = minor variations	C = significant differences

Report Inventory 5.3

A. Accounts Payable Section

your document title
↓

1. Daily listing of payment vouchers prepared. This is used as a control between the Accounts Payable Section and the Treasurer. It is also the basis for posting the subsidiary ledger.

   A B C
   ☐ ☐ ☐ _____

2. Daily listing of Accounts Payable to be Paid.
   ☐ ☐ ☐ _____

3. Purchase Discounts Lost Report.
   ☐ ☐ ☐ _____

4. Vendor Summary Report. This listing is prepared quarterly or annually.
   ☐ ☐ ☐ _____

USE REPORT ANALYSIS FORM

A = essentially similar	B = minor variations	C = significant differences

System Performance Standards 5.3

Units

1. What proportion of the hospital's Payment Vouchers has to be expedited through the Accounts Payable Section to insure a Purchase Discount can be taken?

                          A B

   number per month _____ ☐ ☐

2. What purchase discounts offered are lost?
   dollars per month _____ ☐ ☐

3. How many days does it take to process a vendor's invoice?
   days _____ ☐ ☐

4. What is the percentage of duplicate payments made to vendors?
   percentage _____ ☐ ☐

5. What proportion of duplicate invoices or statements has to be requested from vendors?
   percentage _____ ☐ ☐

6. What proportion of duplicate POs or receiving reports has to be requested from Purchasing or Receiving?
   percentage _____ ☐ ☐

7. What is the current value of days in Accounts Payable?
   current dollar volume of accounts payable divided by total of such purchases times 365 _____ ☐ ☐

USE PERFORMANCE STANDARDS ANALYSIS FORM

A = we have a standard	B = we do not have a standard

System Cost Factors 5.3

What is the average balance of the checking account used to pay accounts payable?

$ _____

USE SYSTEM COST ANALYSIS FORM *(also see Instructions, p. 15)*

System 5.4:
General Accounting

Description 5.4

Notes
↓

The Flow

No other system has as many interface requirements as the General Accounting system. By its very nature, this system must interface with all of the systems of the financial management component as well as with systems from Manpower Management, Materials Management, Facilities and Equipment Planning and Control. Operating under the purview of the Director of Finance's general accounting section, General Accounting makes both summary and special entries for the General Ledger and General Journal, prepares trial balance, makes adjusting entries for periodic statements, and prepares financial reports.

A B C
□ □ □ _____

Practically all departments in the hospital send reports and other documents to General Accounting. These data are the basis for entries into both the General Ledger and the General Journal.

□ □ □ _____

On a monthly basis, this section prepares financial statements for the institution. At a minimum, this involves preparing an earning statement and a balance sheet.

□ □ □ _____

At the end of the year, General Accounting closes the books, prepares year-end financial statements, and prepares the financial reports required by third parties and other outside agencies. Most notable of these reports is the Medicare Cost Report, which the Social Security Administration uses in establishing reimbursement rates for Medicare patients.

□ □ □ _____

General Accounting also furnishes a daily listing of summary and special transactions to concerned elements of the organization, to verify which transactions have been entered into the records.

□ □ □ _____

In addition, periodic (monthly, quarterly and annual) trial balances are prepared. From the trial balances, adjusting entries are prepared and posted.

□ □ □ _____

A = essentially similar   B = minor variations   C = significant differences

Other Revenue

Other revenue activities may exist. Depending upon the extent of these functions within the institution, accounting for them is either centralized in the Director of Finance's Office or scattered throughout the organization.

A B C
☐ ☐ ☐ _____

These revenue activities may be limited to administrative services, like the hospital's cafeteria, and investment portfolio management. On the other hand, they may include the accounting activities for professional buildings owned and operated by the hospital and even activities unrelated to the delivery of health care.

☐ ☐ ☐ _____

Reports

The reports for other Revenue Accounting consist primarily of daily billings for services furnished, records of revenue received from investments, and price listings for services furnished. On a weekly or monthly basis, reports are furnished on aged receivables, bad debts, and the analysis of returns on investments. Status reports on the composition and value of the investment portfolio are also furnished. Finally, status reports on donations and pledges are furnished on a monthly basis.

☐ ☐ ☐ _____

Notes
↓

A = essentially similar   B = minor variations   C = significant differences

340

Flow Chart 5.4

General Accounting

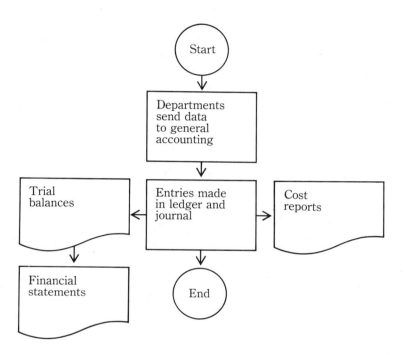

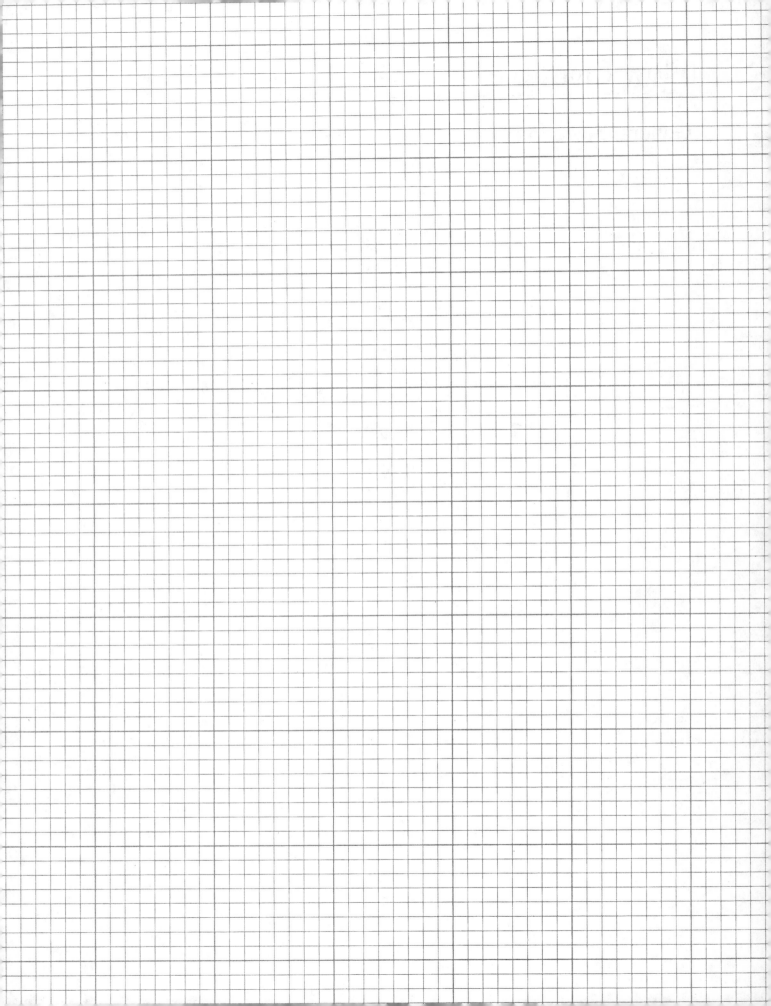

Input Inventory 5.4

A. General Accounting Section

A B C

Memoranda of financial events. ☐ ☐ ☐ _____

B. Business Manager

Summary accounts receivable data. ☐ ☐ ☐ _____

C. Accounts Payable Section

Summary accounts payable data. ☐ ☐ ☐ _____

D. Treasurer

Summary cash transactions data. ☐ ☐ ☐ _____

E. Other Revenue Accounting Section

1. Summary revenue data. ☐ ☐ ☐ _____

2. Summary status data. ☐ ☐ ☐ _____

F. Payroll Section

1. Summary payroll data. ☐ ☐ ☐ _____

2. Summary taxes payable data. ☐ ☐ ☐ _____

G. Inventory Control Section

Physical inventory data. ☐ ☐ ☐ _____

H. Comptroller

1. Chart of accounts. ☐ ☐ ☐ _____

2. Adjustment entry memoranda. ☐ ☐ ☐ _____

I. Director of Donations and Pledges

1. Receipt of donation. ☐ ☐ ☐ _____

2. Receipt of pledge. ☐ ☐ ☐ _____

3. Receipt of payment on pledge. ☐ ☐ ☐ _____

J. Business Office Manager

Bill/Receipt for administrative services.

A B C
☐ ☐ ☐ _____

K. Treasurer

1. Receipt of interest due/dividend paid.   ☐ ☐ ☐ _____

2. Financial investment transaction notification.   ☐ ☐ ☐ _____

L. Cafeteria Manager

1. Summary of cash receipts.   ☐ ☐ ☐ _____

2. Meal charge slips.   ☐ ☐ ☐ _____

M. Other Activity Managers

1. Summary of cash receipts.   ☐ ☐ ☐ _____

2. Bill/Receipt for services.   ☐ ☐ ☐ _____

The number and variety of reports that flow into the General Accounting Section for use in making Ledger and Journal entries vary widely from hospital to hospital. The form on the following page should be used to determine exactly what information General Accounting receives and from where it is received. The code number refers to the code number of the report shown on its Input or Report Inventory Form.   ☐ ☐ ☐ _____

USE INPUT DOCUMENT ANALYSIS FORM

A = same document title   B = minor variations   C = significant differences

GENERAL ACCOUNTING INVENTORY

Name of Report	Report Code	Key Information Report Contains	Who Submits It?	How Often

Master File Inventory 5.4

A. General Accounting Section

1. Chart of Accounts. This specifies what accounts will be used, the amount of detail required, the summary accounts and their method of aggregation.

   A B C
   □ □ □ _____

2. Hospital Cost Report Allocation File. This is used to allocate costs for the annual hospital cost report files.

   □ □ □ _____

3. General Ledger.

   □ □ □ _____

4. General Journal.

   □ □ □ _____

5. Departmental reports.

   □ □ □ _____

B. Director of Finance

1. Donor File. This file is maintained in alphabetical sequence and includes the amount, date, and conditions, if any, for each donation of cash.

   □ □ □ _____

2. Outstanding Pledges File. This file is maintained in alphabetical sequence and includes the total amount of the pledge and the dates and increments of each scheduled payment.

   □ □ □ _____

3. Accounts Receivable – Administrative Services.

   □ □ □ _____

4. Accounts Receivable – Meal Charges.

   □ □ □ _____

5. Accounts Receivable – Other Revenue Activities.

   □ □ □ _____

6. Schedule of Prices of Services – Other Revenue Activities.

   □ □ □ _____

C. Treasurer

1. Investment Portfolio, Master File. This file is maintained in alphabetical sequence of investment (and in chronological sequence when several purchases of the same investment have been made), by investment category (e.g., stocks, bonds, options).

   □ □ □ _____

2. Investment Portfolio, Fund File. This file is maintained in the same sequence as the master file, but is segregated into *separate files* for each donor restricted fund *and* unrestricted fund file.

   □ □ □ _____

3. Interest Income Schedule, Master File. This file is maintained in the same sequence as the Investment Portfolio Master File, for all interest-bearing investments.

A B C
□ □ □

USE MASTER FILE ANALYSIS FORM

A = essentially similar   B = minor variations   C = significant differences

Report Inventory 5.4

A. General Accounting Section

your document title ↓

1. Daily Listing of Summary and Special Transactions. This is used to post entries to accounts and to verify postings of transactions.

A B C
□ □ □

2. Periodic Trial Balance.

□ □ □

3. Annual Hospital Medicare Cost Report Allocations.

□ □ □

4. Monthly financial statements.

□ □ □

5. Yearly financial statements.

□ □ □

B. Director of Finance

1. Daily Listing of Cash Receipts, by Source, by Activity. This is used to post accounting records and verify cash receipts.

□ □ □

2. Daily Listing of Other Revenue, by Source, by Activity. This is used to post accounting records.

□ □ □

3. Price List for Services Offered, by Activity. This is used to disseminate pricing schedules for all services offered in the other revenue area.

□ □ □

4. Aged Accounts Receivable Schedule, by Activity. This is used to analyze credit and collection policies for every other revenue activity.

□ □ □

5. Portfolio Status Report. This monthly report shows the original cost, current market value, earnings, and yield on all currently held investments.

□ □ □

6. Listing of Donations and Pledges Received. This is an information only report published monthly.

□ □ □

7. Listing of Overdue Pledges. This is used for follow-up of outstanding pledges.

A B C

□ □ □

_____

System Performance Standards 5.4

	Units	A	B
1. How much time elapses between the end of a month and the completion of the monthly financial statement?	days _____	□	□
2. How much time elapses between the end of the year and the completion of the yearly financial statement?	days _____	□	□
3. How much time is spent preparing the Medicare Cost Report?	workhours _____	□	□
4. How many adjusting entries have to be made?	number per month _____	□	□
5. How many month-end statements does General Accounting prepare?	number_____	□	□
6. How many responsibility levels are built into the General Accounting System?	(record appropriate number)		
	a. at CEO Level only _____	□	□
	b. down to associate/ assistant administrator _____	□	□
	c. down to Department Head Level but not individual Nursing Stations _____	□	□
	d. down to Department Head Level including reports for each Nursing Station_____	□	□
	e. down to the Section Level _____	□	□
	f. further breakdowns ____	□	□
7. How much does the hospital spend in audit fees?	dollars _____	□	□

System Cost Factors 5.4

1. How many clerical people are employed in General Accounting? $ _____

2. How much time does General Accounting spend in copying reports? $ _____

USE SYSTEM COST ANALYSIS FORM *(also see Instructions, p. 15)*

System 5.5:
Cash Management

Description 5.5

Cash Management is the responsibility of the Treasurer. It encompasses the planning, control, and recording of all cash receipts and disbursements.

A B C
□ □ □ _____

Cash comes into the institution in two ways — currency received and checks received. It leaves in three ways — payroll checks to employees, Accounts Payable checks to vendors, or impress funds.

□ □ □ _____

Currency

Each hospital has at least one Cashier Station. Many have several — in the Business Office, at the ED Desk, in the Outpatient Area, etc.

□ □ □ _____

Each is operated in a similar fashion. At the beginning of each shift, each Cashier signs for a cash box, which contains a fixed amount of money. As cash is accepted, the Cashier records the transaction and issues a receipt. Forms are often designed in such a way that the receipt and transaction record are the same document.

□ □ □ _____

At the end of the shift the supervisor inspects the cash box. The amount it contains should equal the sum of the original amount plus the total value of the receipts.

□ □ □ _____

The supervisor logs the amount received and sends the received cash and the receipts to the Treasurer, who prepares a deposit slip, then sends the money to the bank. The Treasurer also forwards the funds to the appropriate section for posting. Normally, this involves posting payment to patient accounts.

□ □ □ _____

Checks

Checks come to one central receiving point, which usually is part of the Cashier Station. The checks in a single batch are tallied, and a copy of the tally sheet, along with the checks, is sent to the Treasurer, who prepares a deposit slip and sends the money to the bank. In addition, the Treasurer forwards a copy of the tally sheet to the appropriate section for posting. Normally,

---

A = essentially similar   B = minor variations   C = significant differences

this tally sheet contains the name and the amount for checks from private individuals and copies of advice statements for checkes received from insurance companies.

A B C
☐ ☐ ☐   _____

Payroll/Accounts Payable

Payroll sends the Treasurer a report showing how much cash was used in issuing payroll checks. Accounts Payable sends payable vouchers to the Treasurer, who in turn produces checks for vendors.

☐ ☐ ☐   _____

The Treasurer is responsible for recording these takedowns of the hospital's checking account or accounts. Normally, hospitals maintain at least two checking accounts – one for vendors and one for payroll.

☐ ☐ ☐   _____

Cash Management

Cash Management is primarily concerned with reporting the present status of the institution's cash balance in its impressed funds as well as its demand deposit and time deposit accounts. In addition, the Treasurer must have an accurate projection of cash receipts and cash disbursements for the next one to thirty days to insure maximum earnings from idle cash and security from technical insolvency.

☐ ☐ ☐   _____

Daily summaries of cash receipts and cash disbursements insure proper posting in all Journals and Ledgers. These summaries are based on a compilation of cash receipt vouchers and cash disbursement vouchers, which ensures that all the cash received was properly credited. The verification of all disbursements against deposit records and check numbers is an integral part of any cash management system.

☐ ☐ ☐   _____

Reconciliation of the institution's records (daily, weekly, or monthly) with those of the servicing banks or other financial institutions is also a key part of any Cash Management System. Ensuring that all deposits are fully credited, dishonored checks are accounted for and acted upon, and issued checks have cleared, are all key factors in the reconciliation process.

☐ ☐ ☐   _____

Daily forecasts of expected cash receipts, cash disbursements, minimum required balances on a daily basis for the next five to thirty days, and on a weekly or monthly basis for the next thirty to three hundred sixty days, are critical reports to the cash manager.

☐ ☐ ☐   _____

A = essentially similar   B = minor variations   C = significant differences

Flow Chart 5.5

Cash Control

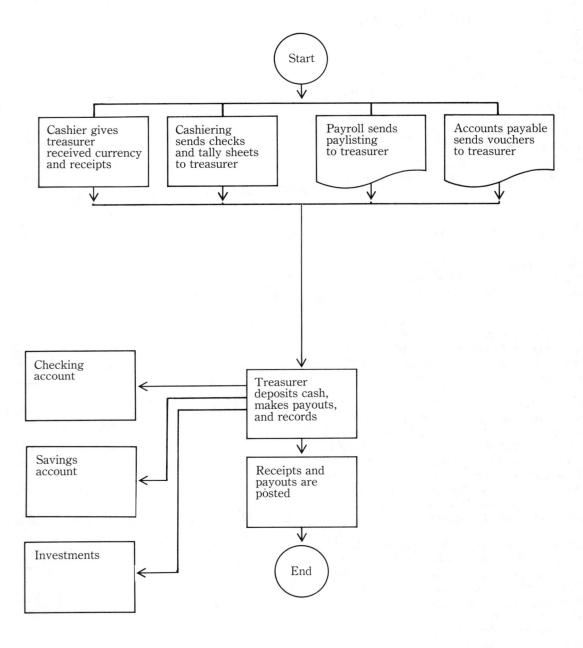

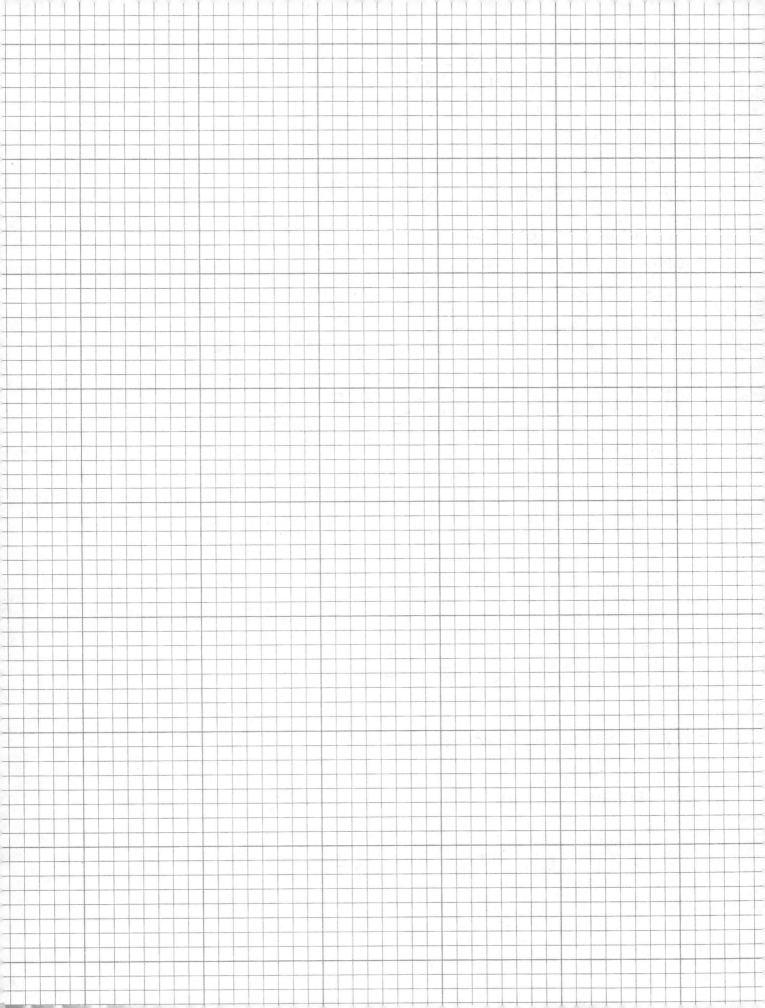

Input Inventory 5.5

A. Treasurer

your document title ↓

     A B C

1. Deposit slips.   ☐ ☐ ☐ _____

2. Bank Reconciliation Statement.   ☐ ☐ ☐ _____

B. Cashier Supervisor

1. Receipts.   ☐ ☐ ☐ _____

2. Check Tally sheets.   ☐ ☐ ☐ _____

USE INPUT DOCUMENT ANALYSIS FORM

A = same document title	B = minor variations	C = significant differences

Master File Inventory 5.5

A. Treasurer

Notes ↓

     A B C

1. Voucher log.   ☐ ☐ ☐ _____

2. Check register.   ☐ ☐ ☐ _____

3. Bank statement.   ☐ ☐ ☐ _____

4. Voucher file.   ☐ ☐ ☐ _____

5. Receipt file.   ☐ ☐ ☐ _____

6. Deposit receipts.   ☐ ☐ ☐ _____

USE MASTER FILE ANALYSIS FORM

A = essentially similar	B = minor variations	C = significant differences

Report Inventory 5.5

A. Treasurer's Office

your document title ↓

1. Daily Listing of Cash Receipts. This is used as a control to ensure accurate posting, verify accounts receivable postings, verify bank deposits, verify receipt totals from cash collection points.

     A B C

☐ ☐ ☐ _____

2. Daily Listing of Cash Disbursements. This is used as a control to ensure accurate postings,

verify accounts payable postings, verify bank
statement reconciliations, verify disbursement
authorizations, and verify total from cash
disbursement points.

A B C

☐ ☐ ☐ _____

your document title
↓

3. Dishonored Check Listing. This is used to
adjust prior postings. It is then placed into
the credit files.

☐ ☐ ☐ _____

4. Daily Cash Summary. This summary listing,
by receipt and disbursement category, shows
beginning and ending balances and is used
for general ledger postings and an end-of-day
status report of cash account balances.

☐ ☐ ☐ _____

5. Cash Forecast. This is used to project cash
receipts and disbursements and determine
idle cash shortfalls above or below minimum
balance.

☐ ☐ ☐ _____

6. Bank Statement Reconciliation Listing. This
is used to record and post cash activities not
recorded elsewhere (e.g., bank service
charges, interest income, interest expense on
line of credits).

☐ ☐ ☐ _____

USE REPORT ANALYSIS FORM

A = essentially similar	B = minor variations	C = significant differences

System Performance Standards 5.5

Units

A B

1. How many days does it take to get cash receipts
deposited from the time the cash or check is received?   days _____ ☐ ☐

2. How many days does it take to prepare, process, and
distribute a check once a properly authenticated
payment voucher or disbursement voucher is received
by the Treasurer's Office?   days _____ ☐ ☐

3. How many errors are made on the daily bank deposit
slips?   number per week _____ ☐ ☐

4. What proportion of the time is the cash balance more
than $100 above or below the minimum cash balance
required?   percentage of days _____ ☐ ☐

5. How many dollars above impressed fund starting
balances are kept in the institution's safe overnight?   dollars _____ ☐ ☐

6. How often is the daily cash forecast more than ±$100
from actual daily ending balances?   number of times per month __ ☐ ☐

7. Does the hospital use a cashbox approach to control
cash at the Cashier Station?   yes or no _____ ☐ ☐

8. How much does the hospital receive in interest revenue?

Units

A B

dollars per year _____ □ □

9. How much does the hospital pay out in interest on short-term loans?

dollars per year _____ □ □

USE PERFORMANCE STANDARDS ANALYSIS FORM

A = we have a standard   B = we do not have a standard

System Cost Factors 5.5

(none)

Personnel Management Systems

System 6.1:
Timekeeping/Payroll
Description 6.1

Collecting payroll information and issuing paychecks is the responsibility of the Payroll Department, which is part of the Business Office. However, Personnel also shares in this responsibility by assuring that accurate records are kept, showing who is on the payroll and what they should be paid. A pay scale is associated with every job title in the hospital. Typically, each scale has an entry rate and several additional steps. The total number of steps and the wage difference between them varies from hospital to hospital.

A B C
☐ ☐ ☐

In some hospitals, almost every job title has its own scale. Other hospitals group job titles into pay scale categories, thereby reducing the total number of scales. For example, Laboratory Technician, Admitting Supervisor, and Unit Secretary may all be considered level T jobs, with every employee in a level T position having the same pay scale.

☐ ☐ ☐

Hiring

When an employee is hired, Personnel sends Payroll a new-hire notification, which includes the employee's name, the number of the position he or she is filling, starting salary, and starting date.

☐ ☐ ☐

A Payroll Clerk uses this information to update the Payroll Master File – a listing showing each employee, the job he or she is filling, current salary, and deductions. This Master File may represent an alphabetical filing of the entire hospital staff or names may be filed alphabetically by department.

☐ ☐ ☐

The Payroll Clerk also updates the department's Table of Organization, prepares a time card for the new employee, and files the new-hire notification.

☐ ☐ ☐

Wage Increases

Personnel also maintains a card file that contains one card per employee, filed chronologically by the date on which the next pay increase for that

A = essentially similar   B = minor variations   C = significant differences

359

employee is due. In most hospitals, employees are considered for pay increases on a yearly basis, with an earlier review common some time during the first year of employment. Prior to implementing the increase, the employee's supervisor evaluates the employee's performance.

A B C
☐ ☐ ☐ _____

Personnel uses the increase-due file to determine when to alert supervisors that evaluations are due. As an employee's card comes up in the file, Personnel sends the supervisor a blank evaluation form and a form on which the supervisor can indicate whether a raise is recommended. This form contains the employee's name, position number, current salary, recommended salary increase, if any, and the date the new salary will take effect.

☐ ☐ ☐ _____

If the supervisor wants to recommend an increase, he or she completes an evaluation, signs this form, and sends it to Personnel. One copy is placed in the employee's file, and another is sent to Payroll.

☐ ☐ ☐ _____

Upon receiving it, a Payroll Clerk updates the Payroll Master File.

☐ ☐ ☐ _____

Paycheck Preparation

The length of the pay cycle – the time between paychecks – varies from hospital to hospital. Payment every two weeks and twice monthly are typical.

☐ ☐ ☐ _____

At the beginning of a cycle, Payroll prepares one time card for each employee. This card contains the employee's name, department, and position number. Payroll Clerks place these cards in holders that are kept next to the time clocks.

☐ ☐ ☐ _____

During the pay cycle, the employees clock in and out, generating a record of hours worked.

☐ ☐ ☐ _____

If, during the cycle, an employee takes a vacation or uses sick time, the supervisor notifies Payroll, stating the employee's name, position number, the dates and number of hours the employee was away from the job, and the reason for the absence. Payroll files these notifications until the end of the pay cycle.

☐ ☐ ☐ _____

If an employee was authorized to work overtime, the supervisor sends an overtime authorization to Payroll. It states when the overtime was worked, how many hours were authorized, and why they were necessary. Typically, a copy of this form goes to the Department Head.

☐ ☐ ☐ _____

A = essentially similar   B = minor variations   C = significant differences

Time cards are not the only method of keeping track of time worked. Some hospitals use time sheets that contain the names of all employees in a given department or section. Each day the supervisor records the employee's arrival time and departure time. Another approach requires the employees themselves to mark down on a time sheet their times of arrival and departure. At the end of the pay cycle, the supervisor sends the time sheet to Payroll.

When a time card system is used, Payroll Clerks pick up old time cards at the end of a cycle and deposit new ones.

A variety of factors come in to play when Payroll Clerks compute an employee's pay for a given cycle. Working from a time card, or other document that tells how many hours an employee worked during a cycle, the clerk first computes the number of hours worked and multiplies that figure by the employee's hourly rate. If the employee used vacation time or sick time, pay for that is computed. The clerk uses the notification forms received from supervisors to determine the amount of sick time and vacation time for which an employee should receive payment. This figure is added to the employee's paycheck.

In addition, the clerk must consider such items as shift differential, holiday pay, and premium pay for weekend work. Some employees also are paid for being on call. The supervisor is responsible for notifying Payroll how often an employee was on call during a pay cycle.

After taking all of this information into account, the Payroll Clerk computes the amount owed to each employee. The clerk enters this amount, along with all of its components, on a work-sheet. In addition, the clerk adjusts the amount of sick time and vacation time the employee has available after accruing and possibly using hours during the particular pay cycle. The sick-time and vacation-time records may be part of the Master File or they may be kept in a separate alphabetical file.

Next, the Payroll Clerk computes the deductions for each employee. These include mandated deductions, such as income and social security taxes, and optional deductions, such as credit-union deposits. All deductions are itemized on the worksheet.

At this point, the department has all the information needed to prepare the employee's paycheck.

A = essentially similar   B = minor variations   C = significant differences

361

In most hospitals, the Payroll Department itself does not compute payrolls and prepare paychecks. Instead, the department prepares the necessary input data and submits these data to a service bureau, which prepares the checks and returns them to Payroll.

A B C
☐ ☐ ☐ _____

In some hospitals, however, a Payroll Clerk does prepare the checks, which usually include an advice statement or stub. Once the checks are prepared, they are signed. In some hospitals, either the Chief Financial Officer or the Chief Operating Officer signs each check. In others, a check-signing machine is used.

☐ ☐ ☐ _____

As part of preparing the checks, the clerk compiles a checks-issued list. For each check, this list shows the check number, the person to whom it was issued, the amount, and, possibly, the amounts withheld for tax purposes.

☐ ☐ ☐ _____

There are several approaches to distributing checks. Some hospitals mail them. Others deposit them in employee bank accounts. Another approach is to have a central location where checks can be picked up. The most common approach is for the supervisors to distribute them.

☐ ☐ ☐ _____

Salaried Employees

For salaried employees, the flow is similar but less complex. There is no need to compute total hours worked, overtime or shift differentials. In addition to the payroll computed for salaried personnel, a confidential payroll is often used which consists of payroll information for executive personnel and salaried physicians. This payroll may be kept "by hand" by a Payroll or Accounting employee. The same detail is required as is needed for the salaried payroll. There may be a separate payroll account for the confidential payroll.

☐ ☐ ☐ _____

Reports

In gathering the information needed to prepare paychecks, Payroll becomes the depository for a large amount of information concerning who is working where and for how long. As a result, Payroll is called upon to supply a variety of management reports. These vary in format, content, and distribution, but basically they are designed to supply the following key pieces of information:

☐ ☐ ☐ _____

1. Hours worked by each employee.

☐ ☐ ☐ _____

A = essentially similar   B = minor variations   C = significant differences

	A	B	C	Notes ↓
2. Overtime hours worked by each employee.	□	□	□	_____
3. Total workhours used by each department.	□	□	□	_____
4. Total wage expenses consumed by each department.	□	□	□	_____
5. Tax withheld for each employee.	□	□	□	_____
Payroll must also supply the Treasurer with reports stating how much wage expense was accumulated by each department.	□	□	□	_____

A = essentially similar   B = minor variations   C = significant differences

Flow Chart 6.1a

New Employees

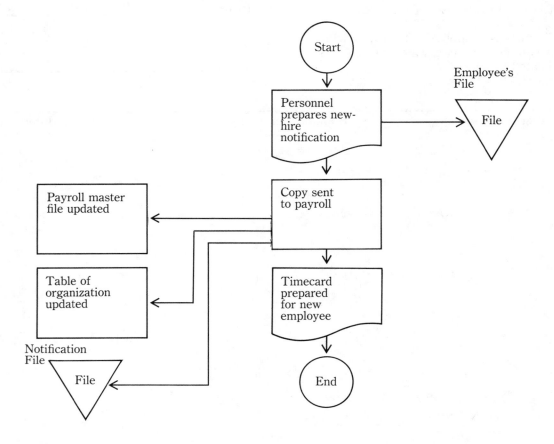

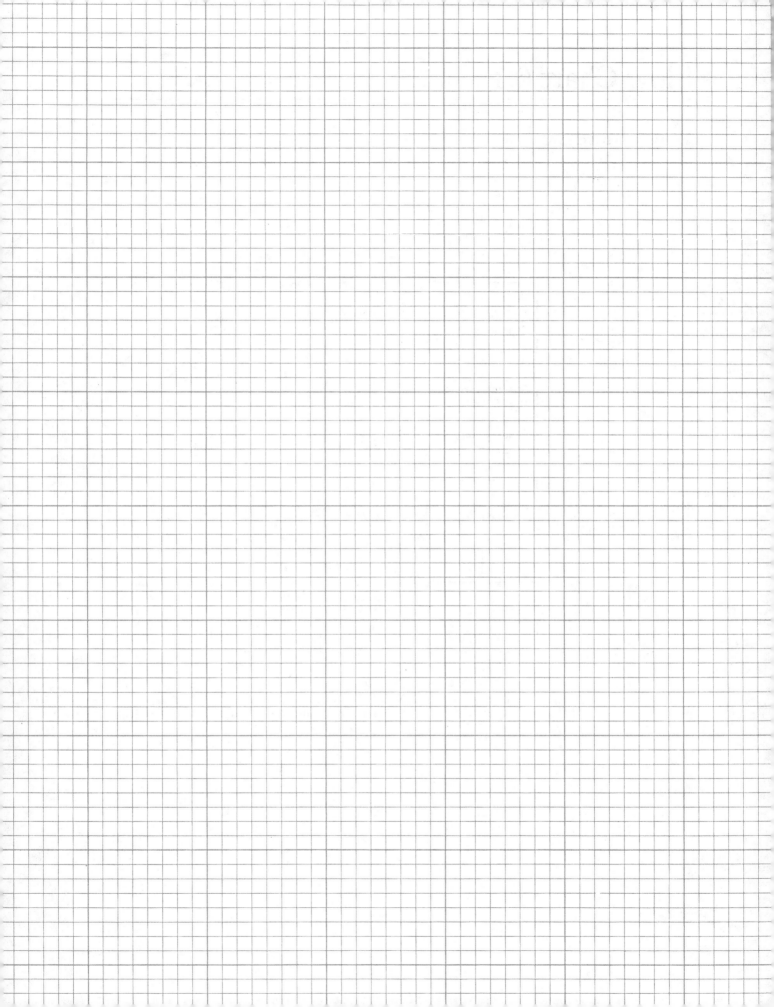

Flow Chart 6.1b

Wage Increase

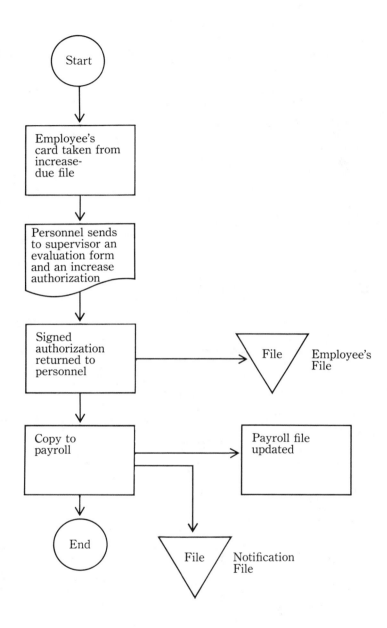

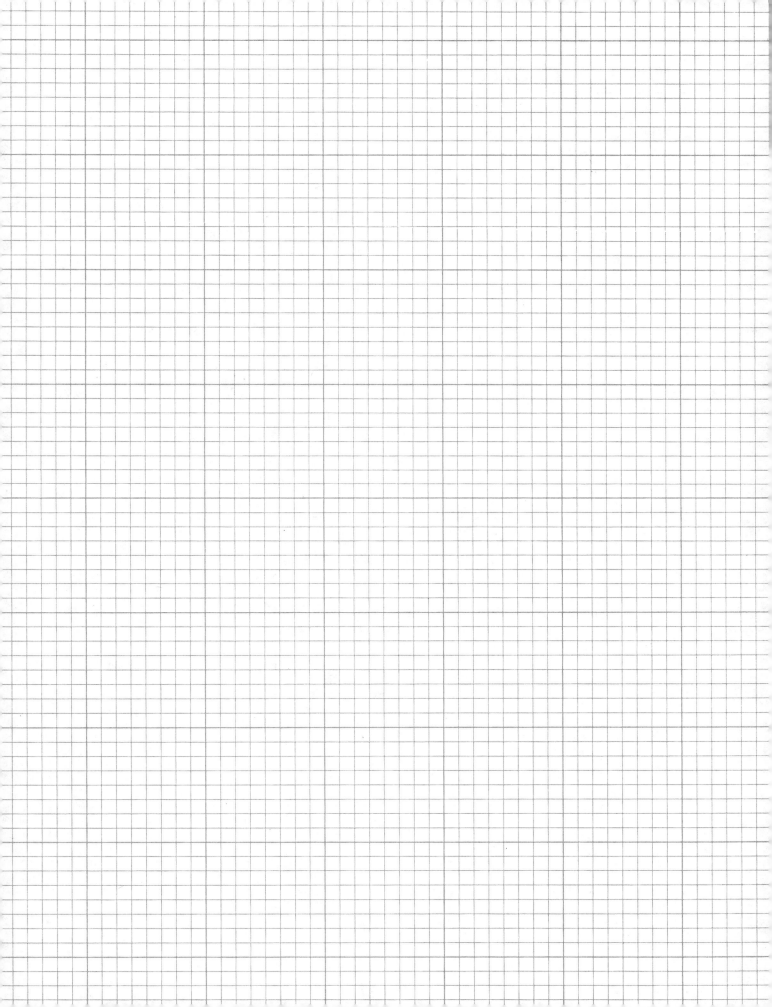

Flow Chart 6.1c

Preparing the Check

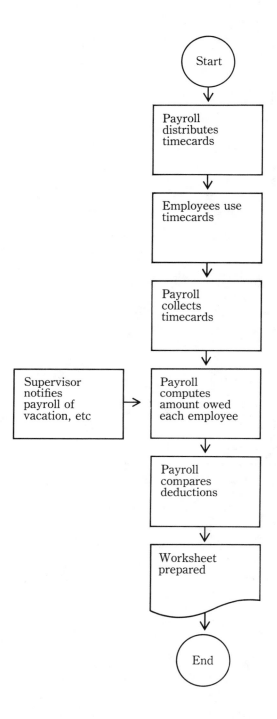

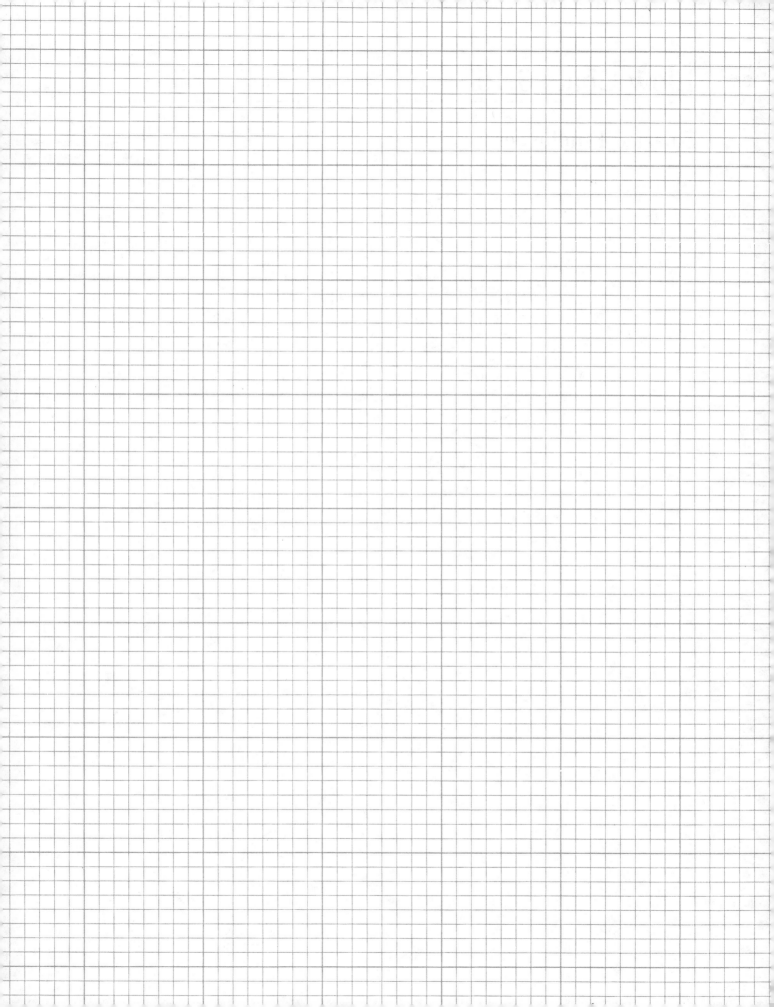

Flow Chart 6.1d

Salaried Employees

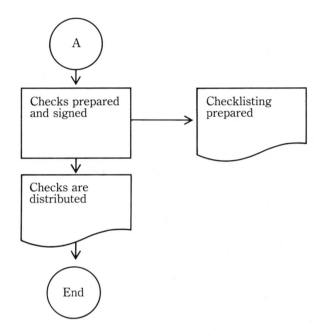

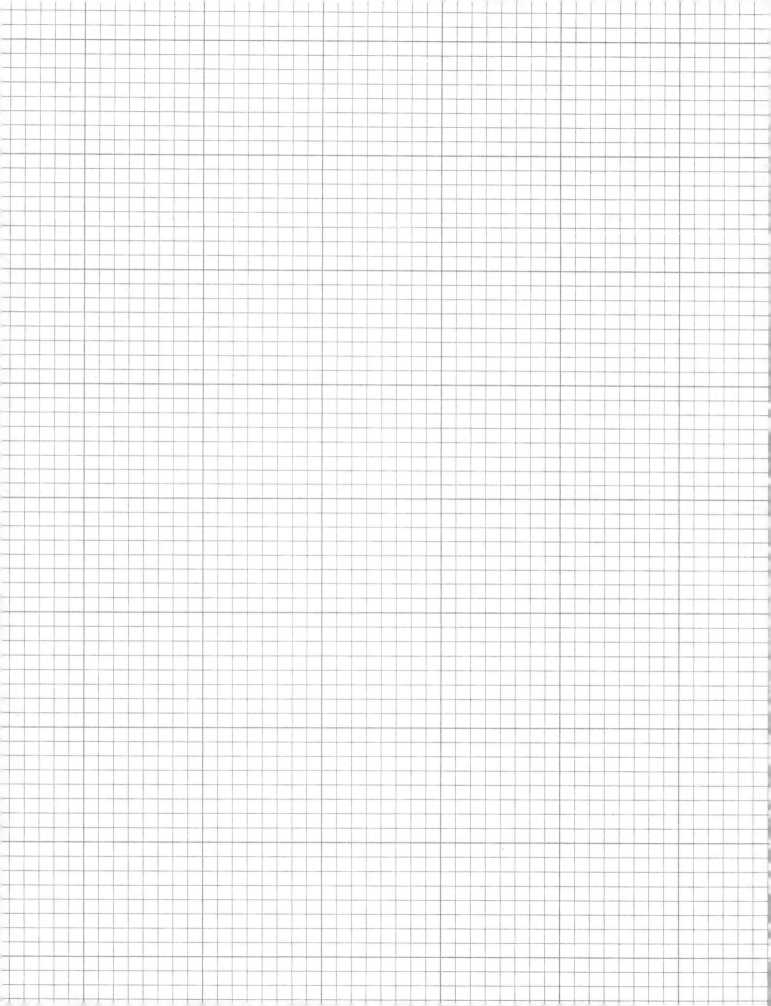

Input Inventory 6.1

A. Payroll Supervisor

your document title
↓

	A	B	C	
1. Time card.	☐	☐	☐	_____
2. Time sheet.	☐	☐	☐	_____
3. Overtime authorization.	☐	☐	☐	_____
4. Notification of sick time, vacation time, and other off-the-job time.	☐	☐	☐	_____
5. New-hire notification.	☐	☐	☐	_____
6. Raise notification.	☐	☐	☐	_____
7. Call-time report.	☐	☐	☐	_____
8. Payroll worksheet.	☐	☐	☐	_____

USE INPUT DOCUMENT ANALYSIS FORM

A = same document title   B = minor variations   C = significant differences

Master File Inventory 6.1

A. Payroll Supervisor

Notes
↓

	A	B	C	
1. Payroll Master File.	☐	☐	☐	_____
2. Notifications of new hires and salary changes.	☐	☐	☐	_____
3. Pay scales.	☐	☐	☐	_____
4. Table of Organization.	☐	☐	☐	_____

B. Personnel Director

	A	B	C	
Date-of-hire file.	☐	☐	☐	_____

USE MASTER FILE ANALYSIS FORM

A = essentially similar   B = minor variations   C = significant differences

Report Inventory 6.1

A. Payroll Supervisor

your document title
↓

	A B C	
1. Check.	☐ ☐ ☐	_____
2. Check stub.	☐ ☐ ☐	_____
3. Workhours report (with wage expense and overtime information).	☐ ☐ ☐	_____
4. Listing of sick time and vacation time available to each employee.	☐ ☐ ☐	_____
5. Taxes withheld from each employee.	☐ ☐ ☐	_____
6. Listing of checks issued.	☐ ☐ ☐	_____

USE REPORT ANALYSIS FORM

A = essentially similar   B = minor variations   C = significant differences

System Performance Standards 6.1

Units

		A B
1. What is the minimum time between the end of a pay cycle and the issuing of paychecks?	days _____	☐ ☐
2. How many checks are prepared incorrectly?	average number per cycle ____	☐ ☐
3. How many pay scales are there?	number_____	☐ ☐
4. How often are time cards lost?	number of times per cycle ____	☐ ☐
5. Are Department Heads required to authorize overtime?	yes or no _____	☐ ☐
6. How much overtime is used?	hours per pay period _____	☐ ☐

USE PERFORMANCE STANDARDS ANALYSIS FORM

A = we have a standard   B = we do not have a standard

System Cost Factors 6.1

1. How much time is spent producing reports? $ _____

2. How much time is spent passing out and picking up time cards? $ _____

3. How much time is spent distributing reports? $ _____

USE SYSTEM COST ANALYSIS FORM *(also see Instructions, p. 15)*

System 6.2: Position Control

Description 6.2

Position control refers to a hospital's ability to define the exact number of people it will employ, establish procedures to assure that this limit is not exceeded, and determine exactly what jobs those employees will do.

A B C
□ □ □ _____

This is a hospital-wide activity, with Personnel having the major responsibility for assuring that the hiring and assigning of new employees is controlled.

□ □ □ _____

Establishing the Program

The key document in position control is the Table of Organization. This lists, in hierarchal order, every position in the hospital as approved by top management. It begins with the position of Chief Executive Officer and shows all those who report to him or her. The next section shows all those positions that are directly under the staffers who report to the Chief Executive Officer. The branching continues until all hospital positions have been included.

□ □ □ _____

Positions are not the same as job titles. Phlebotomist, for example, is a job title. But if a hospital has 15 approved phlebotomist positions, phlebotomist would show up 15 times on the Table of Organization.

□ □ □ _____

To improve control, some hospitals assign a number to each position in order to uniquely identify it. For example, 4-608 could refer to a particular day-shift staff nurse position, while 3-798 could refer to a particular night-shift housekeeper slot.

□ □ □ _____

Each position is associated with a job title, and for each job title there is a job description. The master copy of each description is kept in Personnel with the master copy of the Table of Organization. Additional copies are given to each employee with that title and, also, to each supervisor utilizing those employees.

□ □ □ _____

To control the hiring of new employees, Personnel maintains a position-control file – one card or one folder for each approved position.

A = essentially similar   B = minor variations   C = significant differences

These cards or folders are typically filed by department and by shift. For example, all of Radiology's positions would be in one section, segmented according to shift.

The usual approach to setting up this control file is to use a set of cards laid out in a visible file. Each card has two sections – position information and employee information. The former includes the position name and number, the salary range, the hours, the authority this position reports to, and perhaps some key excerpts from the job description.

The employee section is divided into columns, which are used to write the name of the person currently holding the position, the date the person assumed that position, and the date the person left that position. The last name written in this section is either the person currently in the position or, for a vacant position, the person who last held it.

A termination date written next to the last entry indicates that the position is open.

Hiring

The filling of a vacant position begins when a Department Head submits an employee requisition to Personnel. The Department Head, aware that an employee is leaving, enters that employee's name and position, the position number, and the date the position will be open.

After receiving the requisition, a Personnel Clerk removes the employee's Personnel file and places it in a suspense file. The Personnel Clerk also forwards a copy of the requisition to Payroll so the final checks can be prepared for the employee.

Personnel then begins to seek a replacement. As applicants come to the hospital, they complete an application and have a screening interview with a Personnel Officer. Selected applicants are then scheduled for interviews with the affected supervisor or Department Head. Personnel, in the meantime, checks the applicant's references, work history, and license or certificate if one is needed for the job in question.

When the supervisor hires an applicant, he or she notifies Personnel, which gives its approval. A Personnel file is begun, and the new employee's name and starting date are written onto the position card. Personnel sends Payroll a new-hire notification, containing the name of the

Notes ↓

A B C
□ □ □ _____

□ □ □ _____

□ □ □ _____

□ □ □ _____

□ □ □ _____

□ □ □ _____

□ □ □ _____

A = essentially similar   B = minor variations   C = significant differences

375

new employee, key demographic information, the employee's position number, starting salary, and starting date. A copy of this document is placed in the Personnel file.

A B C
□ □ □ _____

In addition, Personnel initiates a variety of paperwork associated with a new hire – insurance forms, tax forms, etc.

□ □ □ _____

Periodically, a Personnel Clerk reviews the Personnel files held in the suspense file, to assure that employees scheduled to leave the institution actually did.

□ □ □ _____

When an employee does leave, his or her Personnel file is placed alphabetically in a former-employee file.

□ □ □ _____

Additions

During the course of a budget year, a Department Head may need to hire additional staffers. The typical approach for this requires that the Department Head submit a request to his or her Administrative Officer, along with a justification for the new position.

□ □ □ _____

If the Administrative Officer approves, he or she signs the request and forwards it to Personnel. There the Table of Organization is updated; a number is assigned to the new position; a position card is placed in the control file; and the recruiting cycle begins.

□ □ □ _____

Terminating

When an employee is leaving the hospital, he or she notifies his or her supervisor, who then notifies Personnel. An exit interview is scheduled and a final paycheck is prepared.

□ □ □ _____

After the employee has left the hospital, his or her personnel file is moved into the former-employee file.

□ □ □ _____

Flow Chart 6.2

Hiring

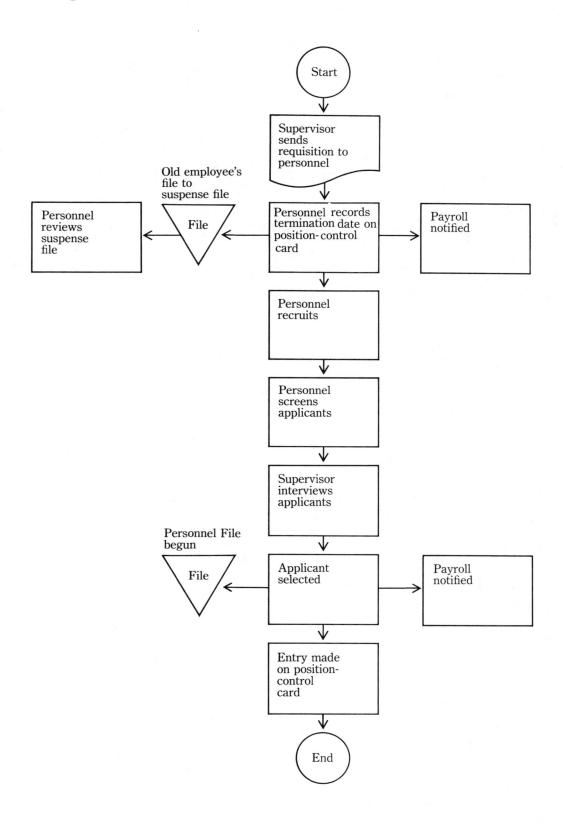

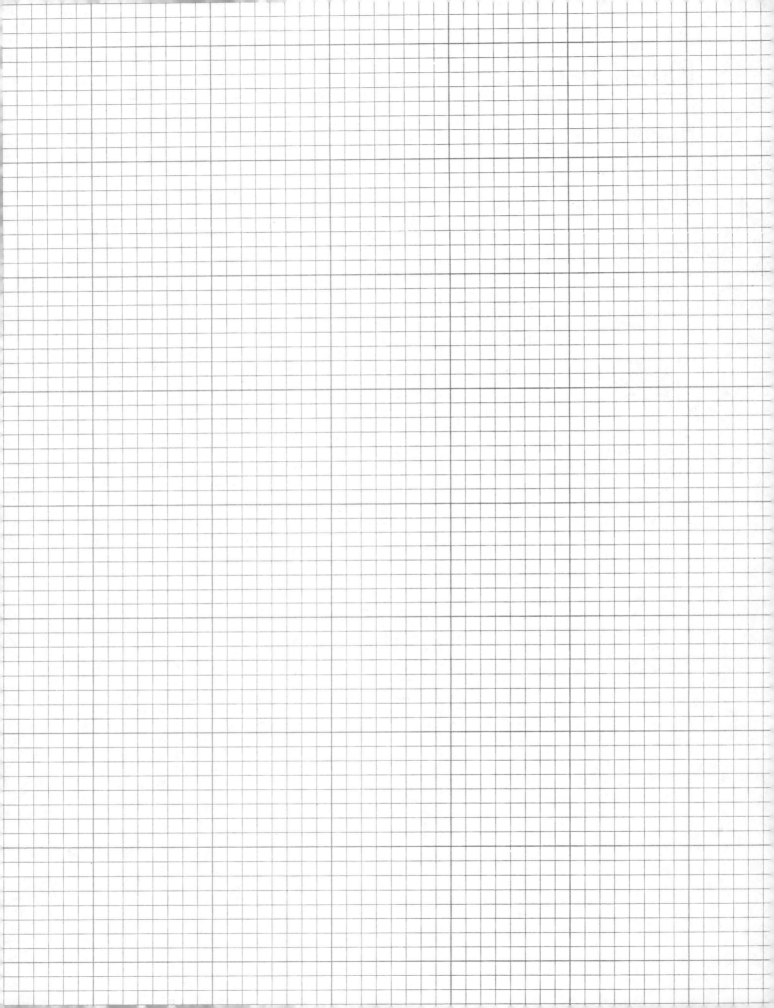

Input Inventory 6.2

A. Personnel Director

your document title ↓

		A	B	C	
1.	Job application.	☐	☐	☐	_____
2.	New-hire notification.	☐	☐	☐	_____
3.	Termination notification.	☐	☐	☐	_____
4.	Position-control card.	☐	☐	☐	_____
5.	Employee requisition.	☐	☐	☐	_____
6.	New-position request.	☐	☐	☐	_____

USE INPUT DOCUMENT ANALYSIS FORM

A = same document title   B = minor variations   C = significant differences

Master File Inventory 6.2

A. Personnel Director

Notes ↓

		A	B	C	
1.	Suspense file/employees leaving.	☐	☐	☐	_____
2.	Table of Organization.	☐	☐	☐	_____
3.	Position-control file.	☐	☐	☐	_____

USE MASTER FILE ANALYSIS FORM

A = essentially similar   B = minor variations   C = significant differences

Report Inventory 6.2

A. Personnel Director

your document title ↓

		A	B	C	
1.	Monthly turnover report.	☐	☐	☐	_____
2.	Listing of new hires.	☐	☐	☐	_____
3.	Updates of Table of Organization.	☐	☐	☐	_____

USE REPORT ANALYSIS FORM

A = essentially similar   B = minor variations   C = significant differences

System Performance Standards 6.2

	Units	A	B
1. What is the turnover rate?	number of employees who terminate yearly divided by average number of full-time-equivalent employees _____	☐	☐
2. How many positions are vacant?	number_____	☐	☐
3. Does Personnel perform screening interviews?	yes or no _____	☐	☐
4. Does Personnel sign off on all hires?	yes or no _____	☐	☐
5. Is there a position-control file and Table of Organization?	yes or no _____	☐	☐
6. How many positions have job descriptions?	number_____	☐	☐
7. How many positions have standards of performance?	number_____	☐	☐
8. What percentage of new employees have had their references checked?	number of hired employees with reference checks divided by total number of new hires_____	☐	☐
9. What percentage of full-time-equivalent personnel are terminated via hospital-initiated action?	percent per year _____	☐	☐

USE PERFORMANCE STANDARDS ANALYSIS FORM

A = we have a standard   B = we do not have a standard

System Cost Factors 6.2

1. What is the budget for Personnel? $ _____

2. How much time do supervisors spend interviewing prospective employees? $ _____

3. How often are people hired without Personnel knowing about it? $ _____

USE SYSTEM COST ANALYSIS FORM *(also see Instructions, p. 15)*

System 6.3:
Evaluation and Training

Description 6.3

The New Employee

Certain procedures are followed in bringing a new employee into an organization. After completing all the necessary paperwork, the new employee goes through an orientation program run by Personnel. The purpose of this program is to familiarize the employee with hospital policies and give general information about the institution.

A B C
□ □ □ _____

Some hospitals supply the Personnel representative conducting the orientation with a checklist. As the Personnel representative reviews key items, he or she puts a check beside them. At the end of the orientation, the Personnel representative asks the new employee to review the list and ask any questions he or she may still have. When all questions have been answered, the new employee signs the checklist, which is then placed in his or her Personnel file.

□ □ □ _____

Next, the employee is taken to his or her supervisor, who conducts a second orientation, this one directly related to the job he or she was hired to perform. The supervisor again reviews the employee's responsibilities and the departmental policies. During this part of the orientation, the employee may be asked to perform the main tasks of his or her job while the supervisor looks on, ready to answer any questions.

□ □ □ _____

For the first several months, the new employee is considered to be on a probationary status. If, at the end of that period, the supervisor believes the employee can perform the job satisfactorily, he or she informs Personnel via a status-change notification. Sometimes the Personnel Department "flags" the new employee's file to alert the supervisor that the probationary period is nearing an end. Many times, however, the probationary status expires at the end of the hospital's stated probationary period without specific action of the supervisor. The employee then automatically goes from probationary to permanent status, and the notification is placed in his or her Personnel file.

□ □ □ _____

A = essentially similar   B = minor variations   C = significant differences

381

Evaluation

Periodically, each employee is evaluated by his or her supervisor. Personnel maintains a card file, with one card for each employee. The cards are filed chronologically, according to the date on which the employee assumed his or her current job.

A B C
☐ ☐ ☐ _____

A Personnel Clerk reviews this file on a weekly basis obtaining the names of all employees who are due to be evaluated. Evaluations are usually performed yearly. The clerk removes the cards of employees whose evaluations are due and places these cards in a suspense file.

☐ ☐ ☐ _____

Personnel then notifies the supervisor that an evaluation is due and sends him or her a copy of the evaluation form. The supervisor meets with the employee and reviews his or her performance. If performance standards have been developed for the position in question, the supervisor uses these standards as a guide during the evaluation process.

☐ ☐ ☐ _____

After the supervisor completes the evaluation and obtains written comments and a signature from the employee, he or she sends the evaluation to Personnel, via his or her Department Head.

☐ ☐ ☐ _____

A Personnel Clerk notes the receipt of the evaluation on the employee's date-of-hire card, replaces the card in the file, and puts the evaluation into the employee's Personnel file.

☐ ☐ ☐ _____

Training

Hospitals engage in a wide range of training programs. There also is great variety in the organizational structures that hospitals set up to control and coordinate their educational activities. The major types of training are:

☐ ☐ ☐ _____

1. Inservice. Training given by hospital personnel and by vendors. Inservice is normally intended to teach employees new procedures or the use of new equipment.

☐ ☐ ☐ _____

2. Special Courses. Formal classroom sessions on specific topics. These courses are given by hospital employees, outside instructors, and staff physicians.

☐ ☐ ☐ _____

3. Affiliation. Hospitals allow schools to bring students into the institution to observe and practice their skills. The schools provide instructors and training coordinators. This

---

A = essentially similar   B = minor variations   C = significant differences

type of arrangement usually involves schools teaching nursing and medical technology.

A B C
□ □ □ _____

4. On-the-job training. Because of the difficulty in hiring experienced personnel, hospitals often set up extended orientation programs that are intended to develop skills in inexperienced employees.

□ □ □ _____

5. Schools. Certificate- or diploma-granting programs run by the hospital itself.

□ □ □ _____

6. Stipends. Training that is done outside the hospital and paid for as an employee benefit.

□ □ □ _____

7. Physician Training. Intern and residency programs.

□ □ □ _____

8. Continuing Education. Programs designed for members of the medical staff.

□ □ □ _____

Typically, the responsibility for educational programs is spread throughout the institution. Among those who may be involved are the Director of Inservice Education, Department Heads, the Director of Personnel, and the Director of Medical Education.

□ □ □ _____

A = essentially similar   B = minor variations   C = significant differences

Flow Chart 6.3

Employee Evaluation

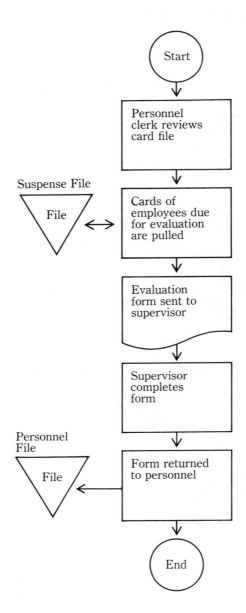

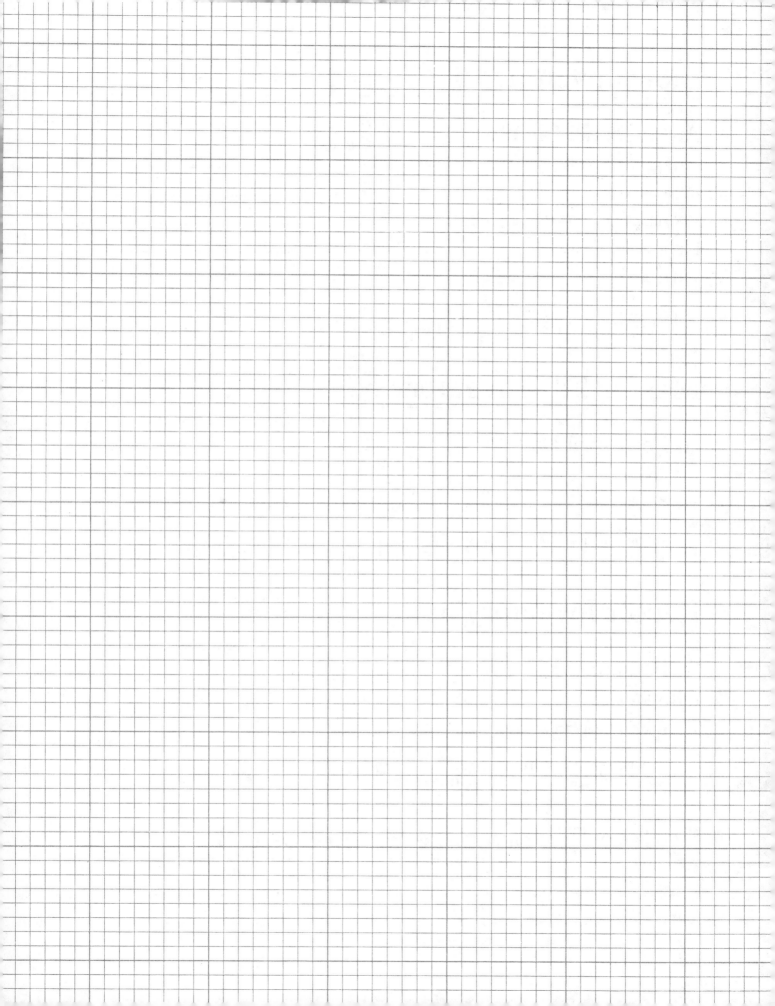

Input Inventory 6.3

A. Personnel Director

your document title
↓

	A	B	C	
1. Orientation checklist.	☐	☐	☐	_____
2. Evaluation form.	☐	☐	☐	_____
3. Notification of status change.	☐	☐	☐	_____
4. Standards of performance.	☐	☐	☐	_____
5. Hire-date card.	☐	☐	☐	_____

USE INPUT DOCUMENT ANALYSIS FORM

A = same document title   B = minor variations   C = significant differences

Master File Inventory 6.3

A. Personnel Director

Notes
↓

	A	B	C	
1. Personnel file.	☐	☐	☐	_____
2. Date-of-hire file.	☐	☐	☐	_____

USE MASTER FILE ANALYSIS FORM

A = essentially similar   B = minor variations   C = significant differences

Report Inventory 6.3

A. Personnel Director

your document title
↓

	A	B	C	
1. New hire list.	☐	☐	☐	_____
2. Training program activity.	☐	☐	☐	_____

USE REPORT ANALYSIS FORM

A = essentially similar   B = minor variations   C = significant differences

System Performance Standards 6.3

		Units	A	B
1. Do standards of performance exist for each job?	yes or no	_____	☐	☐
2. How many evaluations are delinquent?	number	_____	☐	☐

3. How many employees are terminated before the end of
their probationary period?   yearly number_____   □   □

4. How often does Personnel fail to notify a supervisor
that an evaluation is due?   number of times per month __   □   □

5. How many people have responsibility for setting up
educational programs?   number_____   □   □

6. What percentage of employees receive evaluations of
above-average or better?
                                                                                      number of employees with
                                                                                      those ratings divided by
                                                                                      total number of employees __   □   □

USE PERFORMANCE STANDARDS ANALYSIS FORM

A = we have a standard   B = we do not have a standard

System Cost Factors 6.3

(none)

Materials Management Systems

Materials Management Systems
Description

Materials management is more an untried concept than an established approach to hospital organization. The basic idea is to establish one department that has sole responsibility for the flow of material —supplies and equipment—through the institution. The individual heading this department would report to the hospital's Chief Executive Officer.

The department's major responsibilities would be:

A B C

A . Coordinating the review of supply and equipment requests from all other departments. ☐ ☐ ☐ _____

B . Assisting the departments in evaluating different types and brands of supplies and equipment. ☐ ☐ ☐ _____

C . Purchasing. ☐ ☐ ☐ _____

D . Receiving and storing. ☐ ☐ ☐ _____

E . Distributing. ☐ ☐ ☐ _____

F . Maintaining equipment. ☐ ☐ ☐ _____

G . Disposing of equipment. ☐ ☐ ☐ _____

Such a department would encompass all or part of the responsibilities normally held by Purchasing, Central Supply, Pharmacy, Dietary, and Biomedical Engineering.

Most hospitals still maintain the traditional arrangement, although it is not unusual to find Purchasing Departments now called Materials Management.

The traditional organizational structure is the one that will be considered in this section.

A=essentially similar   B=minor variations   C=significant differences

System 7.1:
Capital Equipment

Description 7.1

Equipment is any item that is long lasting (i.e., not consumed in use) and worth more than an amount established by the hospital (usually $100). In contrast, an item that is either consumed in use or worth less than the specified amount is considered a supply.

A B C
☐ ☐ ☐ _____

There are major differences in the purchasing, storing, and delivering of equipment as compared with supplies. Accounting procedures are also different, primarily because equipment is depreciable.

☐ ☐ ☐ _____

Evaluating

The introduction of a piece of equipment into a hospital begins in the department that will be using it. Through a variety of mechanisms – physician suggestions, vendor recommendations, efficiency studies, equipment breakdown, etc. – the Department Head decides to requisition a particular piece of equipment.

☐ ☐ ☐ _____

The Department Head completes an equipment requisition. When this procedure is carried out during the budget preparation process, it goes through the full budget approval process.

☐ ☐ ☐ _____

The requisition contains the name of the equipment needed, the suggested vendor, the approximate cost, and the date by which the item is needed. The requisition also contains the Department Head's justification for the request.

☐ ☐ ☐ _____

The Department Head keeps one copy and sends the other to his or her Administrative Officer, who analyzes the request, considering the following factors:

1. Is the purchase included in the current budget? If not, does the Department Head's justification qualify the item for a nonbudgeted purchase?

☐ ☐ ☐ _____

2. Are additional studies (e.g., use of a consultant, availability of alternatives, or involvement of other departments to be affected by the new equipment) necessary?

☐ ☐ ☐ _____

A = essentially similar   B = minor variations   C = significant differences

The amount of effort put out by the Administrative Officer depends on how much the item costs, whether it is budgeted, and whether it is a replacement. A $500,000 request to begin a new service in Radiology will command much more attention than a budgeted request to replace a $10,000 monitor in the Intensive Care Unit.

Once the Administrative Officer agrees the equipment is needed, the hospital makes a buy-or-lease decision. The major factor influencing this choice is which arrangement better serves the financial needs of the institution. It is a decision that should be made primarily by the Director of Finance.

If the equipment costs more than $100,000 (or some other amount written into state or federal regulations at the time), the hospital must seek approval from the Designated Planning Agency (DPA) – an organization under contract to carry out federal health-planning regulations. Normally, the DPA is a state agency, such as the Public Health Department.

Seeking approval involves completing forms that, in effect, require the hospital to justify the purchase. These forms are submitted simultaneously to the DPA and the Health Systems Agency (HSA). Both evaluate the request. The HSA makes a recommendation to the DPA, which is then responsible for a final decision. This entire procedure is generally referred to as the Certificate of Need (CON) process.

After receiving approval from the DPA, the hospital is ready to make the purchase. Negotiations begin with vendors to obtain the best financial arrangements and to assure that the vendors have a clear understanding of what the hospital wants.

These negotiations result in the selection of a vendor and the development of a written contract or written specifications.

The Administrative Officer then signs the requisition, attaches copies of the supporting documentation, and forwards all of the material to Purchasing.

Ordering

When the Director of Purchasing receives the requisition, he or she completes a PO. This is a multicopy form authorizing the vendor to ship the equipment and send a bill to the hospital.

Notes

A B C

A = essentially similar   B = minor variations   C = significant differences

393

The major information items on the PO are a description of the equipment being ordered, the price, the name and address of the vendor, and the department for which the equipment is being purchased. In addition, the form has a control number, called the PO number. Typically, this control number is preprinted onto the form. The Director of Purchasing is then responsible for accounting for each PO.

A B C
☐ ☐ ☐ _____

After the form is completed, a clerk enters the PO number, the name of the item and vendor, the price, and the date into the PO log.

☐ ☐ ☐ _____

POs have at least six copies. A typical distribution is as follows:

1. One copy goes to the equipment-ordered file in Purchasing, which is kept in numerical sequence.

☐ ☐ ☐ _____

2. One copy goes to the vendor.

☐ ☐ ☐ _____

3. Two copies go to Receiving. In most hospitals, the PO has spaces to note the amount ordered and the amount received. It is common practice to have the amount-ordered section of the Receiving copies blacked out. The purpose of this is to assure that Receiving Clerks will count the amount received rather than relying on the number shown on the PO.

☐ ☐ ☐ _____

4. One copy goes to the department that placed the order.

☐ ☐ ☐ _____

5. One copy goes to Accounts Payable. In most hospitals, the ordering department is charged for the equipment when the order is placed. After assuring that the proper bookkeeping entries have been made, Accounts Payable places the PO in numerical sequence in a suspense file, which is periodically reviewed.

☐ ☐ ☐ _____

Delivery

When the equipment arrives, a Receiving Clerk checks the packing slip and the invoice and makes sure the delivery is accurate. The Receiving Clerk then removes the copies of the PO from the equipment-ordered file, notes what was received, attaches one copy to the invoice and one copy of the packing slip, and sends the material to Purchasing.

☐ ☐ ☐ _____

The remaining copy of the packing slip is placed in Receiving's orders-received file.

☐ ☐ ☐ _____

A = essentially similar   B = minor variations   C = significant differences

The Receiving Clerk then notifies the ordering department that the equipment has been received and makes arrangements for it to be delivered and installed.

A B C
☐ ☐ ☐ _____

When Purchasing receives the material from Receiving, a Purchasing Clerk removes Purchasing's copy of the PO from the equipment-ordered file, attaches it to the other material, and files it in numerical sequence in a to-be-paid file.

☐ ☐ ☐ _____

When all items ordered have been received, one Receiving copy of the PO can be thrown away. If the order is not complete, one copy is returned to Receiving to be placed in Receiving's equipment-ordered file.

☐ ☐ ☐ _____

When the ordering Department Head is satisfied that the new equipment meets specifications, he or she sends an equipment-approval notification to Purchasing. This document should contain the name of item, the PO number, and the Department Head's signature.

☐ ☐ ☐ _____

Upon receiving this, a Purchasing clerk removes the material from the to-be-paid file, detaches the invoice and one Receiving copy, gives these two forms to a supervisor, and files the remaining material in numerical sequence in a Completed PO file.

☐ ☐ ☐ _____

When the supervisor knows that the item has been delivered and is performing according to specifications, he or she then signs the invoice to authorize payment, and sends both forms to Accounts Payable.

☐ ☐ ☐ _____

Property Book

Once a piece of equipment has been received, the Director of Purchasing notifies the Property Book (or Plant Ledger) Manager.

☐ ☐ ☐ _____

This notification is made by having either a special form or an extra copy of the PO set aside for the Property Book Manager.

☐ ☐ ☐ _____

The Manager assigns a number to the new equipment and prepares a label or tag for it. The Manager makes sure this identification document is attached to the equipment, then logs the equipment into the Property Book.

☐ ☐ ☐ _____

The Property Book records each piece of equipment, showing the name and number of the equipment, serial number, date of purchase, price, assigned department, and location.

☐ ☐ ☐ _____

Notes

A = essentially similar   B = minor variations   C = significant differences

Disposal

When a piece of equipment is to be disposed of
because of age, obsolescence, breakdown or
other reason, the Department Head notifies the
Property Book Manager via a disposal-request
form. Since disposal normally results in the
requisitioning of new equipment, a copy of the
disposal request usually goes to the appropriate
Administrative Officer.

A B C
☐ ☐ ☐ _____

Working with the Department Head, the
Property Book Manager determines what should
be done with the equipment – throw it away,
trade it in, or sell it. Once the equipment leaves
the hospital, the Manager records the disposal
date in the Property Book.

☐ ☐ ☐ _____

A = essentially similar   B = minor variations   C = significant differences

Flow Chart 7.1a

Ordering Equipment

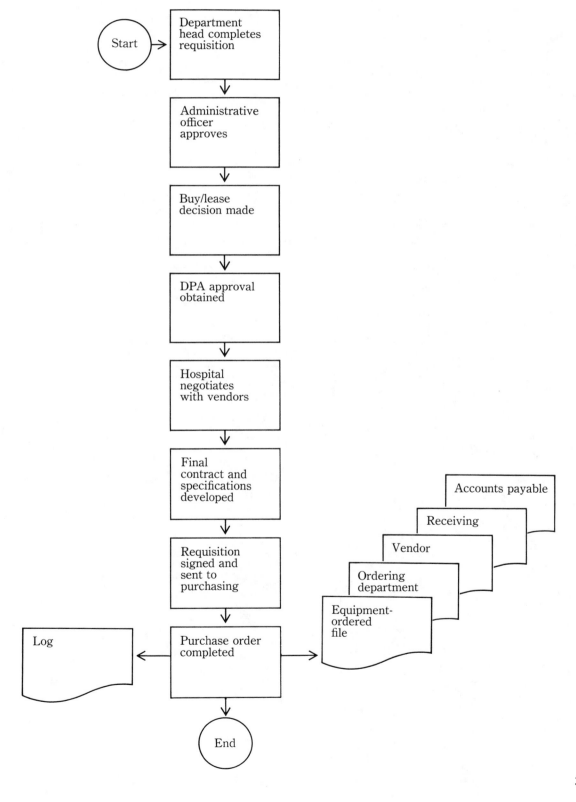

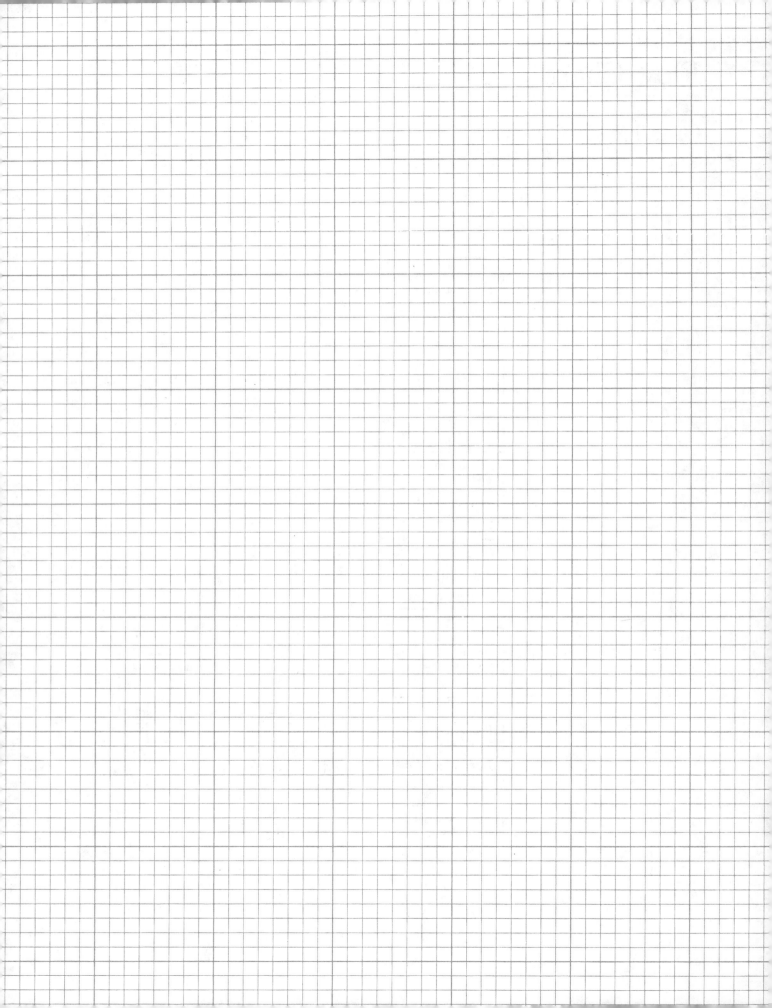

Flow Chart 7.1b

Receiving

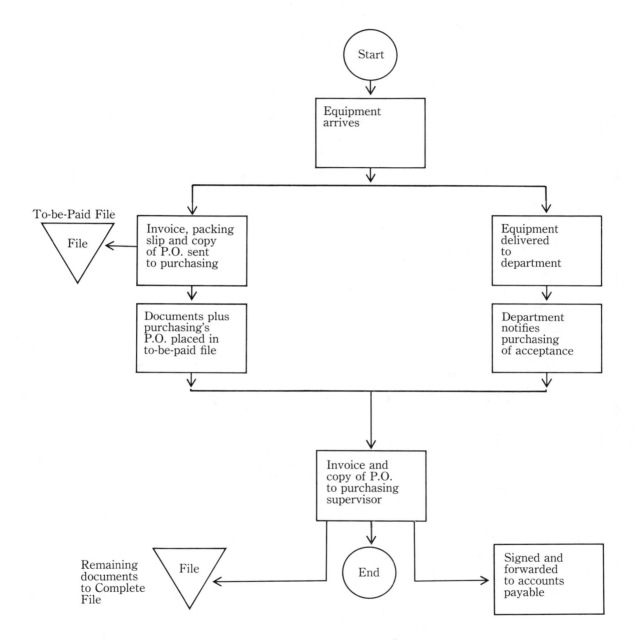

To-be-Paid File

File

Start

Equipment arrives

Invoice, packing slip and copy of P.O. sent to purchasing

Equipment delivered to department

Documents plus purchasing's P.O. placed in to-be-paid file

Department notifies purchasing of acceptance

Invoice and copy of P.O. to purchasing supervisor

Remaining documents to Complete File

File

End

Signed and forwarded to accounts payable

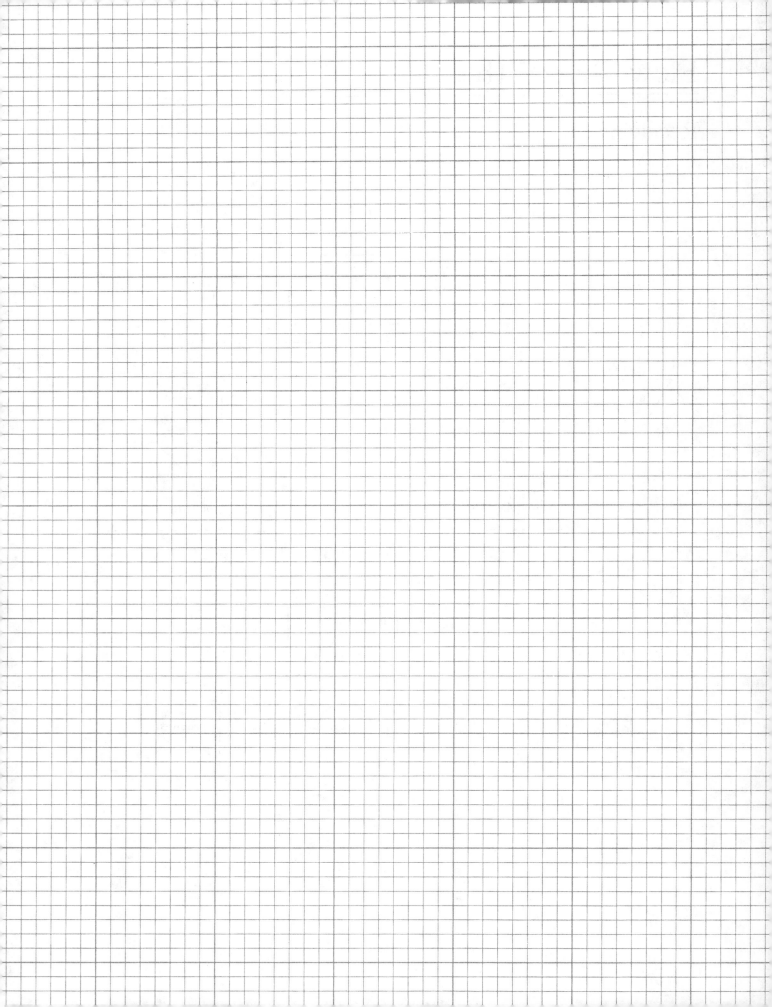

Input Inventory 7.1

A. Director of Purchasing

your document title
↓

A B C

1. Equipment Requisition. □ □ □ _____

2. Purchase Order. □ □ □ _____

3. Equipment-acceptable notification. □ □ □ _____

B. Property Book Manager

1. Identification tag. □ □ □ _____

2. Request for disposal. □ □ □ _____

USE INPUT DOCUMENT ANALYSIS FORM

A = same document title   B = minor variations   C = significant differences

Master File Inventory 7.1

A. Director of Purchasing

Notes
↓

A B C

1. Vendor information. □ □ □ _____

2. Equipment-ordered file (Purchasing). □ □ □ _____

3. Equipment-ordered file (Receiving). □ □ □ _____

4. Log for POs. □ □ □ _____

5. To-be-paid file. □ □ □ _____

6. Completed POs. □ □ □ _____

7. Orders-received file (Receiving). □ □ □ _____

B. Department Heads

Purchase-order suspense file. □ □ □ _____

C. Accounts Payable Supervisor

Purchase-order suspense file. □ □ □ _____

D. Property Book Manager

Property Book.

A B C
☐ ☐ ☐ _____

USE MASTER FILE ANALYSIS FORM

A = essentially similar	B = minor variations	C = significant differences

Report Inventory 7.1

A. Director of Purchasing

your document title ↓

1. Monthly report of equipment ordered and
   equipment received.

   A B C
   ☐ ☐ ☐ _____

2. Monthly listing of outstanding POs.

   ☐ ☐ ☐ _____

B. Property Book Manager

1. Book value of equipment.

   ☐ ☐ ☐ _____

2. Depreciation reports.

   ☐ ☐ ☐ _____

USE REPORT ANALYSIS FORM

A = essentially similar	B = minor variations	C = significant differences

System Performance Standards 7.1

	Units	A	B
1. What is the ratio of leases to purchases?	Purchase price of equipment whose leases began last year divided by dollars spent last year for equipment purchases	☐	☐
2. What is monthly lease expense?	dollars _____	☐	☐
3. How many vendors supply equipment to the hospital?	number in last six months ____	☐	☐
4. How many equipment-purchase decisions are made on the basis of competitive bids?	dollar value of equipment purchased on competitive basis divided by total number of dollars spent on equipment _____	☐	☐
5. Does an attorney review all purchase contracts and leases?	yes or no _____	☐	☐
6. Are POs prenumbered?	yes or no _____	☐	☐

7. Is a PO log maintained?

yes or no _____ ☐   ☐

USE PERFORMANCE STANDARDS ANALYSIS FORM

A = we have a standard   B = we do not have a standard

System Cost Factors 7.1

How many workhours are spent in preparing CON documents? $ _____

USE SYSTEM COST ANALYSIS FORM *(also see Instructions, p. 15)*

System 7.2:
Purchasing and General Stores
Description 7.2

Notes
↓

The focal point of the hospital's supply system is the Storeroom. All supply items that eventually will be distributed to hospital departments are kept in this Storeroom.

A B C
☐ ☐ ☐

The determination on what items the Storeroom stocks and which vendors are authorized as hospital suppliers is made by the Department Heads, the Director of Purchasing, and affected Administrative Officers.

☐ ☐ ☐

All items authorized for stocking are listed in the Supply Catalog, which the Storeroom prepares. This Catalog lists each item by name and Storeroom number.

☐ ☐ ☐

The Director of Purchasing establishes stocking levels, based on historical data or expected usage patterns. In many institutions, this level actually represents two figures – a high and a low. The high is the maximum amount the Storeroom will keep on hand; the low is the level to which the inventory must fall before a reorder is placed.

☐ ☐ ☐

In an ideal situation, a Storeroom would not be needed. Departments would run out of supplies at the same time that replacements were being delivered to Receiving. The actual goal then of the supply-purchasing activity is to minimize Storeroom inventory while ensuring that the number of times the hospital runs out of needed supplies is held to an acceptable minimum.

☐ ☐ ☐

Stocking

For most supplies, the Storeroom maintains an inventory-control card. Along with the name of the supply and its catalog number, this card contains columns for recording transaction date, amount ordered, amount received, amount disbursed, the department receiving the item, and the current on-hand level in the Storeroom. Each time the item is ordered, received, or sent to a department, an entry is made.

☐ ☐ ☐

These cards are filed either alphabetically or by Storeroom number.

☐ ☐ ☐

A = essentially similar   B = minor variations   C = significant differences

This system for keeping Storeroom records is called the perpetual-inventory approach.

Notes
↓

For some Storeroom items, another approach, called periodic inventory, is used. When this approach is used, Storeroom Clerks do not keep a running account to show how much of a given item is on hand. Periodically, a clerk counts the number on hand and records that figure on an inventory-tally sheet. One sheet is kept for each item, and the sheets are filed either alphabetically or numerically. Periodic inventory offers less control and less information, but is less expensive.

Ordering and Receiving

Periodically, a Storeroom Clerk reviews the on-hand level of certain supply items. For items under perpetual inventory, this review amounts to an examination of the inventory-control cards. For periodic-inventory items, the clerk takes a physical inventory.

The clerk completes a Storeroom-to-Purchasing requisition for all items that must be reordered. One copy is placed in a supplies-on-order file. The remaining copies go to Purchasing.

A Purchasing Clerk completes a PO for each item and logs the PO by recording the PO number, the item ordered, the vendor, and the date ordered.

One copy of this order is attached to a copy of the requisition and filed in a supplies-on-order file, with PO number determining the filing sequence. One copy is sent to the vendor. Two copies are sent to Receiving, where they are placed in a supplies-on-order file. One copy is sent to Accounts Payable.

To notify the Storeroom that the item has been ordered, some hospitals include a Storeroom copy in the distribution of their POs. This copy is returned to the Storeroom, where it is filed with the requisition. In other hospitals, the Purchasing Clerk writes the PO number onto a copy of the requisition and sends that copy back to the Storeroom. There, a clerk files this copy and destroys the one originally filed.

When a supply item is received, a Receiving Clerk removes the packing slip and invoice and inspects the package to confirm that the information on the packing slip is accurate. The clerk then removes the two copies of the PO from the file, records the quantity received on

A = essentially similar   B = minor variations   C = significant differences

the copies, and sends them to Purchasing, along with a copy of the packing slip and the vendor's invoice.

A B C
□ □ □ _____

A Storeroom Clerk then takes the items and the remaining copy of the packing slip to the Storeroom. A Storeroom Clerk signs the packing slip, acknowledging delivery of the supplies. The slip is then placed chronologically in a supplies-and-equipment received file.

□ □ □ _____

Meanwhile, at Purchasing, a clerk removes Purchasing's copy of the PO from the supplies-on-order file and matches it with the material received from the Storeroom.

□ □ □ _____

The clerk first compares the amount ordered with the amount received. If the delivery represents the entire order, the clerk enters the date received in the log book. The clerk then attaches the invoice to one of the Receiving copies and gives it to a Purchasing Supervisor. The supervisor inspects the documents, signs one of them, and sends the material to Accounts Payable. The signature authorizes Accounts Payable to pay vendor.

□ □ □ _____

The remaining documentation is placed in chronological order in a Completed PO file.

□ □ □ _____

If the order is incomplete, the Purchasing Clerk makes a partial-delivery notation in the log book and enters the amount received on Purchasing's copy of the Purchase Order. The clerk then attaches the invoice to one of the Receiving copies and gives the material to a supervisor, who signs the invoice and sends the material to Accounts Payable.

□ □ □ _____

The final Receiving copy of the PO is returned to Receiving, where it goes back into the supplies-on-order file. The remaining material is put back into Purchasing's supplies-on-order file.

□ □ □ _____

In the Storeroom, receipt of the supplies is noted on an inventory-control card, if the items are perpetual-inventory supplies.

□ □ □ _____

The supplies are then placed in their proper storage location. If the supplies are periodic-inventory items, they are taken directly to the storage location.

□ □ □ _____

In either case, a Storeroom Clerk removes the requisition for the item from the supplies-on-order file and places it in the supplies-received file.

□ □ □ _____

Requisitioning

When a department needs a supply, a department clerk completes a Storeroom requisition, puts one copy into a suspense file, and delivers the remaining copies to the Storeroom.

A B C
□ □ □ _____

Departments may use one of two types of requisition. For items that must be ordered often, the department may have prepared requisitions with the items' names and catalog numbers preprinted onto a form. In these cases, the clerk simply writes in the amount needed and the date.

□ □ □ _____

For less frequently used items, a general-purpose requisition is used. The clerk must write in the item's name and number on the general-purpose requisition.

□ □ □ _____

When the requisition is received, a clerk obtains the supplies from storage, makes the appropriate entries on an inventory-control card, and has the items delivered.

□ □ □ _____

The courier delivering the supplies obtains the signature of the person accepting them on one copy of the requisition. This is then returned to the Storeroom, where it is filed chronologically by department in a requisition-filled file.

□ □ □ _____

A Storeroom Clerk writes the price of the supplies on the other copy of the requisition and sends it to Accounting so the supply expense can be charged to the appropriate department.

□ □ □ _____

If the requisitioned item is not on hand, the Storeroom sends the department a back-ordered notification and places the copies of the requisition into a back-ordered file.

□ □ □ _____

This file is reviewed daily to determine if the request can be filled.

□ □ □ _____

In issuing supplies, most hospitals try to disburse the oldest items in stock. This minimizes loss due to spoilage.

□ □ □ _____

Catalog Changes

A Department Head normally has the authority to order a supply that is not in the catalog but is needed occasionally.

□ □ □ _____

The ordering procedure is the same except for the fact that a notation is made on the requisition, indicating that a noncatalog item is being ordered.

□ □ □ _____

A = essentially similar   B = minor variations   C = significant differences

If a particular noncatalog item is requested often, the Director of Purchasing may choose to include it in the next catalog. Normally, Storeroom Catalogs are reprinted yearly.

Notes
↓

A B C
☐ ☐ ☐ _____

Physical Inventory

Periodically, Purchasing performs an inventory of the Storeroom. Each item is counted, and the level is compared with levels indicated by inventory-control cards and requisitions.

☐ ☐ ☐ _____

A = essentially similar   B = minor variations   C = significant differences

Flow Chart 7.2a

Ordering and Receiving

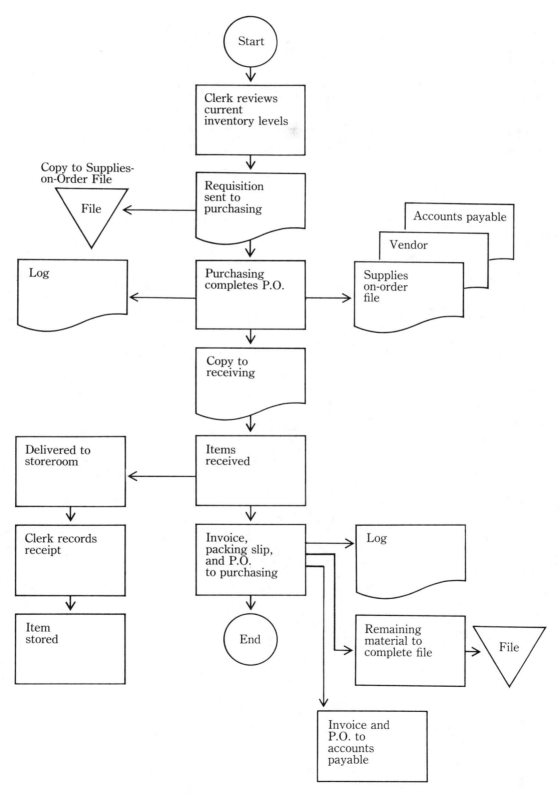

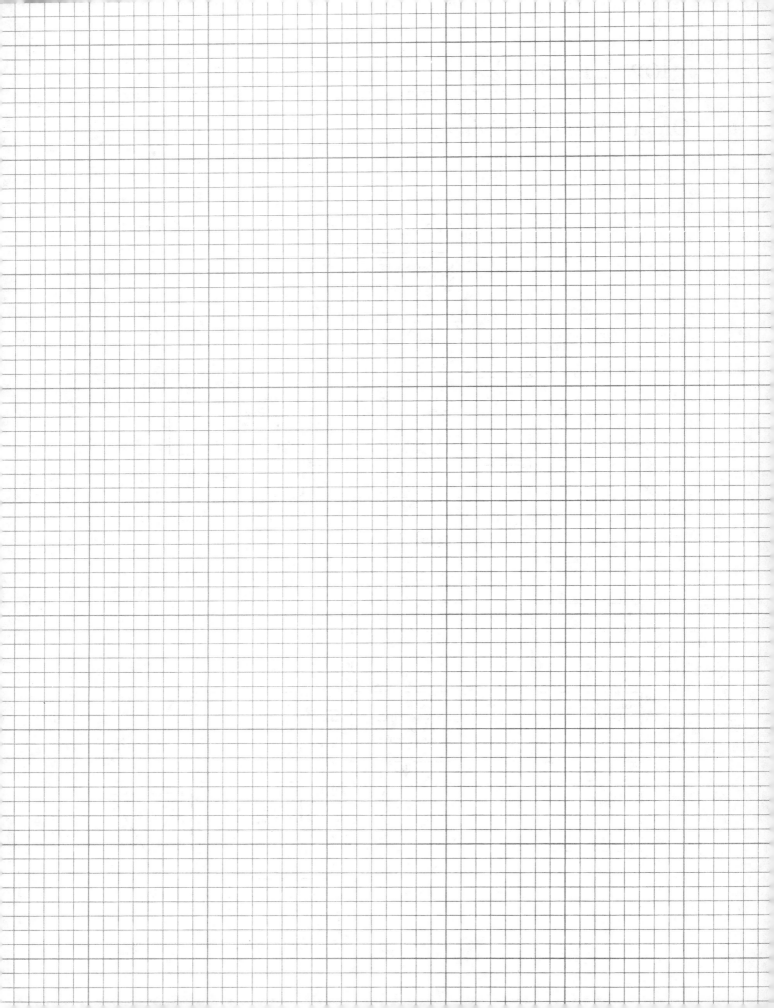

Flow Chart 7.2b

Requisitioning from the Storeroom

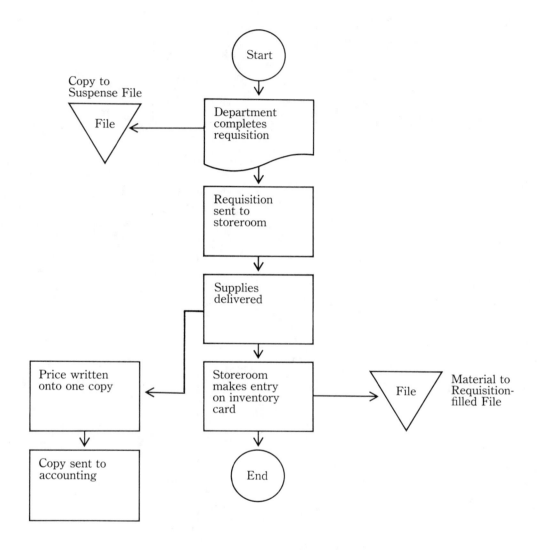

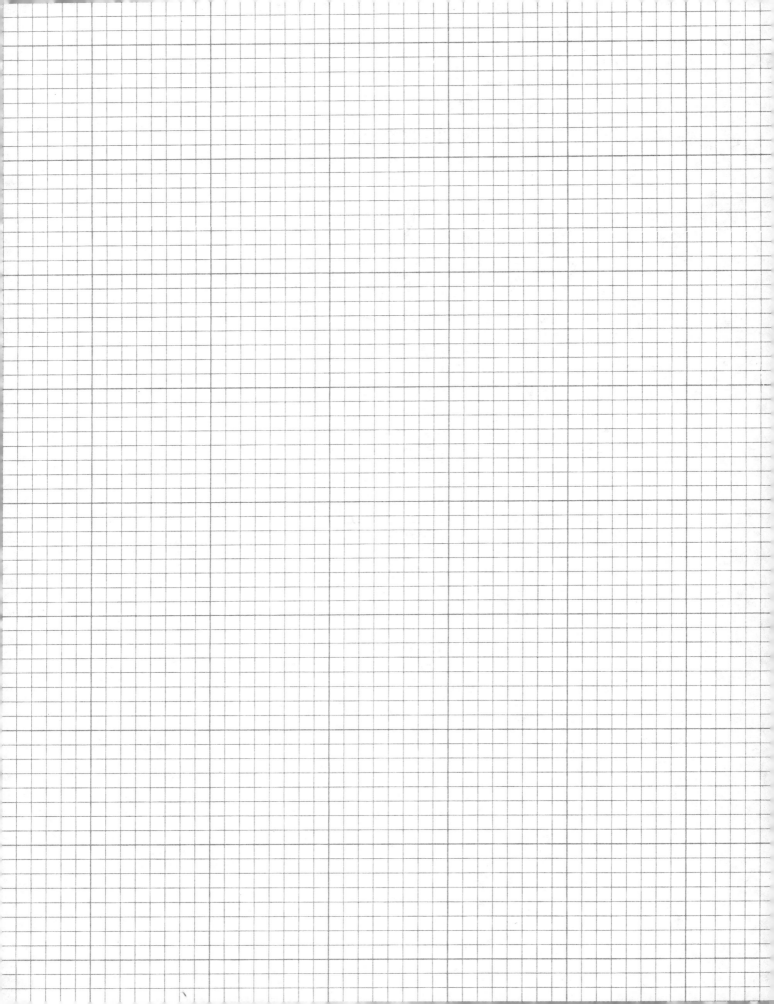

Input Inventory 7.2

A. Director of Purchasing

your document title

A B C

1. Inventory-control card. ☐ ☐ ☐ _____

2. Inventory tally sheet. ☐ ☐ ☐ _____

3. Back-order notification. ☐ ☐ ☐ _____

4. General requisition. ☐ ☐ ☐ _____

5. Preprinted requisitions. ☐ ☐ ☐ _____

6. Storeroom-to-Purchasing requisition. ☐ ☐ ☐ _____

USE INPUT DOCUMENT ANALYSIS FORM

A = same document title   B = minor variations   C = significant differences

Master File Inventory 7.2

A. Director of Purchasing

Notes

A B C

1. Supply Catalog. ☐ ☐ ☐ _____

2. Purchase Order Log. ☐ ☐ ☐ _____

3. Supplies-on-order file (Storeroom). ☐ ☐ ☐ _____

4. Supplies-on-order file (Purchasing). ☐ ☐ ☐ _____

5. Inventory-control file. ☐ ☐ ☐ _____

6. Inventory-tally-sheet file. ☐ ☐ ☐ _____

7. Back-order file. ☐ ☐ ☐ _____

8. Supplies received. ☐ ☐ ☐ _____

9. Requisitions-filled file. ☐ ☐ ☐ _____

B. Department Heads

Requisition suspense file. ☐ ☐ ☐ _____

USE MASTER FILE ANALYSIS FORM

A = essentially similar   B = minor variations   C = significant differences

Report Inventory 7.2

A. Director of Purchasing

your document title
↓

A B C

1. Inventory. ☐ ☐ ☐ _____

2. Monthly report of supplies received and disbursed. ☐ ☐ ☐ _____

B. Bookkeeping

Supply expense by department. ☐ ☐ ☐ _____

USE REPORT ANALYSIS FORM

A = essentially similar	B = minor variations	C = significant differences

System Performance Standards 7.2

	Units	A	B
1. Is there a Storeroom catalog?	yes or no _____	☐	☐
2. How often is it reprinted and revised?	number of months between revisions _____	☐	☐
3. Is each supply assigned a Storeroom number?	yes or no _____	☐	☐
4. How many items does the Storeroom stock?	number _____	☐	☐
5. How much is the inventory worth?	dollars _____	☐	☐
6. How much inventory must be discarded because of spoilage or obsolescence?	dollars each year _____	☐	☐
7. From the time a department orders a supply, how much time elapses until it is delivered?	hours _____	☐	☐
8. How many items are back-ordered?	number _____	☐	☐
9. How often is the Storeroom unable to fill a supply order?	number of times per month __	☐	☐
10. What percentage of items are on perpetual inventory?	number on perpetual inventory divided by total number of types of supplies stores _____	☐	☐
11. Are older supplies dispensed first?	yes or no _____	☐	☐

USE PERFORMANCE STANDARDS ANALYSIS FORM

A = we have a standard	B = we do not have a standard

System Cost Factors 7.2

1. How much space does the Storeroom take up? $ _____

2. How many clerical staffers are employed in Purchasing, Receiving, and the Storeroom? $ _____

USE SYSTEM COST ANALYSIS FORM *(also see Instructions, p. 15)*

System 7.3:
Central Supply

Description 7.3

Notes
↓

The major responsibility of Central Supply, or Central Service, is to provide patient-care supplies and equipment to Nursing Stations and to other clinical areas.

A B C
☐ ☐ ☐ _____

In executing this responsibility, the department performs the following key tasks:

1. Cleaning and sterilizing supplies and equipment.

☐ ☐ ☐ _____

2. Preparing surgical packs.

☐ ☐ ☐ _____

3. Maintaining adequate inventory levels of supply items.

☐ ☐ ☐ _____

4. Delivering supplies and equipment.

☐ ☐ ☐ _____

5. Ensuring that patients are charged for supplies and equipment.

☐ ☐ ☐ _____

6. Coordinating the inservice training needed by Nursing when new equipment and types of supplies are introduced.

☐ ☐ ☐ _____

In addition, Central Supply may perform a variety of other tasks. At many hospitals, relatively minor jobs that do not fit conveniently into any other department seem to wind up in Central Supply. Among the tasks the department may be called upon to carry out are providing courier service (i.e., pick up and deliver drugs, requisitions, written reports, etc.), performing surgical preps, receiving and delivering mail, installing traction, and delivering flowers to patient rooms.

☐ ☐ ☐ _____

Preparing Surgical Packs

Central Supply keeps on hand the linen it needs to make packs.

☐ ☐ ☐ _____

Dirty surgical instruments are either brought to the department by surgical personnel or picked up by Central Supply technicians. The instruments are washed, with special attention given to removing dried blood and other caked-on dirt. Once the instruments are clean, they are sorted and stored.

☐ ☐ ☐ _____

A = essentially similar   B = minor variations   C = significant differences

Each day a supervisor prepares a production schedule. Working from the schedule and written procedures for preparing different types of packs, technicians prepare the needed packs, which are then labeled, dated, and placed in a sterilizer. When the sterilization cycle is completed, the packs are removed and stored. Each day a supervisor inspects the stored packs, sending back for resterilization all of those that are more than a fixed number of days old.

A B C
☐ ☐ ☐ _____

Each day, Central Supply technicians remove packs from the storage area, and deliver them to Surgery and other departments, such as the ED and Obstetrics.

☐ ☐ ☐ _____

The delivering technician gives Surgery and these other departments enough of each type of pack to bring the on-hand supply up to present levels. The technician also notes on a resupply tally sheet how many of each type were delivered to each unit.

☐ ☐ ☐ _____

Sterilizing and preparing packs may not be centralized in Central Supply. In many hospitals, Surgery has its own sterilizing equipment. The amount of sterilization and pack preparation done by Surgery varies from hospital to hospital. In some, Surgery handles the task for the entire hospital. In others, Surgery does only its own pack work.

☐ ☐ ☐ _____

The most common approach is for Surgery to have limited sterilization capability – enough to allow staffers to clean and sterilize small, often-used instruments quickly so that they can be used more than once on the same day.

☐ ☐ ☐ _____

Inventory

Central Supply is responsible for stocking patient-care supplies – both disposable and non-disposable.

☐ ☐ ☐ _____

The common way the department obtains supplies is by ordering them through Purchasing. However, some hospitals allow the department to place its own orders.

☐ ☐ ☐ _____

Central Supply keeps track of on-hand levels of disposable items in one of two ways. For some items, the perpetual-inventory approach is used. Central Supply keeps an inventory-control card for each item it stocks. Each card shows the item, its Storeroom number, and its storage location in Central Supply. The card also has columns for recording transaction information – transaction date, how much was ordered, how much was disbursed and to whom, how much

A = essentially similar   B = minor variations   C = significant differences

was received and at what price, and how much is currently on hand. As an item is ordered, disbursed, or received, appropriate entries are made on the card.

The other approach is called periodic inventory. No running count is kept of the on-hand quantity. As items are needed, they are disbursed; as the supply level becomes low, they are ordered; and as they are received, they are stocked. Periodically, a Central Supply technician makes a physical inventory, recording the amount on hand on an inventory tally sheet. There is one sheet for each item, with columns for writing the date of the inventory and the amount on hand.

On a daily or weekly basis, a Central Supply clerk reviews current stocking levels. A Store-room requisition is completed for each item that must be recorded. One copy is placed in the supplies-ordered file, usually in chronological order. For perpetual-inventory items, the proper notation is made on the inventory control card. The remaining copies of the requisition are sent to the Storeroom.

A Storeroom Clerk prepares the items requisitioned for delivery. The clerk then enters the price of each item onto the requisition. The items and the remaining copies of the requisition are taken by a Storeroom Clerk to Central Supply. There, a clerk signs the requisition to indicate acceptance. One copy is returned to the Storeroom; the other stays in the department.

A Central Supply Clerk makes the appropriate entries on inventory-control records and enters the current price of the item on the inventory-control card, the inventory-tally sheet, or a master-price listing. The pricing information will be used in assigning supply costs to individual departments.

The clerk then removes the copy of the requisition from the supplies-order file, throws it away, and places the copy with the prices in a requisition-complete file. This is kept either chronologically or alphabetically by vendor or by the name of the supply. The supplies are then placed in storage.

Supply Cleaning

Aside from surgical instruments, various reusable supply items, such as syringes and bedpans, are also cleaned by Central Supply.

Central Supply technicians pick up dirty reusables from the Nursing Stations and bring them back to the department for cleaning. They are then placed in storage for further use.

A B C
□ □ □ _____

Floor Stock

Each Nursing Station, as well as other clinical areas, stocks certain patient-care items so they are available for immediate use. Central Supply is responsible for keeping these floor stocks at the appropriate levels.

□ □ □ _____

There are three common ways of carrying out this task – the fixed-stocking-level approach, the exchange-cart method, and the requisition approach.

□ □ □ _____

In some hospitals, each Nursing Station and clinical area is authorized to stock certain items at certain levels. In those institutions, either the fixed-level or the exchange-cart method may be used.

□ □ □ _____

When the fixed-level method is used, Central Supply technicians go to the storage areas of each Nursing Station and clinical area, count the number of each authorized supply on hand, then add enough to the inventory to bring each item up to its preset level. The technicians then record on a daily-delivery sheet how many of each item were added. Typically, one sheet will be completed for each Nursing Station and clinical area each day. These sheets are filed chronologically by station or area.

□ □ □ _____

When the exchange-cart method is used, two supply carts are set aside for each Nursing Station and clinical area. Each day a Central Supply technician takes one cart – stocked to the appropriate level for each item – to each Nursing Station and clinical area. The technician then brings back the other cart, which has been in use for the past 24 hours.

□ □ □ _____

Technicians then restock the cart, recording on a daily-delivery sheet how many of each item are going into the cart.

□ □ □ _____

On the following day, the cycle is repeated.

□ □ □ _____

In the requisition approach, a unit secretary or departmental clerk completes a requisition for any item that a Head Nurse or supervisor believes is falling below acceptable levels. One copy is kept in a suspense file at the station or area. The other copies are sent to Central Supply. The items are sent to the station or area, along with a copy of the requisition. The

---

A = essentially similar   B = minor variations   C = significant differences

person accepting the items signs the requisition, which is then returned to the department, where it is filed chronologically by Nursing Station or area.

A B C
☐ ☐ ☐

Regardless of the method used, a Central Supply technician makes appropriate entries on the inventory-control card of each perpetual-inventory item issued.

☐ ☐ ☐

On a periodic basis (usually monthly), a Central Supply clerk computes the cost of supplies sent to each Nursing Station and clinical area. This expense-by-department figure is sent to the Bookkeeper.

☐ ☐ ☐

Charging

In any one hospital, charges of disposable and nondisposable supplies are generated in the same way. However, among hospitals there are a variety of methods used for charge generation.

☐ ☐ ☐

One common approach is to have the Nurse who is dispensing the supply complete a charge ticket, which shows the patient's name and number and the name of the item used. This ticket is sent to Central Supply, where a clerk enters the appropriate charge. The document is then sent to the Business Office.

☐ ☐ ☐

In many hospitals, the name of the item and the price is preprinted onto a charge form, which is attached to the supply. The nurse enters the patient's name and number, then sends the form to Central Supply. There it is reviewed and sent to the Business Office.

☐ ☐ ☐

Another approach is to use removable labels showing the name and price of a supply. A label is attached to the supply before it is sent to the Nursing Station. When the item is used, the label is removed and stuck onto a charge card containing the patient's name and number. The labels and cards are designed so the card can handle labels for a day's worth of supplies. At the end of a 24-hour period, the cards for all patients in a Nursing Station are removed from their central file and sent to Central Supply for forwarding to the Business Office. A unit secretary then prepares a new charge card for each patient for use in the next 24-hour period.

☐ ☐ ☐

Special Supplies

When a supply that is not part of floor stock is needed, a nurse telephones the order to Central Supply and completes a charge ticket. A Central

Supply courier delivers the item and picks up the charge ticket. Back in Central Supply, a clerk writes the price onto the ticket and forwards it to the Business Office.

A B C
☐ ☐ ☐ _____

Control

Many hospitals use charge tickets to control the dispensing of supplies in order to ensure that a charge ticket has been produced for each supply item dispensed. One way to do this is to compare charge tickets with the listing of supplies issued. They should match.

☐ ☐ ☐ _____

Another approach is to use the charge tickets as requisitions. One item is replaced for each charge ticket received.

☐ ☐ ☐ _____

Equipment

Central Supply maintains a stock of portable clinical-care equipment (e.g., suction machines, monitors, thermal blankets) to be sent to Nursing Stations for the use of individual patients. When a patient no longer needs the equipment, it is returned to the department.

☐ ☐ ☐ _____

In some hospitals, Central Supply keeps a control card for each piece of equipment. For those items in the department, the cards are kept in alphabetical order in an equipment-ready file. Each card contains the name of the item, its daily charge, and its serial number.

☐ ☐ ☐ _____

When a piece of equipment is needed, a nurse completes an equipment requisition and sends it to Central Supply. A clerk enters the date, the patient's name and number, and the patient's room and bed number onto the control card for the desired item. A Central Supply technician takes the equipment to the patient, and the clerk places the control card in an equipment-in-use file.

☐ ☐ ☐ _____

Each day the clerk contacts the Nursing Stations that are using equipment, to assure that all dispatched equipment is still in use. For those items that are still being used, the clerk prepares a charge ticket and sends it to the Business Office. The clerk dispatches a technician to retrieve those items that no longer are needed. When this equipment arrives back in the department, the clerk records the date and transfers the card back to the equipment-ready file. The equipment itself is cleaned and placed in storage.

☐ ☐ ☐ _____

A = essentially similar   B = minor variations   C = significant differences

Dedicated Equipment

It is not unusual for equipment whose use is
chargeable to be assigned permanently to a
Nursing Station.

For these items, the unit secretary prepares a
charge ticket each day. The tickets are sent to
Central Supply for pricing and forwarding to the
Business Office.

Notes

A B C
□ □ □ _____

□ □ □ _____

A = essentially similar   B = minor variations   C = significant differences

Flow Chart 7.3a

Pack Preparation

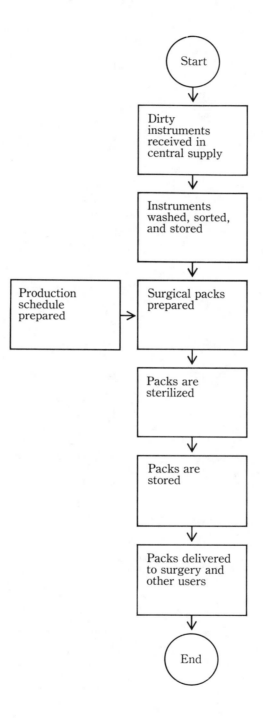

Flow Chart 7.3b

Inventory

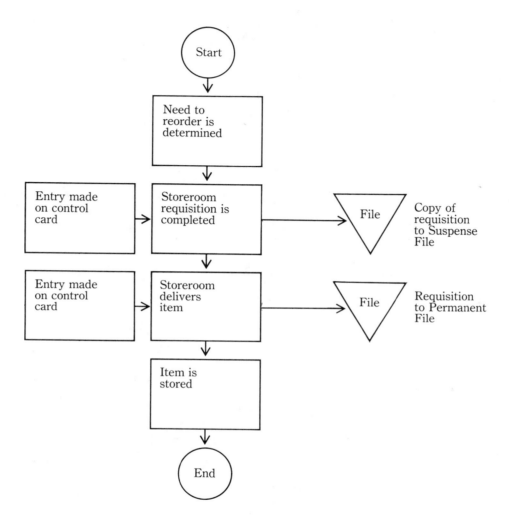

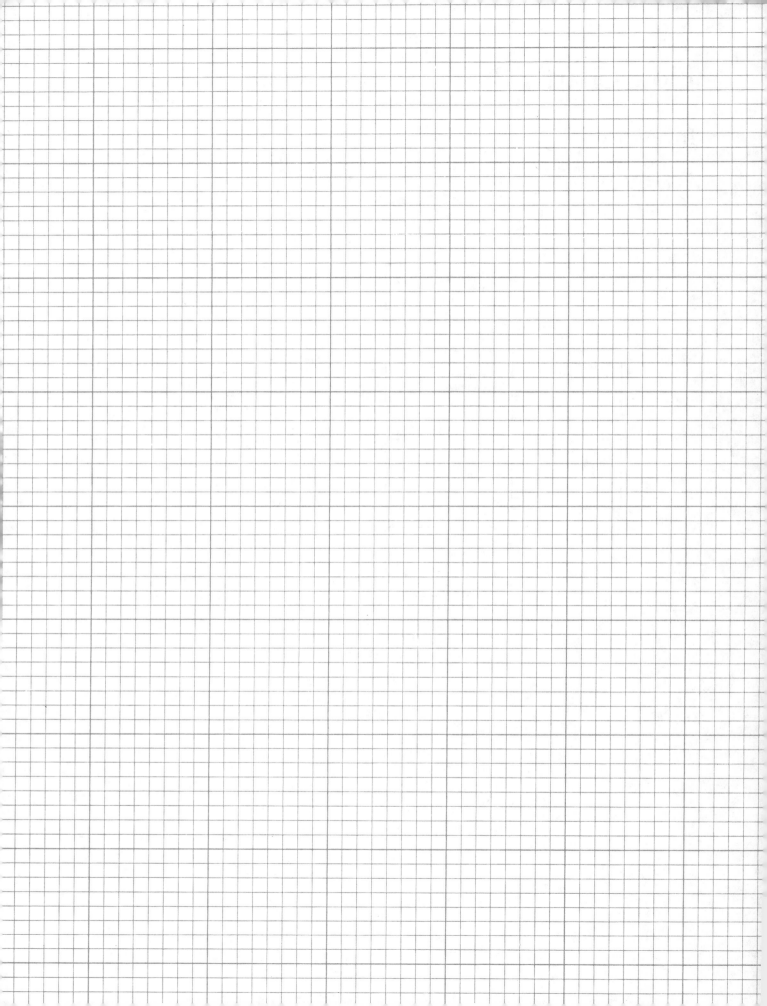

Flow Chart 7.3c

Maintaining Floor Stock

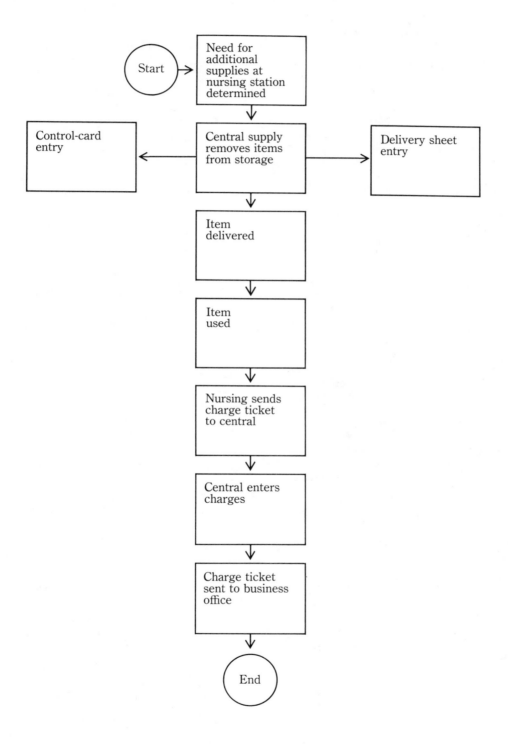

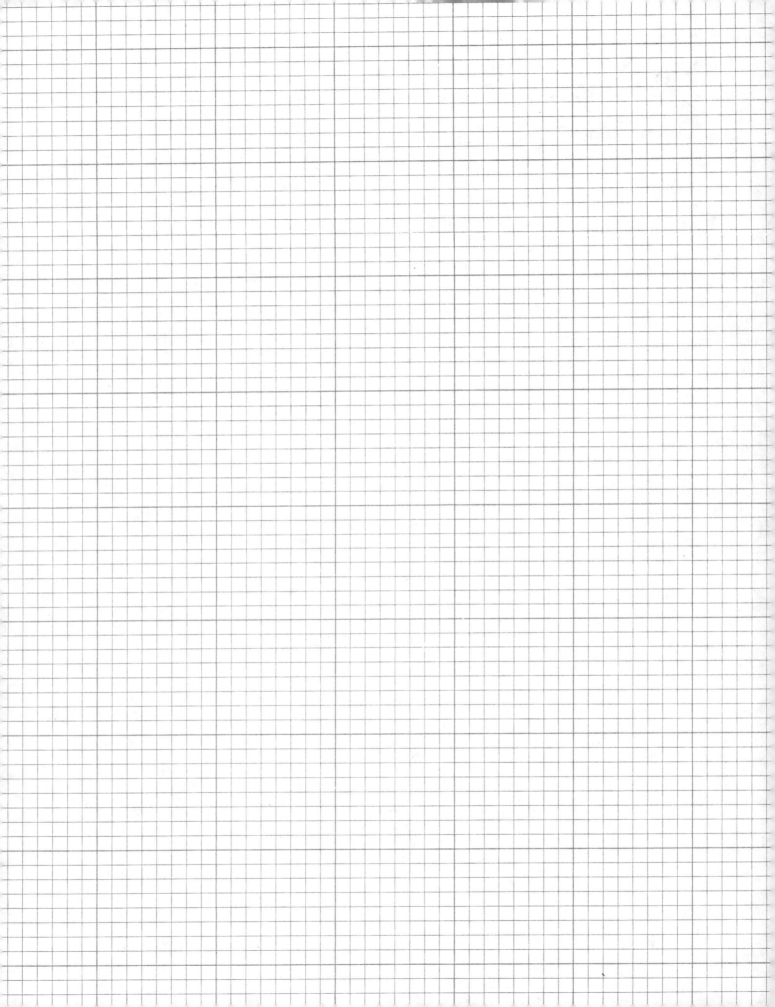

Flow Chart 7.3d

Equipment

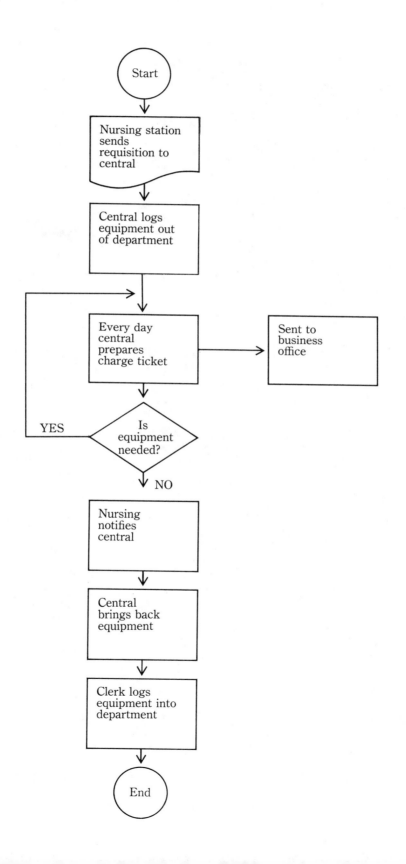

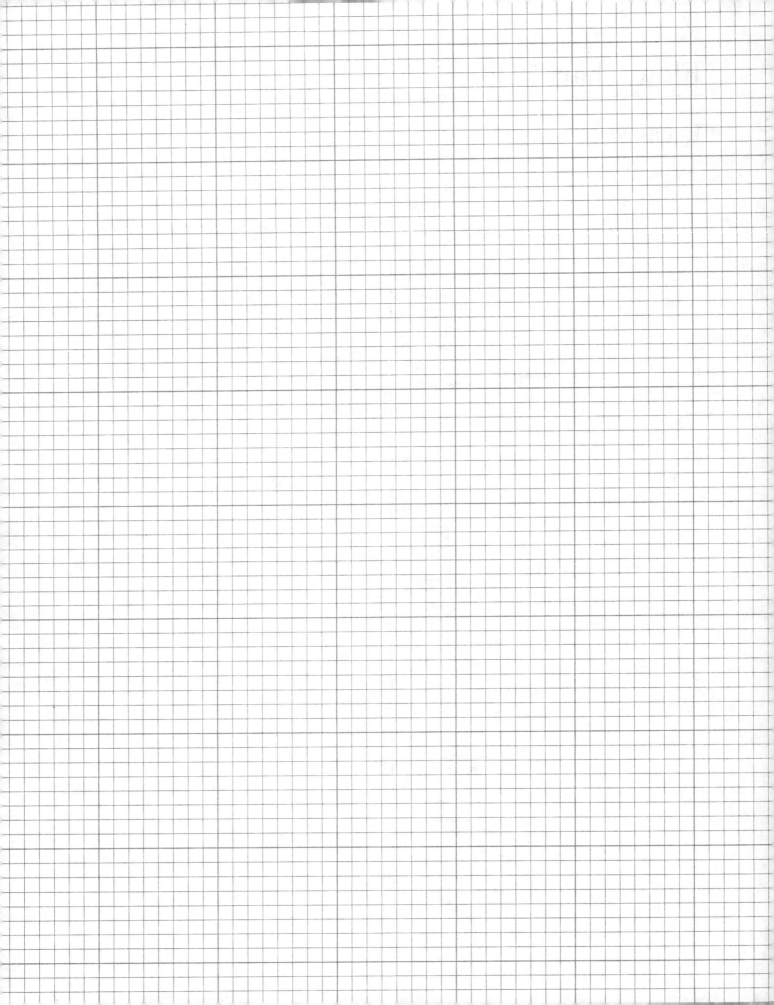

Input Inventory 7.3

A. Director of Central Supply

your document title
↓

A B C

1. Surgical Pack Resupply tally sheet. □ □ □ _____

2. Inventory control card. □ □ □ _____

3. Inventory tally sheet. □ □ □ _____

4. Storeroom requisition. □ □ □ _____

5. Daily supply delivery sheet. □ □ □ _____

6. Supply requisition (sent to Central Supply). □ □ □ _____

7. Special supply requisitions (e.g., preprinted, checklists). □ □ □ _____

8. Supply charge ticket. □ □ □ _____

9. Equipment control card. □ □ □ _____

10. Equipment requisition. □ □ □ _____

11. Equipment charge ticket. □ □ □ _____

12. Charge ticket for dedicated equipment. □ □ □ _____

USE INPUT DOCUMENT ANALYSIS FORM

A = same document title	B = minor variations	C = significant differences

Master File Inventory 7.3

A. Director of Central Supply

Notes
↓

A B C

1. Surgical pack production schedule. □ □ □ _____

2. Procedures for preparing surgical packs. □ □ □ _____

3. Control care file. □ □ □ _____

4. Supply tally sheet file. □ □ □ _____

5. Supplies-ordered file. □ □ □ _____

6. Supplies-received file. □ □ □ _____

7. Daily delivery sheets. □ □ □ _____

8. Listing of floor stock authorized for each Nursing Station and clinical area. □ □ □ _____

	A B C	Notes
9. Equipment-ready file.	☐ ☐ ☐	_____
10. Equipment-in-use file.	☐ ☐ ☐	_____

USE MASTER FILE ANALYSIS FORM

A = essentially similar	B = minor variations	C = significant differences

Report Inventory 7.3

A. Director of Central Supply

your document title ↓

	A B C	
1. Supply costs by department and Nursing Station.	☐ ☐ ☐	_____
2. Monthly activity report.	☐ ☐ ☐	_____
3. Unfilled requisitions.	☐ ☐ ☐	_____

USE REPORT ANALYSIS FORM

A = essentially similar	B = minor variations	C = significant differences

System Performance Standards 7.3

	Units	A B
1. What is the value of the supply inventory on hand?	dollars _____	☐ ☐
2. How often is a piece of equipment ordered that is not on hand in Central Supply?	number of times per month __	☐ ☐
3. How many surgical packs must be resterilized because of high shelf life?	number of resterilizations per week _____	☐ ☐
4. How often is a needed pack unavailable in Surgery?	number of times per month __	☐ ☐
5. How often must surgery be delayed until a pack can be prepared or instruments can be resterilized?	number of times per month __	☐ ☐
6. Are there written procedures for preparing packs?	yes or no _____	☐ ☐
7. What is the number of types of supplies stored in Central Supply?	number_____	☐ ☐
8. How often is the Storeroom unable to deliver a requested supply immediately?	number of times per week____	☐ ☐
9. What is the value of floor stock authorized for a general Nursing Station?	dollars _____	☐ ☐
10. Does Nursing prepare a charge ticket for every chargeable supply issued?	yes or no _____	☐ ☐

432

11. How often do Nursing Stations run out of supplies?

	Units	A	B
	number of times per week____	☐	☐

12. Once a supply is dispensed, how much time elapses before a charge ticket arrives in the Business Office?

hours_____   ☐ ☐

13. Are supplies delivered checked against charge tickets prepared?

yes or no _____   ☐ ☐

14. When a supply is ordered by telephone, how long does it take to deliver it?

mean time in minutes_____   ☐ ☐

15. Once a requisition for equipment is received, how much time elapses before it is installed?

minutes_____   ☐ ☐

16. What is the percentage margin generated by supplies?

annual cost of chargeable
supplies divided by annual
supply revenue _____   ☐ ☐

USE PERFORMANCE STANDARDS ANALYSIS FORM

A = we have a standard   B = we do not have a standard

System Cost Factors 7.3

1. How many sterilizers does the hospital have? $ _____

2. In how many different departments are these located? $ _____

3. Who authorizes switches from nondisposable to disposable supplies? $ _____

4. How much area is used by Central Supply for storage? $ _____

5. How much time do nurses spend filling out supply charge tickets? $ _____

6. How accurate are the charges recorded on charge tickets? $ _____

USE SYSTEM COST ANALYSIS FORM *(also see Instructions, p. 15)*

Facilities and Equipment Management Systems

System 8.1: Work Orders

Description 8.1

Notes ↓

When repairs or renovations are needed in a given area, the Head of the affected department completes a work order. This multicopy form states what is being requested and its priority (e.g., high, routine, low). The Department Head signs the form, keeps one copy for the suspense file, and sends the remaining copies to Maintenance.

A B C
□ □ □ _____

When emergency repairs are needed, Maintenance is contacted by telephone. The work is done as soon as possible, and the paperwork is completed later.

□ □ □ _____

In nonemergency cases involving large investments of time or money, hospital policy usually dictates that the administrative offices in charge of the department requesting the work sign the work order before it is sent to Maintenance.

□ □ □ _____

When the work order arrives at Maintenance, a clerk assigns it a number and logs it. The clerk removes one copy of the form and files it numerically in a work-in-progress file. The remaining copies go to the supervisor, who schedules the work, assigns personnel to carry it out, and designates one person to be the team leader. The team leader receives a copy of the work order.

□ □ □ _____

The team leader investigates the request, plans the team activities, and draws the needed supplies from Maintenance's storeroom. When the storeroom clerk issues the supplies, he or she records the work order number on storeroom's listing of supplies issued.

□ □ □ _____

The team then begins work on the project, with the leader keeping a record of the number of hours worked by each person.

□ □ □ _____

When the job is completed, the supervisor inspects the work. The team leader then records on the work order the total hours worked by each person, the date the project began, and the date the job was completed.

□ □ □ _____

The team leader turns the work order in to the maintenance clerk, who files it in a temporary

---

A = essentially similar   B = minor variations   C = significant differences

437

work-completed file. This file contains copies of the work orders for all jobs completed that month.

A B C
☐ ☐ ☐ _____

The clerk then records the completion of the job in the log and destroys the copy of the work order that is in the work-in-progress file.

☐ ☐ ☐ _____

Monthly Report

At the end of the month, the storeroom clerk gives the maintenance clerk a list of all supplies issued that month, categorized by work-order number. This list also contains prices for the supplies.

☐ ☐ ☐ _____

To obtain wage expenses, the maintenance clerk goes to the temporary work-completed file. Using these work orders and the Storeroom report, the maintenance clerk prepares a report showing what work was done for each department and what the supply and wage expenses were for those jobs. One copy of this report is filed in Maintenance. Another copy goes to the Business Office.

☐ ☐ ☐ _____

The work orders from the temporary file are kept in numerical sequence in the permanent work-completed file.

☐ ☐ ☐ _____

A = essentially similar   B = minor variations   C = significant differences

Flow Chart 8.1

Work Order

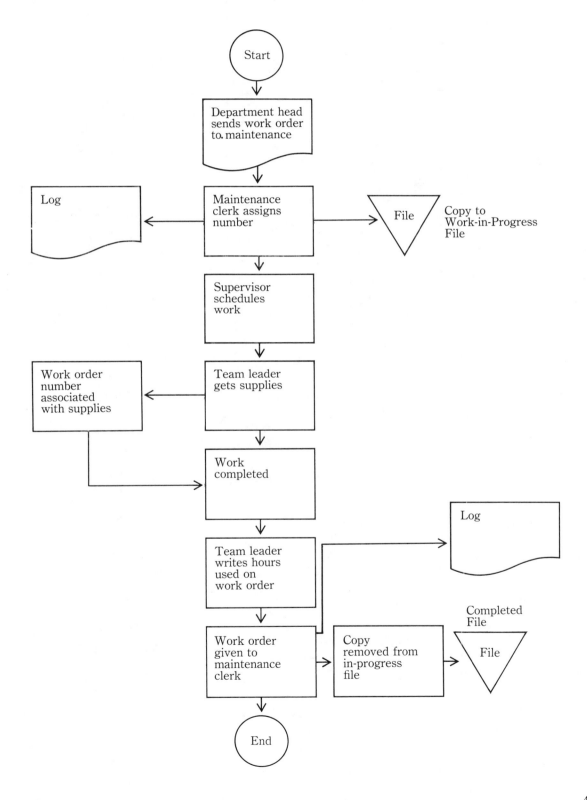

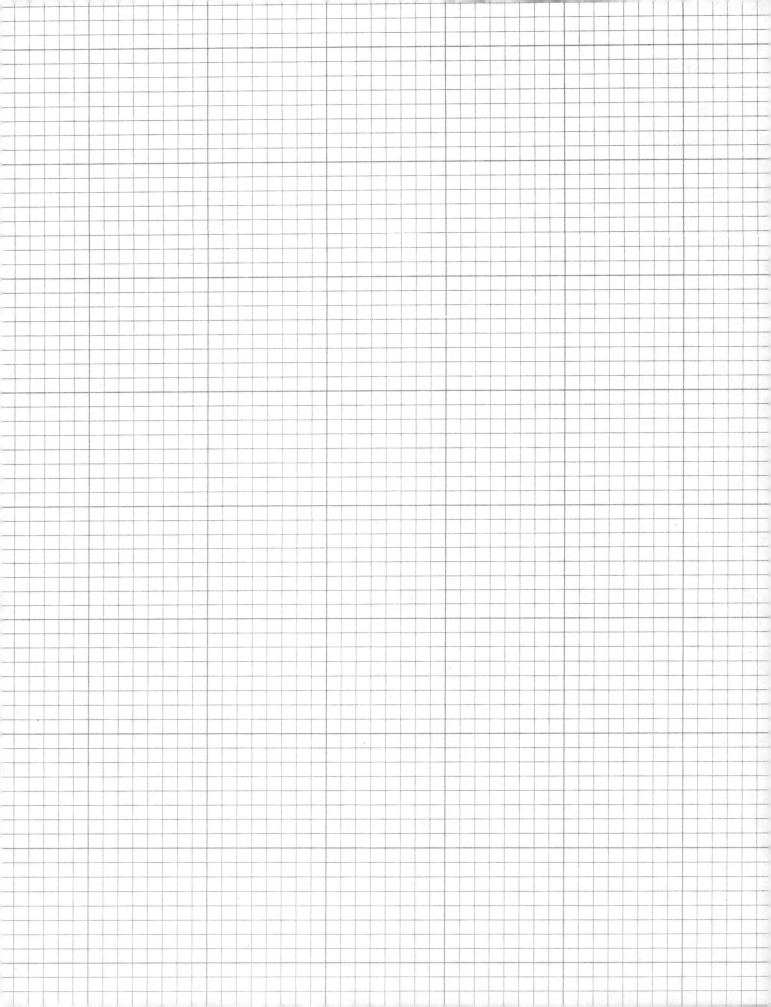

Input Inventory 8.1

A. Maintenance Supervisor

your document title
↓

          A B C

1. Work order.   ☐ ☐ ☐ _____

2. Supplies-issued sheet.   ☐ ☐ ☐ _____

USE INPUT DOCUMENT ANALYSIS FORM

A = same document title   B = minor variations   C = significant differences

Master File Inventory 8.1

A. Maintenance Supervisor

Notes
↓

          A B C

1. Log.   ☐ ☐ ☐ _____

2. Work-in-progress file.   ☐ ☐ ☐ _____

3. Temporary work-completed file.   ☐ ☐ ☐ _____

4. Permanent work-completed file.   ☐ ☐ ☐ _____

5. Schedule.   ☐ ☐ ☐ _____

USE MASTER FILE ANALYSIS FORM

A = essentially similar   B = minor variations   C = significant differences

Report Inventory 8.1

A. Maintenance Supervisor

your document title
↓

          A B C

1. Storeroom report of supplies issued.   ☐ ☐ ☐ _____

2. Monthly report of work done for each department.   ☐ ☐ ☐ _____

USE REPORT ANALYSIS FORM

A = essentially similar   B = minor variations   C = significant differences

System Performance Standards 8.1

Units

			A	B
1. How much time elapses between the preparation of a work order by a Department Head and the dispatching of a team to perform the work?	hours_____		☐	☐
2. How many work orders are in the work-in-progress file?	number_____		☐	☐
3. How long does it take to complete a work order?	days (equal to the average age of work orders in the work-in-progress file) _____		☐	☐
4. How many emergency jobs does the department do?	number of emergency calls divided by total number of work orders received per month _____		☐	☐
5. How many work orders are delayed because of a lack of supplies?	number per month _____		☐	☐

USE PERFORMANCE STANDARDS ANALYSIS FORM

A = we have a standard   B = we do not have a standard

System Cost Factors 8.1

1. How many clerical staffers work in Maintenance? $ _____

2. Does the department have a method of keeping track of where employees are and what they are doing? $ _____

USE SYSTEM COST ANALYSIS FORM *(also see Instructions, p. 15)*

System 8.2:
Scheduled Maintenance
Description 8.2

Notes
↓

Maintenance is responsible for performing scheduled, cyclic maintenance on the hospital buildings, many pieces of major equipment, and components of such vital building systems as the air conditioning/heating network.

A B C
☐ ☐ ☐ _____

Scheduled maintenance can be anything from a visual inspection to a complete rebuilding.

☐ ☐ ☐ _____

Hospitals use a variety of approaches to handle scheduled maintenance. Most involve establishing two files – one an information file, the other a tickler file.

☐ ☐ ☐ _____

The information file has a separate folder for each piece of equipment or building component requiring scheduled maintenance. The label on the folder gives the item's name, serial number, and location. The folder itself contains vendor literature and procedure sheets explaining how to perform scheduled maintenance. These sheets are often in the form of checklists.

☐ ☐ ☐ _____

The tickler file is a card file. It has a card for every item requiring scheduled maintenance. Each card contains the item's name, serial number, and location, as well as a brief description of the item's scheduled maintenance program (e.g., quarterly visual inspection, change filters once a year). The card also has space to record when scheduled maintenance was performed and by whom. The last entry in this section should be the date of the next scheduled maintenance. When that day arrives and the maintenance is performed, this fact is recorded next to the date, and the next due date is written on the following line.

☐ ☐ ☐ _____

These tickler cards are filed chronologically according to the date of the next scheduled maintenance.

☐ ☐ ☐ _____

Each day a maintenance clerk removes all tickler cards for the next day's scheduled maintenance. The clerk prepares a scheduled maintenance work order for each job, assigning each a number and logging it in the scheduled maintenance log book.

☐ ☐ ☐ _____

A = essentially similar   B = minor variations   C = significant differences

443

The clerk removes one copy of the work order and places it in numerical order in the work-in-progress file.

A B C
☐ ☐ ☐ _____

The clerk then obtains a checklist for the job from the alphabetical file and attaches the checklist to the appropriate work order. This material is sent to a supervisor, who schedules the job and assigns maintenance personnel to it.

☐ ☐ ☐ _____

The supervisor keeps one copy of the work order and gives the other, along with the checklist, to the maintenance team leader.

☐ ☐ ☐ _____

The leader inspects the area where the maintenance is to be performed, then reviews the checklist. Next, the leader obtains the needed supplies from the maintenance storeroom. The storeroom clerk records the supplies issued and the number of the job for which they were drawn.

☐ ☐ ☐ _____

The assigned maintenance team performs the scheduled task and returns to the department. The leader records on the work order the number of hours required of each team member. The leader completes the checklist and signs it. Both documents are returned to the maintenance clerk, who logs the completion of the job, returns the checklist to the alphabetical file, records the completion of the job on the tickler card, and enters the next scheduled maintenance date on the tickler card before refiling it. Finally, the clerk removes the copy of the work order that has been in the work-in-progress file. The work-order copy received from the team leader is placed in a completed-job file. This file is organized by month in numerical sequence.

☐ ☐ ☐ _____

Outside Contractors

Maintenance itself does not perform all scheduled maintenance. Some work is done through contracts with outside firms. The tickler file should also contain cards for these jobs, with each card noting the name of the outside contractor who is responsible.

☐ ☐ ☐ _____

When the maintenance clerk takes these cards from the file, he or she gives them to a supervisor who determines if the scheduled services were actually rendered. If they were, the supervisor notes the completion on the tickler card, writes down the next scheduled maintenance date, and returns the card to the clerk for filing.

☐ ☐ ☐ _____

Flow Chart 8.2

Scheduled Maintenance

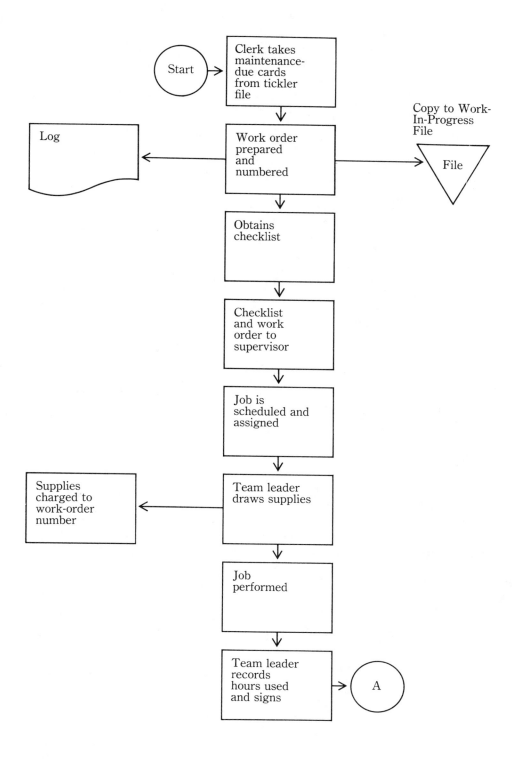

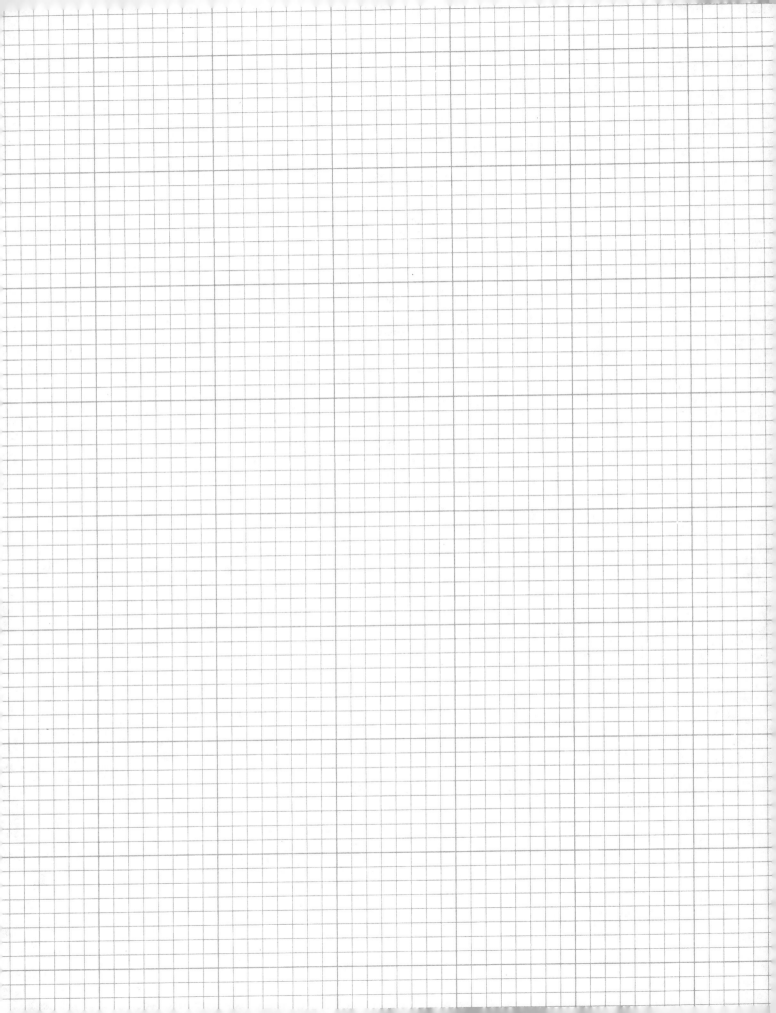

Scheduled Maintenance, continued

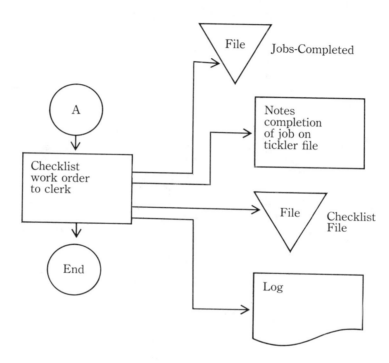

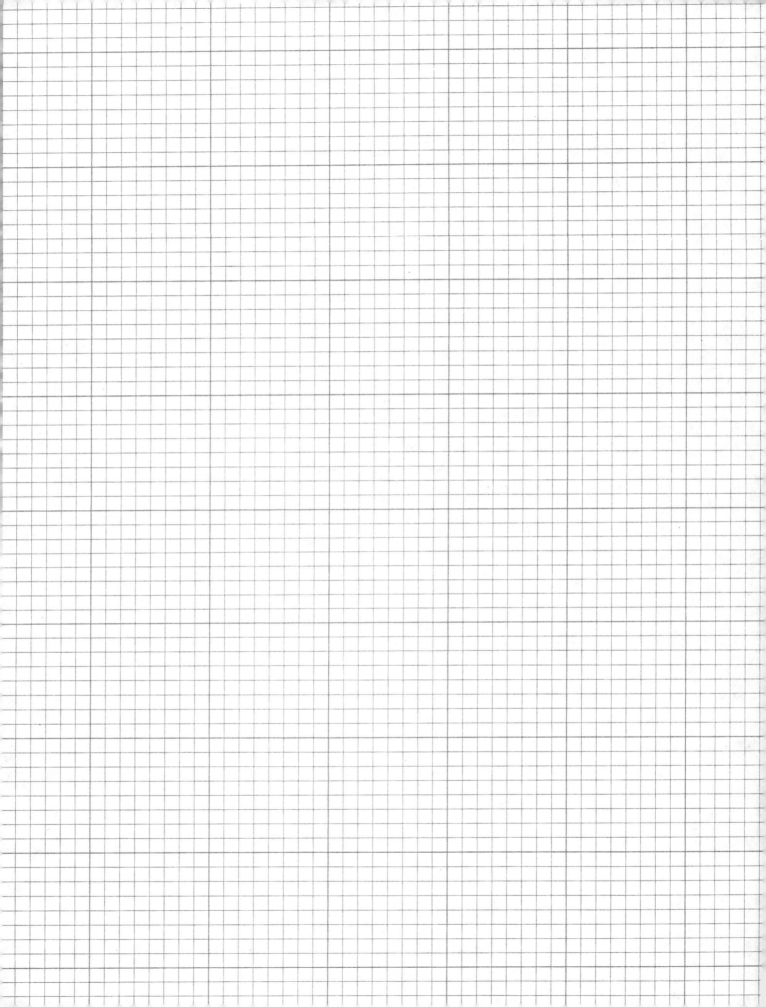

Input Inventory 8.2

A. Maintenance Supervisor

your document title
↓

A B C

1. Scheduled-maintenance work order. □ □ □ _____

2. Procedures/checklists for scheduled
   maintenance. □ □ □ _____

USE INPUT DOCUMENT ANALYSIS FORM

A = same document title   B = minor variations   C = significant differences

Master File Inventory 8.2

A. Maintenance Supervisor

Notes
↓

A B C

1. Alphabetical file for equipment and
   components needing scheduled maintenance. □ □ □ _____

2. Tickler file. □ □ □ _____

3. Work-in-progress file. □ □ □ _____

4. Completed-job file. □ □ □ _____

5. Scheduled-maintenance log. □ □ □ _____

USE MASTER FILE ANALYSIS FORM

A = essentially similar   B = minor variations   C = significant differences

Report Inventory 8.2

A. Maintenance Supervisor

your document title
↓

A B C

1. Activity report. □ □ □ _____

2. Monthly report by job number recording
   supplies used and hours worked. □ □ □ _____

USE REPORT ANALYSIS FORM

A = essentially similar   B = minor variations   C = significant differences

System Performance Standards 8.2

Units

1. What proportion of the total workhours worked by Maintenance is devoted to scheduled maintenance?

    hours worked per month on scheduled maintenance divided by hours worked overall _____

    A   B
    ☐   ☐

2. How many items receive scheduled maintenance?

    number_____

    ☐   ☐

3. How much is spent for scheduled maintenance service contracts?

    dollars _____

    ☐   ☐

4. Does Maintenance charge other departments for scheduled maintenance work?

    yes or no _____

    ☐   ☐

5. Do other departments participate in the scheduled maintenance program?

    yes or no _____

    ☐   ☐

6. How far behind schedule is the hospital in performing scheduled maintenance?

    days _____

    ☐   ☐

7. Does the hospital have written checklists for scheduled maintenance?

    yes or no _____

    ☐   ☐

USE PERFORMANCE STANDARDS ANALYSIS FORM

A = we have a standard   B = we do not have a standard

System Cost Factors 8.2

1. What special tools must the hospital buy to perform scheduled maintenance? $ _____

2. How much time do maintenance personnel spend doing clerical tasks? $ _____

3. How many breakdowns occur on items that are maintained on a scheduled basis? $ _____

4. Does the hospital have a separate biomedical-engineering section? $ _____

USE SYSTEM COST ANALYSIS FORM *(also see Instructions, p. 15)*

Management Planning and Control Systems

System 9.1:
Internal Management Reporting

The generation and flow of management information vary widely from hospital to hospital. In many situations, there is no formal management reporting process. Report generation has evolved with little consideration given to the question of who needs what information when.

The following charts list key items of information that could be of use to a hospital's Chief Executive Officer (CEO). For each item of information, ask the CEO the following questions:

A. Do you receive this information?

    1. Yes
    2. No

B. How often do you get this information?

    1. Daily
    2. Weekly
    3. Bimonthly
    4. Monthly
    5. Quarterly
    6. Yearly
    7. On request
    8. On an exception basis

C. Is the current information compared with historical data?

    1. Yes
    2. No

D. Is the current information compared with budget information or other standards?

    1. Yes
    2. No

E. Who supplies the information?

    1. Administrative Officer who reports to the CEO
    2. Personnel
    3. Medical Staff
    4. A Clinical Department
    5. Medical Records
    6. Fiscal Affairs
    7. Admitting
    8. Nursing
    9. Other Department
    10. Outside agency

F. How old is the information when you get it?

    1.   Less than one day old
    2.   Less than one week old
    3.   Less than two weeks old
    4.   Less than one month old
    5.   More than one month old

G. What is the name of the report that contains the information?

Internal Management Reporting Evaluation

INFORMATION	A. Do you receive this information? (1. Yes, 2. No)	B. How often do you get this information? (1. Daily, 2. Weekly, 3. Bimonthly, 4. Monthly, 5. Quarterly, 6. Yearly, 7. On request, 8. On an exception basis)	C. Is the current information compared with historical data? (1. Yes, 2. No)	D. Is the current information compared with budget information on other standards? (1. Yes, 2. No)	E. Who supplies the information? (1. Administrative Officer who reports to the CEO, 2. Personnel, 3. Medical Staff, 4. A Clinical Department, 5. Medical Records, 6. Fiscal Affairs, 7. Admitting, 8. Nursing, 9. Other Department, 10. Outside agency)	F. How old is the information when you get it? (1. Less than one day, 2. Less than one week, 3. Less than two weeks, 4. Less than one month, 5. More than one month)	G. What is the name of the report that contains the information?
1. Days in Receivables							
2. Amount of cash on hand							
3. Inpatient revenue per patient day							
4. Outpatient revenue per visit							
5. No. of admissions							
6. Census							
7. Length of stay							
8. No. of accounts that are more than 90 days old							
9. No. of accounts turned over to a collection agency or otherwise written off							
10. No. of incident reports submitted							
11. Percentage of accounts that are selfpay							
12. No. of days to produce a bill from time of discharge							
13. No. of records being held in Medical Records for a final diagnosis and physician signature							
14. Return on outside investments							
15. Collection rate							
16. Total revenue							
17. Major equipment purchases to be made in next 60 days							
18. Major one-time expenditures to be made in next 60 days							
19. Projects that are behind schedule							
20. Mean hospital salary							
21. Mean hospital salary for the community							
22. Wage expenses by department							
23. Hours worked by department							
24. Supply expense by department							

Internal Management Reporting Evaluation, continued

A. Do you receive this information?
1. Yes
2. No

B. How often do you get this information?
1. Daily
2. Weekly
3. Bimonthly
4. Monthly
5. Quarterly
6. Yearly
7. On request
8. On an exception basis

C. Is the current information compared with historical data?
1. Yes
2. No

D. Is the current information compared with budget information on other standards?
1. Yes
2. No

E. Who supplies the information?
1. Administrative Officer who reports to the CEO
2. Personnel
3. Medical Staff
4. A Clinical Department
5. Medical Records
6. Fiscal Affairs
7. Admitting
8. Nursing
9. Other Department
10. Outside agency

F. How old is the information when you get it?
1. Less than one day
2. Less than one week
3. Less than two weeks
4. Less than one month
5. More than one month

G. What is the name of the report that contains the information?

INFORMATION
25. No. of unfilled positions
26. Turnover rate
27. Absentee rate
28. Expense for equipment leases
29. Nursing workhours per patient day
Revenue/expense ratio for:
30. Radiology
31. Laboratory
32. Respiratory Therapy
33. Pharmacy
34. EKG
35. Nuclear Medicine
36. Physical Medicine
37. Time since last disaster drill
38. Time since last test of emergency power supply
39. No. of physicians on staff
40. No. of general practitioners
41. Mean age of medical staff
42. Revenue generated by each physician
43. Interest expense paid
44. Pounds of linen cleaned per patient day
45. Value of Storeroom and Central Supply Inventory
46. No. of requisitioned items not in stock (i.e., back-orders)
47. No. of autopsies
48. Percentage of dismissals with lengths of stay exceeding hospital standards
49. No. of emergency room visits
50. No. of operations
51. Margin
52. Invoices past due

The CEO may get reports other than those listed in column G of the preceding section. On the following chart, list those reports with the following information:

A. What is the name of the report?

B. How often do you receive it?

    1. Daily
    2. Weekly
    3. Bimonthly
    4. Monthly
    5. Quarterly
    6. Yearly
    7. On request

C. Who supplies the report?

    1. Administrative Officer who reports to the CEO
    2. Personnel
    3. Medical Staff
    4. A Clinical Department
    5. Medical Records
    6. Fiscal Affairs
    7. Admitting
    8. Nursing
    9. Other Department
   10. Outside agency

Supplemental Report Inventory

A. What is the name of the report?

B. How often do you receive it?
1. Daily
2. Weekly
3. Bimonthly
4. Monthly
5. Quarterly
6. Yearly
7. On request

C. Who supplies the report?
1. Administrative Officer who reports to the CEO
2. Personnel
3. Medical Staff
4. A Clinical Department
5. Medical Records
6. Fiscal Affairs
7. Admitting
8. Nursing
9. Other Department
10. Outside agency

458

System 9.2:
External Reporting

Each hospital has a variety of reports that it submits to outside agencies. For the CEO and other administrative officers, compile a list of all reports sent by the hospital to outside agencies. Ask the following questions about each report:

A. What is the name of the report?

B. What type of agency receives it?

    1.   Hospital association
    2.   Local government agency
    3.   State agency
    4.   Federal agency other than HEW
    5.   HEW
    6.   HSA
    7.   Other inspection agency
    8.   Medical agency (AMA, etc.)
    9.   Other

C. How often must the report be submitted?

    1.   More frequently than monthly
    2.   Monthly
    3.   Quarterly
    4.   Yearly
    5.   Less frequently than yearly
    6.   On demand

D. How many workhours are needed to prepare the report?

    1.   Less than 1
    2.   Less than 10
    3.   Less than 40
    4.   Less than 80
    5.   Less than 160
    6.   More than 160

E. Which department is responsible for submitting the report?

    1.   Administration
    2.   Medical Staff or Medical Affairs
    3.   Medical Records
    4.   Personnel
    5.   Fiscal Affairs
    6.   Nursing
    7.   Clinical Department
    8.   Other nonclinical department

External Report Inventory

A. What is the name of the report?

B. What type of agency receives it?
1. Hospital association
2. Local government agency
3. State agency
4. Federal agency other than HHS
5. HHS
6. HSA
7. Other inspection agency
8. Medical agency (AMA, etc.)
9. Other

C. How often must the report be submitted?
1. More often than monthly
2. Monthly
3. Quarterly
4. Yearly
5. Less frequently than yearly
6. On demand

D. How many workhours are needed to prepare the report?
1. Less than 1
2. Less than 10
3. Less than 40
4. Less than 80
5. Less than 160
6. More than 160

E. Which department is responsible for submitting the report?
1. Administration
2. Medical Staff or Medical Affairs
3. Medical Records
4. Personnel
5. Fiscal Affairs
6. Nursing
7. Clinical Department
8. Other nonclinical departments

Selected References

Austin, Charles J. and Greene, Barry R. "Hospital Information Systems: A Current Perspective." *Inquiry,* June 1978, pp. 95–112.

Austin, Charles J. *Information Systems for Hospital Administration.* Ann Arbor, Michigan: Health Administration Press, 1979.

Austin, Charles J. "Planning and Selecting An Information System." *Hospitals,* October 16, 1977, pp. 95–100, 202.

Bingham, J. E. and Davies, G. W. P. *A Handbook of Systems Analysis.* New York: John Wiley & Sons, 1972.

Carlsen, Robert D. and Lewis, James A. *The Systems Analysis Workbook.* Englewood Cliffs, New Jersey: Prentice Hall, 1973.

Davis, Samuel and Freeman, John R. "Hospital Managers Need Management Information Systems." *Health Care Management Review,* Fall 1976, pp. 65–74.

Fitzgerald, John M. and Fitzgerald, Ardra F. *Fundamentals of Systems Analysis.* New York: John Wiley & Sons, 1973.

Garrett, Raymon D. *Hospitals—A Systems Approach.* Philadelphia: Auerbach Publishers, 1973.

Giebink, Gerald A. and Hurst, Leonard L. *Computer Projects in Health Care.* Ann Arbor, Michigan. Health Administration Press, 1975.

Gillette, P. J.; Rathburn, P. W.; and Wolfe, H. B. "Hospital Information Systems." *Hospitals,* Part I, August 16, 1970, pp. 76–78; Part II, September 1, 1970, pp. 45–48, 110.

Grams, Ralph R. *Problem Solving, Systems Analysis and Medicine.* Springfield, Illinois: Charles C. Thomas, 1972.

Griffith, John R. *Quantitative Techniques for Hospital Planning and Control.* Lexington, Massachusetts: Lexington Books, 1972.

Hammon, Gary S. "Planning and Involvement are the Words to Remember for an In-house Computer System." *Hospital Financial Management,* February 1974, pp. 38–42.

Herzlinger, Regina. "Management Noninformation Systems in Health Care Organizations." *Health Care Management Review,* Spring 1976, pp. 71–76.

Hospital Financial Management Association. *The State of Information Processing in the Health Care Industry.* Chicago: The Association, 1976.

Koza, Russel C., ed. *Health Information Systems Evaluation.* Boulder, Colorado: Colorado Associated University Press, 1974.

Levey, Samuel and Loomba, N. Paul. *Health Care Administration: A Managerial Perspective.* Philadelphia: J.B. Lippincott, 1973. Note particularly Chapter 8, "Health Information Systems."

Matthews, J.B. "Planning for Hospital Information Systems." *Modern Health Care,* December 1975, pp. 36–38.

McFarlan, F. Warren and Nolan, Richard L., eds. *The Information Systems Handbook.* Homewood, Illinois: Dow Jones-Irwin, 1975.

Murdick, Robert G. and Ross, Joel E. *Introduction to Management Information Systems.* Englewood Cliffs, New Jersey: Prentice Hall, 1977.

Schmitz, Homer H. "A Protocol for Evaluating Hospital Information Systems." *Hospital and Health Services Administration,* Winter 1977, pp. 45–56.

Sheldon, A.; Baker, F.; and McLaughlin, C.P., eds. *Systems and Medical Care.* Cambridge, Mass.: MIT Press, 1970.

Shuman, Larry J.; Speas, R. Dixon, Jr.; and Young, John P., eds. *Operations Research in Health Care.* Baltimore: John Hopkins University Press, 1975. See particularly Chapter 11, "Information Systems" by Ronald L. Gue and John R. Freeman.

Solomon, Irving I. and Weingart, Laurence O. *Management Uses of the Computer.* New York: Harper & Row, 1966.

Stimson, David H. and Stimson, Ruth H. *Operations Research in Hospitals: Diagnosis and Prognosis.* Chicago: Hospital Research and Educational Trust, 1972. Note particularly "Computer Applications and Total Hospital Information Systems," pp. 26–35.

United Hospital Fund of New York. Chapter 2, "An Administrator's Survey of Systems Concepts." In *A General Systems Approach to Hospital Management and Organization.* New York: The Fund, 1971.

Yasaki, E.K. "Wide Variety of Computer Bases Systems Available to Hospitals." *Datamation,* March 1975, pp. 115–121.

Index

About the Authors

Trained as both an engineer and a hospital administrator, Owen Doyle is currently Director of Management Systems at Miami Valley Hospital, in Dayton, Ohio; the Vice President of a hospital consulting firm, Administrative Health Management; and an Assistant Professor at Xavier University in the graduate program in Hospital and Health Care Administration. He received his B.S. degree in Electrical Engineering from Notre Dame, his M.S. in Biomedical Engineering from Drexal University and his M.H.A. from Xavier University. He is co-author of *Systems Analysis Workbook.*

Charles J. Austin is Vice President and Professor of Management at Georgia Southern University in Statesboro. He was Dean of Graduate Studies and Professor of Health Care Administration at Trinity University, San Antonio, Texas. He received a B.S. degree from Xavier University, an M.S. in Health Administration from the University of Colorado, and a Ph.D from the University of Cincinnati. Dr. Austin is the author of *Information Systems for Hospital Administration.*

Stephen Tucker is Professor and Chairman of the Department of Health Care Administration at Trinity University in San Antonio, Texas. Before going to Trinity University, he was Associate Professor in Hospital Administration at Xavier University and Associate Director of Harrisburg Hospital in Harrisburg, Pennsylvania. He holds a B.A. from Dartmouth, an M.B.A. from Xavier, and he received a D.B.A. from George Washington University in 1970. Dr. Tucker had a WHO Fellowship for the study of the National Health Service in Great Britain.